Back to the Dance Itself

D1614550

Back to the Dance Itself

Phenomenologies of the Body in Performance

Edited with Essays by

SONDRA FRALEIGH

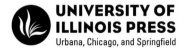

**UNIVERSITY OF
ILLINOIS PRESS**
Urbana, Chicago, and Springfield

∞ This book is printed on acid-free paper.
Printed and bound in Great Britain by
Marston Book Services Ltd, Oxfordshire

Library of Congress Cataloging-in-Publication Data
Names: Fraleigh, Sondra Horton, 1939– editor.
Title: Back to the dance itself: of the body in performance / edited
    with essays by Sondra Fraleigh.
Description: Urbana: University of Illinois Press, [2017] | Includes
    bibliographical references and index.
Identifiers: LCCN 2018012523| ISBN 9780252042041 (cloth : alk.
    paper) | ISBN 9780252083730 (pbk. : alk. paper)
Subjects: LCSH: Dance—Philosophy. | Dance—Social aspects. |
    Phenomenology.
Classification: LCC GV1588.3 .B33 2017 | DDC 792.8—dc23
LC record available at https://lccn.loc.gov/2018012523

Ebook ISBN 970-0-252-05078-7

Dedicated to Maxine Sheets-Johnstone,
for her initiation of the phenomenology of dance
and her unwavering influence on studies
of movement and the body

Coming to know the world in a quite literal sense means coming to grips with it—exploring it, searching it, discovering it in and through movement. There is no human culture in which movement is not epistemologically central in this way. There is, indeed, no culture in which movement is not our mother tongue.

—Maxine Sheets-Johnstone, *The Primacy of Movement*

Our own body is in the world as the heart is in the organism: it keeps the visible spectacle constantly alive, it breathes life into it and sustains it inwardly, and with it forms a system.

—Maurice Merleau-Ponty, *The Phenomenology of Perception*

Subjectivity in its grip upon it of course changes nature, but alters nothing of the unity of nature as core in its own ontological form.

—Edmund Husserl, *Sixth Cartesian Meditation*

Contents

List of Illustrations

Color Insert

Acknowledgments

We wish to thank Maxine Sheets-Johnstone for her original work, *The Phenomenology of Dance*, first published in 1966 and republished in 2015 by Temple University Press as a fifty-year anniversary edition. This is the book that initiated studies in phenomenology of dance and stirred wider interest in philosophical studies of movement. Our book expands Sheets-Johnstone's theme of dance as a created form of movement and other key themes of her work as it also takes a turn toward performance through various current forms of dance, including site-specific work, and delineates several phenomenologies.

We acknowledge the support of our families, friends, and colleagues in bringing this book to light, and also the dancers, performers, and photographers who lend this book their talent through interviews, conversations, and visual images.

By now, phenomenology has a rich history in perspectives on dance, somatics, and performance. We are happy to be able to add to this experiential path of inquiry and appreciate those who have contributed to its development. Many of them are quoted in *Back to the Dance Itself*.

Author Biographies and Places

We pause in arabesque here at the beginning, scrolling through landscapes, cities, and several countries as background to our text. Anticipating its plurality of lifeworld and lived experiences in performance, short place statements follow individual biographies below.

Karen Barbour, PhD, is an associate professor in the School of Arts' at the University of Waikato, New Zealand. Her teaching and research focuses on embodied ways of knowing, particularly feminist choreographic practices in dance, site-specific, digital dance, and pedagogical movement contexts. Her book publications include *Dancing across the Page: Narrative and Embodied Ways of Knowing* (2011) and *Ethnographic Worldviews: Transformations and Social Justice* (Rinehart, Barbour, and Pope 2014). Karen is editor of the journal *Dance Research Aotearoa*, presents regularly at international dance conferences, and has published her writing in a range of books and journals. Karen has completed certification with Eastwest Somatics Institute, is a yoga teacher, and has been the recipient of a Fulbright Travel Award (2006). She has presented site-specific and place-responsive seasons of dance in the Hamilton Gardens Arts Festival over many years.

Places: Karen was born and grew up in Te Puku o Te Ika a Maui (the central north island) of Aoteaora (New Zealand) in Te Moana Nui a Kiwa, (the South Pacific Ocean). She lives her life in Aotearoa with her partner and son, and it is the complexities of being Pākehā (New Zealander with Scottish and Canadian ancestry) and living in relationship with Māori (indigenous peoples) and the lands of Aotearoa that has shaped her most profoundly.

Christine Bellerose (Cricri) is a Québecois movement artist and researcher. Her journeys from musician, costume maker, clown, responsive technology dancer, and playwright have matured into simple solo-explorations in the wild. Today she dances forms of butoh, durational performance art, and somatic arts with nature's elements and cultural artifacts. Eastern-Western cosmologies permeate her art and research. Christine completed her classical music studies at the Conservatoire de musique classique du Québec. A grant from the Canadian South East Asian Foundation allowed her to contribute to Dr. Vu Thi Thanh Huong's body language project, with the Centre for Linguistics and Vietnamese studies in Hanoi. In Beijing, she founded Homônumos—the art, literature, philosophy, and science multilingual magazine. Her project, "Performative Listening of Métis Artifact," funded by the Canada Council for the Arts, led to her current doctoral research in Dance Studies at York University (Toronto, Canada) on the significance of the body as site-of-research. She is assisting archival/embodied research, "Collective Historical Acts of Social Memory," funded by the Social Science and Humanities Research Council, with Dr. Norma Sue Fisher-Stitt and Carol Anderson, on the National Choreographic Seminars (1978–1991).

Places: Christine was born in cosmopolitan Montréal and moved at an early age to beautiful and forested Gatineau (Québec, Canada)—foreshadowing her life with one foot in the urban jungle and the other in the wild. Early, too, Christine dipped in mixed-cultural environments, their deepest imprint, and her life in a Qing Dynasty village bordering Beijing, where elderly women with bound feet mixed with contemporary artists of a new generation. She knew at the time this living situation was going to be the most amazing and unique story of her life.

Robert Bingham, MFA, PhD, lives in Philadelphia, where he teaches dance at Temple University and elsewhere. For over twenty years, he has been a professional dance artist, scholar, and educator whose choreography has been presented throughout North America. He is a Fulbright Scholar Award recipient (Berlin, 2013) and was a Visiting Artist in Dance at Alfred University (2005–2012). Robert has extensive training in somatic modalities, which inform his dancing, teaching, and writing. He is a certified yoga instructor (Integral Yoga Institute, 1996) and Registered Somatic Movement Therapist/Educator (Eastwest Somatics Institute, 2003). He studied with butoh artist Diego Piñon in the United States and Mexico. His chapters on dance, somatics, and ecology appear in *Moving Consciously* (UIP, 2015), *Dance and the Quality of Life* (Springer, 2018), and *Oxford Handbook of Improvisation* (OUP, 2018), and he is a guest coeditor of *Choreographic Practices* (Spring 2018).

Robert has been a presenter at arts conferences in the United States, United Kingdom, Mexico, and Germany.

Places: Robert was born in Boston and has spent much of his adult life in New York and Philadelphia. For twelve years he lived in western New York, including six in the village of Alfred. His research in dance and movement processes has taken him to northern India, Berlin, Germany, and the deserts of Southwest Utah. All of these places live in his dances, writing, and environmental activism.

Karen E. Bond, PhD, is associate professor and chair of dance at Temple University. She was formerly senior lecturer and coordinator of dance education and research at the University of Melbourne where she developed Australia's first master's level courses in dance. At Temple, she teaches graduate courses in philosophy of dance education, dance pedagogy, and first-person research methodologies (phenomenology, autoethnography, autobiography), as well as foundations of dance education for BFA dance majors. She was an inaugural recipient of the Congress on Research in Dance's Graduate Research Award (1990), which was presented to her by professor Sondra Fraleigh, CORD's president at the time. More recently, she was the inaugural recipient of the Outstanding Dance Education Researcher Award (2012) from the National Dance Education Organization (NDEO). She has presented papers and workshops in Australia, Brazil, Canada, Denmark, Finland, Jamaica, Japan, The Netherlands, New Zealand, Saipan, Singapore, Taiwan, and across the United States. Known for her research into participant experiences and meanings of dance, spanning education, community arts, performance, and therapy, Karen holds an enduring commitment to supporting and illuminating the dance of childhood.

Places: Born and raised in suburban Chicago, Karen completed undergraduate studies in Ohio and Washington, D.C. She then danced up and down the West Coast for six years before vaulting the Pacific to Australia, a time and place that continues to live in her memory and dreams. After two decades, in 2000 she returned to the United States to live and work in the city of Philadelphia.

Hillel Braude studied medicine at the University of Cape Town Medical School and obtained a PhD in philosophy cum laude with The University of Chicago's Committee for the History of Culture. Hillel completed postdoctoral fellowships in neuroethics with McGill University's Biomedical Ethics Unit and Religious Studies Faculty. His awards include a Mellon Foundation-University of Chicago Dissertation-Year Fellowship and a European Neuroscience Network Visiting Exchange Grant (ENSN) at the Center for Subjectivity Research, University of Copenhagen. Besides his passion for somatics, Hillel's multidisciplinary research interests include neuroethics, phenomenology, dance studies, cognition, and clinical reasoning. In addition to numerous journal articles, he is the author of *Intuition in Medicine: A Philosophical Defense of Clinical Reasoning* (University of Chicago Press, 2012). As a certified Feldenkrais practitioner, Hillel complements his theoretical research with hands-on work in neurorehabilitation (2013) and specializes in working with infants with neurodevelopmental problems. He is currently director of research at the Mifne Center for the treatment of infants with autism and their families. Hillel lives in a small yishuv in Israel with his wife, Ita, and two children Ariel Ziv and Libi.

Places: Hillel lives and works in the North of Israel. He grew up in Johannesburg, South Africa, and is fortunate to have lived in many other cities that have shaped his persona, including Cape Town, London, Chicago, Paris, Montreal, Copenhagen, and Jerusalem.

Sondra Fraleigh is professor emerita of dance at the State University of New York (SUNY Brockport), a Fulbright Scholar, and the award-winning author of eight books. *Moving Consciously: Somatic Transformations through Dance, Yoga, and Touch* (2015) and *BUTOH: Metamorphic Dance and Global Alchemy* (2010) are both published by the University of Illinois Press. Earlier books include *Dancing Identity: Metaphysics in Motion* (2004); *Dancing into Darkness: Butoh, Zen, and Japan* (1999); *Researching Dance: Evolving Modes of Inquiry* (1998); and *Dance and the Lived Body* (1987), the featured book for the American Society for Aesthetics, Eastern division (1987). Her book on the founders of Japanese butoh, *Hijikata Tatsumi and Ohno Kazuo* (2006), is with Routledge Press, and in 2008, she published *Land to Water Yoga* on somatic yoga and infant movement development. She also has numerous chapters in books on culture, aesthetics, ecology, and cognitive psychology. Sondra was chair of the Department of Dance at SUNY Brockport for nine years, and later head of graduate dance studies and also selected by SUNY as a universitywide Faculty Exchange Scholar. She received the Outstanding Service to Dance Award from CORD in 2003. Her choreography has been seen in New York, Germany, Japan, and India. She was a teaching fellow for several months at Ochanomizu University in Tokyo and at the University of Baroda in India. Sondra is the founding director of *Eastwest Somatics Institute* for the study of dance, yoga, and movement, www.eastwestsomatics. com (accessed January 11, 2018).

Places: After retirement from university life, Sondra returned to Southwest Utah to the colored canyons, vast deserts, and alpine mountains where she was born. Of the many places she has lived, she remembers the deep snows

*of Montana; teaching in Japan while making friends through butoh and Zen;
surviving illness during her months of lecturing and choreographing in India;
appreciating the hardships and brilliance of Indian women; living seventeen
years in San Francisco and loving California wines; teaching thirty-three years
in New York while soaking-in the arts. And not to forget, growing up on a cattle
ranch in Utah in what was then one of the most remote areas of the United
States.*

Kimerer L. LaMothe is a dancer, philosopher, scholar of religion, and
award-winning author of five books, including *Nietzsche's Dancers: Isadora
Duncan, Martha Graham, and the Revaluation of Christian Values* (Palgrave
Macmillan, 2006), and *Why We Dance: A Philosophy of Bodily Becoming* (Columbia. 2015). After earning a masters from Harvard Divinity School and a
doctorate from Harvard University, Kimerer taught for six years at Brown
University and then at Harvard, where she also directed the undergraduate
program in the Comparative Study of Religion. She has received yearlong
fellowships from the Radcliffe Institute for Advanced Study and the Center
for the Study of World Religions; and she has choreographed and performed
three solo dance concerts: *Genesis* (2001, 2009), *On Fire* (2004), and *The
Ever Unfolding Present* (2016). In 2005, Kimerer and her musician partner
followed a dream to a retired dairy farm in upstate New York where they
live with their five children, ages seven through twenty-one. Together, the
family performs concerts of music and dance. When not writing or dancing, Kimerer helps her children take care of their two horses, two oxen, two
cows, four cats, twenty-two hens, and large vegetable garden.

*Places: Born in New York City, and raised in Concord, Massachusetts, Ki-
merer spent fifteen years in the environs of Harvard University before moving
with her husband and children to a farm in upstate New York where she now
gleans inspiration amid ninety-six acres of rolling hills, open meadows and
thick forests, two ponds, and a small stream.*

Joanna McNamara, PhD, is a contemporary choreographer, dance filmmaker, and scholar with an interest in capturing the convergence of relationships and activities reflective of Detroit and other urban landscapes.
Her dance films have been presented in conjunction with the Manhattan
Contemporary Chamber Ensemble at Carnegie Hall (2014 and 2016), at the
International Video Dance Festival in South Korea (2015 and 2016, 2017), at
the Detroit Dance City Festival, on CTN-TV Ann Arbor, and in a variety of
other regional and national venues. Joanna's dance film *LANDcakeLOCK*,
which was made for Moving24FPS, was awarded Audience Choice and presented as part of Detroit's Cinetopia Film Festival (2017). Along with Marcus

White/White Werx, she curates and directs *Screen. Dance. Now.*, a festival bringing feature dance films, national and international short dance films, workshops, and panel discussions to Michigan. She has served as dance critic for *Ann Arbor News*, and a feature writer for *Detroit Metro Times* and has several publications in the area of hermeneutic phenomenology. Joanna is creative director of JMc/PRODUCTIONS, and is a professor in the School of Music and Dance at Eastern Michigan University.

Places: Joanna was born in Los Angeles and grew up thirteen miles northeast of downtown L.A. in Arcadia, California, in a neighborhood of domesticated horses, goats, Chinese Silkie chickens, geese, dogs, ducks, and cats. She and her young pals studied, rode horses and bikes, danced, and did cartwheels on the lawn. As soon as they could drive, they went to Los Angeles and Pasadena for everything else. For thirty-two years she has lived in Michigan, mostly in a neighborhood of wild deer, fox, raccoons, skunks, squirrels, and Red-bellied Woodpeckers, forty-three miles west of Detroit. She and her adult pals teach, dance, write, sometimes ride bikes and horses, but don't do cartwheels on the lawn. She goes to Detroit or back to Los Angeles for anything else. Her stopping points between Arcadia, California, and Ann Arbor, Michigan, include Santa Cruz, the Bay Area, and Denton, Texas. Her points of inspiration: Europe, Russia, Tibet, China, and South Korea.

Vida L. Midgelow, dance artist/academic, lives in the middle of England with her teenage daughter. She has over 20 years experience of teaching and researching dance, and her creative work sits comfortably at the interface of theory and practice. Recent performance works include *Skript* (2013, NottDance Festival), and *Stratch* (2016, Nottingham Contemporary Gallery). Her movement and video work has been shown internationally, and recent essays include "Some Fleshy Thinking" (OUP, 2015) and "Creative Articulation Process" (CAP) (Intellect, 2014). She is currently editing the *Handbook on Dance in Improvisation* (OUP, forthcoming) and is the lead researcher for the Artistic Doctors in Europe project (Erasmus plus funding). She also undertakes dramaturgical and consultancy roles. Extending these interests, Vida coedits the hybrid peer-reviewed journal, *Choreographic Practices*, developing new approaches to dance writing, with particular attention to the evocation of the embodied experience of dancing.

Places: Vida lives in the middle of England and works in London. As such, she spends too much time driving on fast-moving roads and sitting in front of a laptop. Making space to attend to the sensate present is an important antidote to the punishing effects of her long-distance commuting and enables embodied ways for her to engage in the professional world. She was born close to where she now lives and spent some years in Florida. She also spends time regularly in rural Pennsylvania and north Auckland to be with her sisters and travels extensively for work, recently in New Zealand, Brazil, China, and Taiwan. Places that resonate with her are sited in learning: the creative, physical, and critical practices that have been absorbed into the flesh and bones of who she is.

Ami Shulman studied dramatic arts at the University of the Witwatersrand where she was awarded the Amanda Holmes Prize for choreography (1997). Her work as a performing artist, choreographer, and movement director has brought her to work with the Cirque Du Soleil; the GoteborgsOperans Danskompani; the National Ballet of Canada; Compagnie Marie Chouinard; the DanceOn Ensemble Berlin; Ballet British Columbia, and the Shakespeare Theatre Company, which earned her a Helen Hayes Award for Choreography (2016). Ami's unique approach to pedagogy in movement and dance has been enhanced by her work as a certified Feldenkrais practitioner and she has been invited to teach at the Juilliard School; Jacob's Pillow; the Alvin Ailey School; and the National Theatre School of Canada, among others. Ami has collaborated with many artists, including large-scale multimedia productions with Butch Rovan and Mouvement Perpetuel, which have been presented internationally. She is currently based in Berlin where she performs, directs, teaches, and writes.

Places: Ami's hometown of Johannesburg, South Africa, touched her deeply with its stories of humanity. Her passion for movement has given her the privilege of living and working around the world. The cities that have left an imprint on her life are Montreal, Amsterdam, New York, San Diego, and Berlin.

Amanda Williamson is a senior lecturer and course leader for dance at The University of Gloucestershire. Her PhD is in the study of spirituality in the field of Somatic Movement Education and Therapy. Her research is interdisciplinary and transdisciplinary in approach, rooted in cultural studies, religious studies, spiritual feminism, phenomenology, and new materialism. Amanda is founding editor of the peer review journal, *Journal of Dance, Movement and Spiritualities*, and editor of *Dance, Somatics and Spiritualities: Contemporary Sacred Narratives* at Intellect Press. She is currently publishing the edited feminist anthology *Spiritual Herstories: Call of the Soul in Dance Research* with Intellect Press.

Amanda grew up in the small fishing village of Mullion in the '70s and '80s in Cornwall, always by, or on, or in the sea. The salty mythological cliffs and ocean surrounding Cornwall inspired her movement and spirituality. Since then, she has lived in different cities in the United Kingdom but spent a large amount of time training in Massachusetts and working in New York, where her deepest friendships developed and her love for somatics consciousness deepened. The beauty of Massachusetts deepened her connections between spirituality and somatics movement; this personal and academic relationship became her vocation as she moved into her 40s.

Back to the Dance Itself

An Introduction

SONDRA FRALEIGH

In what ways can the several methods and lifeworlds of phenomenology illuminate dance and performance? Our book brings this question to the page for dancers, performers, and arts-identified readers interested in the study of experience and performative writing. Various approaches have common threads that define them as phenomenological, as this volume explores.

Back to the things themselves is the clarion call of phenomenology through its beginnings in Edmund Husserl. *Things* are the *phenomena* of consciousness, the identifiable experiential contents—including feelings, observations, performances, happenings, and possibilities. Phenomenology begins with experience. Rather than attempting to observe objects as external "things in themselves," phenomenologists hold that we first experience the world as it appears in subjective life, and that such experiences can be described and shared. In this book we speak to specific experiences of dance and performance as objects of art and theater, intentionally created acts and events, and as processes founding descriptions, values, and theories. We also write in the belief that the methods and insights of phenomenology can actively engage with an area of prime social concern for dance and performance: the environmental world.

As editor, I summarize author contributions and specific approaches in this introduction, also providing a brief account of phenomenology that I will greatly expand in the first two chapters. The terms "dance" and "performance" cover a wide range of phenomena, and thus we delimit our work here at the beginning. *Back to the Dance Itself* is concerned with dance and performance as modes of creativity and cultural productivity, and also with ways of knowing emerging from performative and somatic processes relative to world and nature. Somatic phenomena go back to *soma*, most simply the personal body as regulated and sensed relationally (Fraleigh 2015, xx–xxiv). Soma, lifeworld, and nature are defined in Chapter 1, as key concepts of our text.

In view of particular dance genres and performance styles, we speak to current theater forms of modern/contemporary dance, dance improvisation, somatic modes, durational performance art, cultural hybrids, urban movements, screen dance, butoh, children's dance in education, and site-specific performances. We study these up close in light of body, soma, and experience, which is the distinct venture of phenomenology. The founder of phenomenology, Edmund Husserl, first articulated the somatic basis of movement relative to world and body—which is also a major theme for us.

Following Husserl, French philosopher Merleau-Ponty also presented an integrative view of world and body, as he says in *Phenomenology of Perception*:

> Our own body is in the world as the heart is in the organism: it keeps the visible spectacle constantly alive, it breathes life into it and sustains it inwardly, and with it forms a system. (2012, 235)

Turning toward concrete matters of experience, combined perspectives of German phenomenology and French existentialism continue into this century. Sarah Bakewell's recent book, *At the Existentialist Café* (2016), features French existentialists in conversation with each other as they unravel the intellectual conundrums of German phenomenology. Our book shifts the conversation toward performance arts through the usefulness of phenomenology and existentialism, even as Bakewell refreshes these schools of thought in current discourse.

Outgrowths of phenomenology are rooted in Husserl's philosophy, now differentiated and widely applied in the arts, social science, psychology, somatic studies, ecology, ethnology, epistemology, medicine, and religious studies. Contemporary phenomenology moves outside of disciplinary boundaries, as insights first arising in philosophical phenomenology have expanded to a range of concerns, branching into several *phenomenologies*. I delineate these as central to this volume. All phenomenologies study experience, but from differing vantage points. The full potentials of phenomenology for dance and performance inspire the work of our authors.

Our text is addressed to an inclusive audience concerned with the arts and philosophies of the body. Because phenomenology, as it emerged throughout the twentieth century, was one of the first nondualistic philosophies of the body in the West, it is of special significance for dance and performance. Its influence in theorizing topics of bodily being and becoming, particularly for movement arts, continues into the present century, now with approaches that are friendly to ecological concerns. Themes of becoming and incompletion enter into phenomenology, and because of this, its methods are ongoing, as we consider.

Before foregrounding the essays of this collection, I provide a thumbnail sketch of the phenomenologies that propel them, further defining these contextually in the first and second chapters. Since my first study of phenomenology in 1970, I have discovered that it is not a unified field, but quite diverse and rich in perspectives that can be divided into several distinct categories or forms—even more, perhaps, than I identify here and through a recent article, "Phenomenologies in the Flowing Live Present" (2016). Initially a philosophy of the twentieth century, phenomenology in this century flourishes in a plurality of methods and distinct but overlapping forms.

Thumbnail of Phenomenologies

Philosophical phenomenology is basic and emphasizes suspension of judgments in order to apprehend the obvious that is obscured by ordinary perceptions. *Transcendental phenomenology* is expansive and illuminates our primordial belonging to world and spirit. *Existential phenomenology* is oriented toward lived experience, conceiving the self in relation to others and the more-than-human lifeworld. *Heuristic phenomenology* is oriented toward process, exploration, and discovery, also extending human development beyond the individual in transpersonal and somatic psychology. *Hermeneutic phenomenology* is concerned with meaning; it is interpretive, contextual, and sometimes performative. *Ecological phenomenology* harks back to nature and the environing lifeworld. *Performative phenomenology* crosses between art and philosophy, suggesting that varieties of phenomenology can advance textual instances of performance to inspire performances in the arts. *Neurophenomenology* is a recent mode of inquiry at the intersection of neuroscience and phenomenological studies of embodied enaction, and as a science of the responsive body, greatly benefits dance studies.

Book Sections and Chapters

Part I, *World as Body*, explores intersections of dance with varying worlds of experience, also demonstrating the convergence of phenomenology with contemporary environmental studies. The world we sense around us also moves in and through us, making us part of itself. Chapter 1, "Phenomenology and Lifeworld," is Sondra Fraleigh's thematic expansion of phenomenology. This foundational chapter speaks to topics of *lifeworld* and *the lived body* as key concepts of the text and to *the study of experience* in phenomenology. As a primary category of phenomenology, lifeworld develops ways of understanding the world through experience and environment, ways that directly relate to the body in dance and performance. Fraleigh continues with Chapter 2, "Branching into Phenomenologies," further explaining the multiple perspectives, distinct styles, and approaches of phenomenology that she introduced in the thumbnail earlier. Our authors develop these varied phenomenologies throughout the book.

Robert Bingham extends ecological themes in Chapter 3, "Improvising Meaning in the Age of Humans." His chapter asks how dance, as a practice and generator of theory, might be mobilized as a response to environmental crisis. In response, Bingham writes a phenomenological account of a monthlong interview he conducted in 2015 with Sondra Fraleigh, engaging her as a dance scholar who articulates connections between somatic and ecological consciousness. The interview, which integrated dancing, shared personal histories, and theoretical reflections on dance and embodiment, expanded ideas Fraleigh had developed in earlier publications, reframing them in the stark light of environmental crisis, current theory, and related aesthetic practices. Bingham's chapter draws from these conversations, heuristic phenomenology, and new physics, and from a specific "place dance" experience in Snow Canyon in Southwest Utah. This concluding chapter of Part 1 extends discourse on dance from continuums of body-mind to interrelationships of body-mind-environment.

Part II, *Performing Life and Language*, begins with Vida Midgelow's Chapter 4, "Improvisation as Paradigm for Phenomenologies." In a sleight of hand, Midgelow replaces the word *phenomenology* with *improvisation* while exploring the intersection between these two practices. Focusing on improvisation based in Skinner Releasing Techniques that are broadly somatic in approach, Midgelow goes beyond illuminating dance improvisation through phenomenology to turn instead to a consideration of improvisation as methodological paradigm for phenomenologies. She distinguishes embodiment as a mode of presence and engagement with the world, using dance-rich experiential language in harmonizing perceptual experience with cultural practice.

Chapter 5, "Falling in Love with Language," is by Amanda Williamson, whose writing bridges between dance and language in somatic studies where participants are encouraged to write, speak, or paint from a felt sense of movement. She shows how the embodied, poetic, and aesthetic hermeneutics established in movement-based somatics flow between kinesthetic feelings and language formulation. Language and experience, she says, are implicated in, but cannot replace, one another. She draws upon transpersonal psychology and heuristic phenomenology in illuminating somatic dance experiences focused on aesthetic appreciation of language. Philosophies of somatic awareness in dance, Williamson demonstrates, can attend to the spiritual life of language and the healing power of words. Using insights from Carl Jung through James Hillman and Eugene Gendlin, this chapter observes a love for alchemical and imaginal dance and language—where language, soul, and image are required to counteract abstractions of conceptual thought.

In Chapter 6, "Living Phenomenology," Sondra Fraleigh suggests that life itself is a performance when we look at it that way. Performances, she says, exist in the actions we take on purpose, arising in chunks of time and overlapping spaces that draw particular notice. To bring consciousness to a process or event, to live and perform as one intends, is not that unusual. We make choices daily that affect those around us and ripple out into the world. Fraleigh holds that when we are aware of our chosen actions, we can sometimes see with distance and, in seeing, recognize ourselves. Her chapter suggests tenuous exchanges in existential performances, noticing how perceptual qualities mix affectively, as in music and dance. Her affective language melds common tones in life's incomplete performances. In the somatic fray—listening and distance, touch and matter, love and ambition, worlding and suffering, freedom and gravity, dream and strangeness, lateral mindfulness and metamorphosis—fold into story, dance, and weightlessness.

Part III, *Body and Place*, begins with Chapter 7, "As the Earth Dances: A Philosophy of Bodily Becoming," by Kimerer LaMothe. At the outset, she asks what difference it would make to her dancing and thinking about dance and religion if, on a daily basis, she attended to the experiential shift she values so highly of being moved in and by nature? Her chapter outlines a philosophy of bodily becoming that emerges from her life on a farm and new perspectives on dance that rural life provides. Remaining faithful to the earth, she builds on these perspectives in developing an ecokinetic phenomenological approach to the study of dance designed to help illuminate and mobilize the vast knowledge embedded in dance traditions across cultures and throughout history. LaMothe advances theoretical, practical resources for how to create life-enabling relationships between more than human others and ourselves.

In the next chapter, Joanna McNamara reveals Detroit as a city of arts in transition. Her screen dance of the aesthetic revivals of Detroit—*Jitdance: Detroit Redux*—shows how place and body perform meaning in tandem. Chapter 8, "Filming Jitdance: Detroit Redux," is named for, and is about, this multilayered project, particularly the porous lifeline connecting body to landscape and how a city constantly exceeds its own boundaries thanks to the reciprocity between body and place. McNamara's chapter brings the city of Detroit into a wide circle of inquiry through a hermeneutic study that regards both text and process. The screen dance at the center of the chapter is made in collaboration with Haleem "Stringz" Rasul, Detroit-Jit dancer, choreographer, and company director of Hardcore Detroit. "Haleem's 'Jit dance' is surely the homegrown dancing body of Detroit," says McNamara. Her study reports that dance and filmmakers working in Detroit are not alone in their efforts. All over the city the arts are flourishing and artists working. Artists continue to arrive from around the world to live and work in Detroit or just browse and spend time in this compelling environment where rent is cheap and property inexpensive. McNamara's chapter yields a fascinating experiential aesthetics of Detroit and a vivid sense of place rebuilding through her first-person participant study of dance in relation to film and environmental/architectural art.

Chapter 9 shifts place and perspective toward the East in portraying *ma*, a concept of space-time permeating traditional Japanese fine arts and reappearing in contemporary butoh, the dance form originating in post–WWII Japan, now migrating as a performance perspective adopted by a number of theater art practitioners outside of Japan. In this chapter, "Being *Ma*: Moonlight Peeping through the Doorway," Christine Bellerose explores liminal experience at the nexus of *ma* and the lived body. She further describes *ma* as experienced relative to aesthetic intent in performance. Being Québecoise and also a longtime resident of Beijing, Bellerose says her "*id* and social construct," her own history, is in essence one of space-time transience. Ethnographically, She sees how her personal journey accords with *ma* and, when combined with the Sartrean existential and antiessentialist position that "existence precedes essence," affords an affective, reflexive and embodied research methodology. This chapter's study of *ma* is a simple tribute to a distinct form of space and time that understands the body-as-event. Bellerose considers *ma* as a philosophy of dance and an agent of cultural knowledge. In Japan, kami, the divinities that permeate the cosmos, are involved in productions of *ma*, relating space-time to objects in nature such as pine trees, bamboo shoots, and plum flower trees. Kami also favor cone-shaped sand piles, as often staged in butoh. In its extensive ecology, *ma* lives in a spatial and temporal language that links kami to dance as to humans and the more-than-human world. As Bellerose puts it: "That is *ma*. Unseen, but not unknown."

Part IV, *Questions of Self-Knowing*, asks how we come to know ourselves through dance and performance and how meaning is embodied in the life-world at various stages of life and in contexts of gender. Asking "What If" in a distinctive analysis of dance through transcendental phenomenology, philosopher Hillel Braude and dancer/choreographer Ami Shulman write Chapter 10 as a collaborative venture. In their study, "'What if . . .': A Question of Transcendence," they find that *Free Phantasy Variations* (FFV) represents a relatively neglected component of Husserl's phenomenological methodology. Yet, arguably, FFV is the fundamental method of *eidetic* description, even more than the famous phenomenological *reduction* and *epoché*. Husserl claimed in his *Cartesian Meditations* that FFV is "*the fundamental form of all particular transcendental methods . . .* [and gives] the legitimate sense of a transcendental phenomenology" (1960, 72) Through their analysis, Braude and Shulman emphasize that the correlation of dance and performance with *FFV* grounds phenomenological exploration in the lifeworld, the realm that people inhabit through the body rather than simply becoming a free-floating act of consciousness unmoored from its human and earthly origins. The relation between the invited sense of possibility in *Free Phantasy Variations* and Husserl's concept of "*I can*" provides the central pivot for this philosophically challenging chapter. The phenomenology of dance pioneered by Maxine Sheets-Johnstone, to whom this book is dedicated, rings throughout.

Expanding questions of self-knowing, in Chapter 11, "'Me, a Tree:'": Young Children as Natural Phenomenologists," Karen Bond explains dance and dancing to adults through children's captioned drawings in dialogue with autobiographical reflection and selected phenomenologies. All the children's drawings were created in response to an experiential prompt immediately after sessions of improvisational creative dance. Bond demonstrates how the dances and drawings of young children can ground philosophy in the specifics of practice. She follows Merleau-Ponty who sees the child as a "natural phenomenologist" deeply connected to experience. Acknowledging the full complexity of the three philosophers highlighted in this chapter—Leonard C. Feldstein, Max van Manen, and Maurice Merleau-Ponty—Bond considers how children's lived experience, drawings, and utterances about dancing might illuminate empirical and philosophical ideas. Ultimately, this chapter is a heuristic project, noting van Manen's emphasis on "reflective open attention" that seeks to uncover meaning before naming and analysis occur.

Young children's spontaneous dance drawings offer such openings to meaning with children's lived-experience descriptions of dancing, shedding light on the relation between experience and representation.

In Chapter 12, Karen Barbour explores the intersection of phenomenology with epistemology and feminism. At the root of existential philosophy, Simone de Beauvoir asserted that phenomenology had developed specific ways of knowing and a descriptive method that resonated with many feminist concerns; specifically, it refuted rationalism and objectifying mind-body dualism, focusing instead on embodied affective forms of experience. In this final chapter, "Dancing Epistemology, Situating Feminist Analysis," Barbour traces the weavings of philosophical and feminist engagements in phenenology that inspire dance scholarship and illustrate embodied epistemology within dance performance. She shows how feminist phenomenology provides a clear rationale for investigating embodied ways of knowing specific to dancers themselves, and also their relationship to others and to the ecology of the planet through moving. Barbour's chapter considers the phenomenological notions of bracketing and variation, and of lifeworld and presence in dance performance. She draws predominantly on feminists who have extended phenomenological work, including Simone de Beauvoir, Maxine Sheets-Johnstone, Iris Marion Young, Ann Cooper Albright, and Sondra Fraleigh. Using self-evidence throughout the chapter, she reflects on the lessons that breath and movement offer—juxtaposing descriptions of somatic phenomena with epistemological foundations of the text—where feeling and knowing coalesce. Her homeland of New Zealand sounds distinctly through phenomenological descriptions.

To learn more about the authors and their varied backgrounds, see the author biographies at the front of the book.

I

World as Body

1

Phenomenology and Lifeworld

SONDRA FRALEIGH

Phenomenology first evolved as a specialized branch of philosophy that studies consciousness and experience. In this, it is straightforwardly simple, but not always easy to understand. It encourages the first person voice to emerge at certain points, and its spiraling inward toward pre-reflective awareness is well worth understanding. The phenomenological concept of pre-reflective awareness holds that experiences have subjective, immediately embodied qualities, which we could also call phenomenal or lived qualities. Pre-reflective awareness is "being aware" of what it is like to feel a particular way. Dancing and performing have unique perceptual features in pre-reflective life, different from running or standing still, for instance. Feelings of nervousness, depression, or elation also have unique subjective (or lived) qualities. We might just think of pre-reflective awareness as self-awareness; yet, at the same time we live through an experience, layers of consciousness connect us to a world beyond self—*the lifeworld*—configured in the kinesthetic field of bodily self-awareness.

Body, self, and world are inextricably entwined. This is where phenomenology gets interesting. It views self as part of the world and otherness, even as otherness and world are entwined with the self in unfolding relationships, as we will explore. Attitudes to the body condition these relationships. *World* is an imprecise term that in everyday vernacular can mean planet earth and everything on it, human race, society, parts of these, and a path of decision; it can also mean universe, life, and everything about it, experiences of world, or perhaps a general area of activity (like "dance world," typically used loosely). *World* is a big word to say the least. Edmund Husserl used the more philosophically precise, yet still wide, term *lifeworld*—as envisaged reciprocity of body, psyche, culture, and the natural world, describing the body as "a point of conversion" (1952, 297–299). Later, Maurice Merleau-Ponty broke new ground in his use of the term *chiasm* to describe bodily capacities of perceptual reversibility relative to the outside world. Chiasm describes the body as *a crossing over*, "the intertwining" of phenomena such as touching and touch, the visible and the invisible, body and world (1968, ch. 4).

Lifeworld is central to phenomenology, and it continues to accrue meaning in a variety of contexts. We bring it to considerations of dance and performance in our book with the understanding that phenomenology can be life changing. It has developmental benefits in teaching suspension of judgment and questioning assumptions. Its methods pay close attention to experience, showing how intentional attunement grounds perceptual processes and knowledge. It can be applied to many areas of study, focusing on the potentials of a theme while not depending on established theory. If it doesn't begin with theories, its diverse works often make insightful discoveries and develop new theories.

Next, we expand *lifeworld and the lived body* as related key concepts of our text, while the last part of this chapter concerns *the study of experience* central to phenomenology.

1. Lifeworld and Lived Body

Lifeworld (*lebenswelt*) is defined from several perspectives in Husserl's *Ideas II*—a work penciled in manuscript in 1912, published posthumously in 1952 and, in 1989, translated into English. Lifeworld is an inclusive concept that characterizes experiences of the everyday communicative personal world and the normalized world—also extending to the natural environing world, the intuitive world, and the affective aesthetic world of sense and culture. Husserl critiqued the objective orientations of the natural sciences as the only way of knowing (1989, 383–390). He presents the natural lifeworld as "a world of naturalized realities united with the body as a single psycho-physical thing," but the body he envisions more fully is experienced thematically and with complexity from various "horizons" or "attitudes" (1995, 164–165). Lifeworld is constituted in at least five layers or horizons of experience, and some of these divide further. Our book gives voice to various lifeworlds of dance and performance, including interpersonal and intersubjective communication, intuitive understanding, affective experience, somaesthetic or somatic experience, ecological consciousness, self-understandings, everyday understandings, sociality, and contributions of science.

Lifeworld is sometimes hyphenated in English, as "life-world." It connects the sensed world of substance and form with the formless mysteries of life, the seen with the unseen in experience. As the root expression of lifeworld, "life" is a noun, but scientists Margulis and Sagan say that life functions "more like a verb"—repairing, maintaining, re-creating and outdoing itself (1995, 14). Lifeworld as a concept has unity and multiplicity, worlding within and distantly outward. Thus, it moves: the intricate material phenomena of bodily life extend out interactively toward the environmental world and cycle back in. The breath evidences such cycles.

Husserl originally spoke of the environing natural world. *Our book speaks specifically about nature in light of place*: wilderness places and cultivated ones, barren landscapes, desolate and verdant ones, seascapes, canyon lands, and more. We also turn toward the built (and rebuilt) world of city life. Phenomenologist Edward Casey speaks of nature in experiential terms of "place worlds" (2003, 194), environments that produce specific atmospheres and experiences. Authors of this book benefit from his definition. Specific places and cultures animate performativity and facilitate particular dance experiences.

As lived, nature and culture converge in body and consciousness, as we just considered with Husserl and Merleau-Ponty. Current imperatives of nuclear and climate crisis forge in us a new ethic in respect to nature. We can no longer afford the privileged interpretation of nature as a social construction, or the belief that nature is outside of us. We reject the destructive tendencies of both biological and social determinism. As sociologist Anna Yeatman observes, sociology elaborates the category of the social inclusively, where nature is interpreted as a residual and limiting term in social theory (1990, 287). In seeking to valorize agency and sociality, one can make the mistake of totalizing it. We take the position of phenomenology, which from its be-ginning studies things-in-relation and delineates relational embodiment of humans as part of the world's body—both natural and sociocultural beings. I develop this perspective in earlier works on phenomenology of dance rela-tive to mythology (1987) and metaphysics (2004).

We gain central lessons in phenomenology from Husserl. He taught that we constitute the world in our disposition toward it: "human subjects are only in the world by the fact that, as bearers of world-consciousness, they produce the sense, world, for themselves at every moment" (1995, 166). But this doesn't mean that nature is a fiction, just that it discloses itself to humans in relation to perception and direction of intention. Husserl's ontology does not separate human subjectivity from nature but notices its influence and limits: "subjectivity in its grip upon it changes nature, but alters nothing of the unity of nature as core in its own ontological form" (1995, 189).

Nature is both vast and immanent. As stone and flesh, it appears in many faces and places, and its very marks are life and change. It might live in romantic poetry, but science also explains it, and increasingly in terms of species cooperation. In his book, *The New Wild: Why Invasive Species Will Be Nature's Salvation* (2015), Fred Pearce, noted environmental scientist, shows that "alien" forces and species over time assist in repopulating and sustaining wilderness, advancing the idea that the alien and the native are not necessarily competing. They also cooperate. Many scientists refute the popular notion of survival of the fittest, viewing it as a misinterpretation of Charles Darwin's work. Lynn Margulis and Dorion Sagan in *Microcosmos: Four Billion Years of Microbial Evolution* conceive of evolution in amicable terms. Evolution as violent competition among species and individuals gives way to new views of cooperation, interaction, and mutual interdependence. "Life did not take over the globe by combat, but by networking" (1986, 14–15). In *The New Biology: Discovering the Wisdom in Nature*, Robert Augros and George Stanciu see harmony in nature: "Life works with the environment, not against it. . . . Every living thing is beautifully attuned to its environment" (1988, 138–139).

Likewise, for Husserl, *empathy*, intersubjective mutuality, is a cohesive aspect of experience established dispositionally. Sensuous-intuitive experiences are "dependent on each other" for their content (1989, 179). Thus, connectivity can be cultivated relationally through the body: in our case, through dance and performance, *as lifeworlds are constituted and shared anew through affective reciprocity*. I come by this understanding directly through participation in several movement arts, ranging from modern to contemporary dance through theater performances and somatic studies. I learn further through Husserl that affectivity (psychic life) in itself is individually conditioned, but not entirely: "To each Body for itself there pertains the person's entire psychic life, grasped in empathy" (1989, 176). I shine my curiosity and experience empathy in my connections to others and the world I perceive; I cultivate these somatically (affectively) in dancing and performing with others and through an ethics of relational attentiveness. How I pay attention to the world in its multiplicity has ethical implications. In attending through performance, I can dance toward the earth with gratitude.

*   *   *

Our book gives particular consideration to *the creative lifeworld of making and doing* that phenomenology continues to study through Husserl's influence (see Plate 1). We extend this to the interactive shared world that Husserl articulated in *Sixth Cartesian Meditation*, his work with Eugen Fink in the latter part of his life. Husserl prepared his textual notations and original appendixes for this book over a period of years (as late as 1933–1934) in a rich variety of topics concerning the world of practical life, ecology, culture, and history (1995, xiv, 181–192). The English translation became available in 1995. As a famous Jewish philosopher living in Germany during the rise of Hitler, Husserl accomplished his last works under the threat of anti-Jewish Nazi doctrine. He died in 1938. In his 1936 publication, *Crisis*, he continued to evolve lifeworld meanings (1970).

I call phenomenological inquiry *tabula rasa thinking*. This is the kind that begins with a clean slate and thus allows one to enter a discovery mode of performance and thinking. Phenomenology of any kind is a study of oneself in transition, as in self-referential moments of dancing. It admits the subjective place of the author in dancing, performing, and writing. Still more philosophical foci entail how we humans are situated in the world together, as our authors explore from several vantage points.

It bears repeating from the introduction that this book is concerned with dance and performance as forms of creativity and cultural productivity and also with ways of knowing emerging from specific performative and somatic processes. The latter originate from *soma*, most basically the personal body as regulated and sensed relationally (Fraleigh 2015, xx–xxiv). Because Husserl understood body, soma, and motility as crucial in constituting human consciousness of the lifeworld, his work resonates with somatics as a field of studies and practices. It is significant for concepts of creativity that Husserl brackets (questions and suspends) *activity* as the sole means of cultural productivity. Regarding how consciousness works, he sees *receptivity* as an overlooked constituent of *productivity* (Fink and Husserl 1995, 51). Further, he holds that the productivity of culture involves "high amounts of creativity" (Zahavi 2003, 154). Performative philosophies like that of Deleuze and Guattari provide still more possibilities, as we develop more fully in Chapter 2.

We know by now that Husserl's work as well as the later work of existential phenomenology has traveled cross-culturally. Influences on Japanese phenomenology stand alongside unique Japanese conceptions of the body, now made available in English by Shigenori Nagatomo (1992). Robert Bingham, who has studied with Nagatomo, explores his work in Chapter 3. I integrate views from Japanese phenomenology in *Dancing Identity* (2004, 26–31) and in *BUTOH: Metamorphic dance and global alchemy* (2010, 47, 65–79).

LIFEWORLD, VOICE, AND CURIOSITY

The kind of phenomenology in play depends on who is exploring and questioning, and how they orient their quest. Philosophers, historians, and other theorists write about art and performance from the outside, unless they are also artists or performers. Artists who study philosophy have a ringside seat, especially through phenomenology and applied aesthetics, and they can use this to advantage. In straddling fields of dance and philosophy, I have felt responsible to voice dance experiences through describing the dancer's point of view. If dancers don't do this, then who will? When I write, I ask myself if I can provide examples of what I'm talking about, either from my experience as a dancer and performer, or through describing a performance I've witnessed. *Dance and the Lived Body* (1987) is a descriptive aesthetics with examples of many dances from modern/postmodern and ballet genres. Four of my books on butoh and other dance forms also describe performances extensively, many of them as experiential records (1999, 2004, 2006, 2010). Theory can be dry when it is never applied to actual events and experiences. As phenomenological verification, descriptive examples serve as tests of theory, and they come in a variety of voices, both participatory and observational.

Phenomenology takes form through voice. The initial inquiry is about *phenomena*, another word for *things*, as they arise in consciousness. When we consider dance as a phenomenon and ask, "What is this thing?" or we write about particular dances or performance experiences, we can ask who we are in the picture. Are we speaking with the dancer's voice, that of the audience, or that of the choreographer? Are we speaking broadly beyond concrete manifestations and envisioning ontological essence? Is the voice intimate and local, or is it cast widely to capture the nature of an event? Is the mode of writing interactive, definitional, provocative, or is it seeking to state a principle? Is the writer describing a developmental process or a theatrical performance? Is her perspective cultural? Is it critical or political? When I practice phenomenology—in writing, teaching, and performing—I often ask myself what part of me am I channeling, and can I conjure sensitivities that move my consciousness beyond the limits of my conditioning? In such ways, phenomenology is a self-study, as it develops voice and curiosity.

Readers will recognize various voices among authors in this collection. Each author has a unique style, sometimes overlapping kinds of phenomenologies. In editing the book at hand and writing this first chapter, I have discovered a dynamic and flexible field of phenomenological practices. I also see how the *tenets* of phenomenology can be voiced in media other than words: in dance and music, drawing and visual art, not to mention theater, poetry, somatic movement arts, photography, film, and artists' papers. But this doesn't mean that anything goes. Phenomenology in its study of experience, does not throw reason out the window. Indeed, it wants reason and language on its side. Nevertheless, creativity in the arts often arrives through unconscious, irrational substrata. In Amanda Williamson's Chapter 5, we see how spontaneous visual art from a somatic sense of moving leads toward language, and in Karen Bond's Chapter 11, we witness how dance drawings of children converge with language in a fundamental way.

Somatic movement methods are new partners of the Western arts. Phenomenology supports somatic methods in dance and movement studies through common narratives and theoretical meeting points. I have written more technically about movement-based somatics and phenomenology in my recent book with other contributors, *Moving Consciously* (2015), a book that views somatics as "phenomenology in action" and an approach to personal and professional development applied widely in movement arts, pedagogy, and psychology. Somatics and phenomenology give voice to many of the same principles, as Vida Midgelow's Chapter 4 shows. In principle, both fields attune to the body and let go of assumptions. They both develop a tabula rasa approach to lived time, body, and lifeworld, wiping the slate clean in order to rid the psyche-soma of limiting habits.

The suspension of unquestioned standards in learning processes would be one way of moving past habits and common patterns of dualistic thinking. In methods of phenomenology, *bracketing is a tabula rasa way* of looking at what is taken for granted and preparing for new insight. This is also a matter of finding voice through the power of *both-and inclusive thinking*, as I explain soon. Phenomenologists, like somatic improvisers, invite surprise in the form of unexpected ideas or insights. In finding voice, they both seek "the flowing live present," the experience of present time that Husserl wrote of in his mature years (Bruzina 1995, xiv). This book in your hands has a chapter by Kimerer LaMothe who gives voice to "a philosophy of bodily becoming," valorizing the power of presentness through risk and discovery to broaden the meaning of dance in relation to the earth and world of rural life.

Legitimacy of voice arrives through curiosity in all forms of phenomenology. Curiosity is also basic in dance making, as in improvisation and performance, and it can lead to discovery. The measure of voice in both phenomenology and performance will be found in how we respond, how we keep trust with challenges that arise, what we learn and share, and most assuredly the extent of curiosity we develop as a result. Curiosity grows itself, glowing more brightly through use. In my case, it has carried me into cross-cultural studies through Japan, India, and Germany with specific interests in World War II. I was born in 1939, the year that Hitler invaded Poland, thus my life has been colored by the long-lasting effects of this war, and I have also been curious to understand it from the side of Japan, particularly the war's intersection with butoh, the postmodern dance of Japan. I wrote a Japan-centric account through the lens of my own experiences of nuclear fallout from testing at Frenchman's Flat in Nevada ("Nuclear Fallout and Butoh Invalids," in *Dancing Identity* 2004, 170–183).

Being in unfamiliar circumstances has taught me how culture, time, and place shape experiences. Like phenomenology itself, the unfamiliar often appears through curiosity, but what does one do with it? This is the creative and informative question of searching and writing-into one's experience. Writing in a particular social or political area neither redeems nor disqualifies the author, nor does the experiential voice. What matters is the soundness of the research. There are several avenues toward knowledge. Phenomenology enlarges the narrative-room and space-stage of performance research and dance studies—as an experiential avenue appreciating the complexities of cultures while not reducing them in the process. I appreciate the power of people across wide spectrums of experience to understand each other. The arts, particularly through the expressive immediacy of dance and performance, have such powers. Cross-cultural hybrid aesthetics in the dance of Peiling Kao of the University of Hawaii attest this, as also the dance of Nathalie Guillaume, born in Haiti and living in the United States. Her dance on female divinity unites aesthetics of somatically conceived dance with sensitivities of the African diaspora and Buddhism. *Dancing with the Wind*, her dance in Plate 2, is part of a visual album she is developing to explore Haitian Vodou in its healing forms. She says, "It mirrors African dance from ancient Egypt and Asian expressions from Kabuki in Japan, which I tie into one word "AFRIKASIA" (email communication, August 22, 2017).

THE LIVED BODY, BOTH-AND THINKING, AND WE-LIFE

Dance is immediately enacted nonverbally, while phenomenology offers a philosophy of the body relative to the lifeworld, and is a venture in language and discovery. I am fascinated by the intersection of nonverbal creativity with verbal discourses of embodiment. Amanda Williamson's Chapter 5 shares this fascination. The juncture of language with movement has a somatic component, emphasizing our immediate perceptions of self, or at least this is the supposition. What we call "self" is not bound to individuality and ego. In phenomenology, the self is understood as dynamic and morphic, which doesn't mean that a person doesn't have what neurobiologist Antonio Damasio calls a "material me," a "social me," and a "spiritual me" (2012, 24–25). From my perspective, I would add a somaesthetic "experiential me" and a kinesthetic "moving me," as also a cognitive "knowing self." It is significant that these are descriptive levels of self and not the whole orchestra. Self is ultimately not a thing but "a dynamic process," as Damasio teaches (175) congruent with phenomenology.

Through Husserl's foundational phenomenology, "self" is complex. The body shapes our perceptions of world and otherness and is the basis of self-understanding as founding a sense of our own existence. Husserl distinguishes our embodied fullness as *leib* (in German), or *the lived body*. Phenomenology of the body through his later work explains that "we perceive the lived body but along with it also the things that are perceived 'by means of' it" (quoted in Zahavi 2003, 105). The subjective relationship between body, self, and world is active, both *immanent* as inward looking, and *transcendent* relative to the external world (Fink and Husserl 1995, 158–159). Self is "interwoven" with the world (192). Husserl progressed toward a growing recognition of the intersubjective world and the *lifeworld* (*lebenswelt*). The world is already transcendentally constituted, according to Husserl, and it is up to us to catch up with it.

This is not a private world but a communal one. Life in its myriad meanings is important in Husserl's inclusive discussions of self-awareness, other-awareness, and awareness of the world, shifting away from the self toward a more-than-human ethic. All animals live their bodies, and the body of the world is also alive. Self is not an alone state; it manifests relationships and perceptual multiplicities that can be made explicit in performance, as Noyale Colin describes in "Becoming Plural" (279–296). As living our bodies, we are implicated in the lifeworld, and our being implicated moves both ways: the lifeworld also implicates us. Otherness and lifeworld are "baked into" human life, if you will. Husserl puts this well: "Human life is we-life" in a cultural and environing world constantly in motion. Further, our shared life is impelled: all human life holds "striving toward satisfaction," and in this, "a striving for happiness" (1995, 192).

In the wake of his teachers Husserl and Heidegger, Emmanuel Levinas underlines our subjective responsiveness to each other, providing a particular critique of Heidegger's theoretical ontology of being. Subjectivity, Levinas argues, is (or ought to be) primarily ethical, not theoretical. Our responsibility for the other orients our subjectivity by giving it a meaningful direction (1974, ch. 4). Levinas maintains that subjectivity is conditioned by *empathy*

in responsibility for others. Both-and thinking and Husserl's characteriza-
tion of we-life include possibilities of manifold responsive feelings toward
others, as concerns the topics of this book.

We-life is not simply a matter of human interrelations, but involves the
natural world as well. Value theorist Paul Taylor in *Respect for Nature*, puts
it this way:

> Environmental ethics is concerned with the moral relations that hold between
> humans and the natural world. The ethical principles governing those rela-
> tions determine our duties, obligations, and responsibilities with regard to the
> Earth's natural environment and all animals and plants that inhabit it. (1986, 3)

Indeed, empathic resonance through self-other relations, in collective
community sharing, and in respect for nature is an intrinsic (experiential)
purpose of dance and performance. Is this true of all dance and performance?
I'm not sure it is, especially if I think of more commercial dance. As an experience of we-life, dance relates us to others and to earth on several levels,
as our authors explore. I don't suggest direct kinesthetic correspondence
or always-harmonious rapport. In their works, artists conceive alterity in a
variety of modes, also establishing diverse relationships with audiences and
environmental nature. We dance for ourselves, but also for and with others,
and we are always in some manner relating to surrounding environments,
whether manufactured, cultivated, or wild.

Responsivity to the manifold lifeworld in the arts evinces ethical orientations. What we pay attention to matters. I seek *a relational ethics of attention*, an ethics I pursue extensively in "Canyon Consciousness" (Bond, ed.
forthcoming). Dancing with others and paying attention to the environing
world puts the ethical ventures of art into play. We dance with nature—the
land and its elements, the animals and plants—through our own natures,
and nature answers back. We might wonder whether nature cares. I think it
does. We are as much nature as anything else and entwined with all life. The
ethics of intersubjectivity implicit in Merleau-Ponty's works is explored by
Anya Daly, as she shows how the interdependence of self, other, and world is
affirmed in his *relational ontology* and is markedly different from traditional
ethics founded on the assumptions of dualist or monist ontologies (2016).

Husserl's flowing phenomenology of both-and thinking and we-life precedes Merleau-Ponty, and it also anticipates the process philosophy of Gilles
Deleuze through his collaborations with psychoanalyst Felix Guattari in
the latter half of the twentieth century. Deleuze and Guattari speak to affective "becomings," specifically in a tripartite section of *A Thousand Plateaus*:

"Becoming-Intense, Becoming-Animal, Becoming-Imperceptible" (232–309). They see continuities between earth, animal, and human life: "What we are talking about is not a unity of substance but the infinity of the modifications that are part of one another on this unique plane of life" (254). They theorize movement itself as an imperceptible becoming. With others in this book, I recognize how movement becomes real in the melodic line we hear, in the doing of performance, in a dancing body or dropping leaf.

Phenomenology bubbles up in movement, eventually taking shape through words and ideas, or in performances. Body and *motility* (the ability to move) are foundational in phenomenology. Husserl underlines moving features of the lived body at the heart of the lifeworld and flowing life of experience. His voicings of "lifeworld" and "lived body" concepts are not exact; they are perspectival and morphic for a reason:

> Husserl employs a distinction between *morphological* and *ideal* essences. If we take our point of departure in the perceptual world, and if we investigate the objects we are normally surrounded by, be it utensils such as knives, pens, or glasses, or natural objects such as birds, trees, or stones, they are all characterized by an essential vagueness, and our classification of these objects are, by nature, approximative. If we seek to impose on the phenomena of the lifeworld the exactness and precision that we find in, say, geometry, we violate them. (Zahavi 2003, 130)

What Husserl posited as the lived body is wholly embodied in the lifeworld, made of movement and gifted with ability, ongoing, morphic, and connected to the earth as also the making and doing of human productions. In differing states of flow and becoming, lifeworld includes traditions and normalized activities of dance and performance, and it also *brackets* these (sets them aside) in creative departures. Art evolves through change. It is one of the primary ways we witness our being here and excavate new ways of being in the world.

Through the lens of experience, perspectives of phenomenology speak to somatic states of change and becoming—to a "moving I" and a "moving we"—to "moving with world and nature" and "moving as one." In phenomenology and somatic practices, the body is known through mindful self-awareness, while at the same time being outwardly aware of others and specific environments. Husserl studies how soma expands from self-awareness toward we-life. Like the smooth, open-ended nomad thought of Deleuze and Guattari (1994), Husserl's view of the lived body is also somatically morphic and inclusive. But his style is very different. Here is Husserl on body and movement about eighty years earlier than the performativity of Deleuze and Guattari: "Each movement of the body is full of soul, the coming and going, the standing and sitting, the walking and dancing, etc. Likewise, so is every human performance, every human production" (1989, 252). We consider the morphic performative style of Deleuze and Guattari in Chapter 2.

2. To Study Experience

We have said that phenomenology is the study of experience. Accordingly, is it essentially descriptive and experiential? Or is it highly theoretical?

In manifesting a spectrum of styles and methods, it is both-and, as we show throughout our book. Phenomenology is not purely personal, as is sometimes believed; nor is it a form of *solipsism*—the notion that it is impossible to share knowledge between people or across cultures because the separate self is the only reality. On the contrary, the goal of phenomenology is to move past the personal and toward shared understandings. In this, it advances in two directions, intuitively inward through experiential descriptions and objectively outward toward theory, seeking basic understandings underlying localized instances (Lawrence and O'Connor 1967, 8–9). The basics would be what Husserl called "things in themselves," *phenomena* (objects of perception, the known or noticed). I was taught early on in dance scholarship that nothing is universal. Now I don't believe this. Art exists for increasing understanding, even across cultures, as difficult as this may sometimes seem. Does universality mean understood by everyone, everywhere in the same way? This would seem impossible, and also undesirable. Phenomenology is neither grandly universal nor relativist in radical terms. Its imperative is the study of experience and the discernment of possibility, as it looks toward change and lifeworld connectivity. Self in phenomenology is at root a relational concept; what can seem a separate self is already interactive through reciprocities of nature, culture, and consciousness. Living beings are in exchange: "they all share a common past" (Margulis and Sagan 1995, 4).

As a philosophy, phenomenology develops a nondualistic view of embodiment. Bodymind unity is a principle that runs throughout, a principle now supported in neuroscience and stated well in Damasio's many works beginning with *Descartes' Error* (1994). Phenomenologists explain that body and mind cannot be integrated, because they are not separate to begin with. Body/mind separation, or mind-body duality was Descartes' error. This is an important realization for dance because it creates an appreciation for the intrinsic wholeness of the person, including our intercorporeal connections with each other and the more-than-human lifeworld.

When we bifurcate, we can manipulate. Seeing the mind as the engineer of the body creates a dominator mentality of mind over matter, culture over nature. We see this in suppression of the material body considered inferior, and consequentially in exploitation of the earth, viewed instrumentally as resource for human use. It will take a long time to erase the dualistic language of body and mind as distinct entities in common discourse and in the teaching of dance and movement somatics. We humans are embodied as one with the world. Body, mind, and spirit are convenient language forms, even marketing clichés. We live them as embodied pervasive qualities. Just because we have words for them doesn't mean they are standalone aspects of our living reality. Husserl's works offered a powerful refutation of dualisms, including that of self and other.

Self is identification. Perhaps we are too preoccupied with self. Our aim should be more comprehensive and less ego-centered. When I taught in Japan, students suggested a theme of "body as spirit." Now it seems a natural meme to me. Bodily cultivation in Asia is a spiritual endeavor. Our being in the world is all-encompassing. The body doesn't end with the skin; it exudes *ki*, the invisible energy that unites all life. Japanese phenomenology accounts for this (Nagatomo 1992).

We can acknowledge, however, that feelings of separation and confusion are real. These are explained by existential phenomenology as *lived dualisms*. Feelings of ambiguity, disturbance, or isolation are common, as are depressive states. But such states do not signal that the mind and body are in conflict; rather, the mental and physical implicate each other, inescapably. Feelings of lack and hurt are real, as are illness and loss, and they can adversely influence lives.

Fortunately, life is also shaped autobiographically over time through positive creative processes. I grew up on a ranch in Southwest Utah in one of the most remote and poorest areas of the United States at that time. I didn't experience myself as impoverished, however. I read a lot and played piano and organ. In looking back on a lifetime of dancing, music, and books, I now understand how I came to my current life of teaching and scholarship, just as past experiences of rural life prompt my returning home to the earth wherever I am. I have never worked on a factory floor, but I have taught those who have and am rewarded now in my somatics practice in teaching people from many walks of life.

We undergo the processes we ourselves set in motion and are created and changed by them. We are formed through our performances, particularly the daily rituals. The living tension at the center of phenomenology acknowledges that spark glowing in each person that wants to realize more of itself. The way we spend our time, move our thoughts, and perform our dances eventually settles into the way we breathe and communicate.

* * *

As a research paradigm, phenomenology represents a form of *qualitative inquiry* distinct from quantitative inquiry developed in science. Quantification through employment of statistics in the physical and social sciences is just one way of looking at knowledge, and not the only way. Husserl's *Crisis* (1970) was an extensive critique of science as the only valid form of knowledge. *Researching Dance* (1999), which I edited with Penelope Hanstein, takes up this issue for dance, providing a broad view of qualitative research methods of history, culture, philosophy, and ethnography, also including quantitative scientific methods of kinesiology.

Through its various perspectives, phenomenology investigates individual and intrapersonal lifeworlds, also accounting for cultural and ecological worlds. It stems from the study of experience, not through navel gazing, but with bodies of knowledge extending over more than a century. Human experience of a more-than-human world becomes increasingly important in our times. *Intersubjectivity* is a key concept of phenomenology, delineating what passes between people experientially and how community arises, while also voicing our human responsibility to the larger world.

Seeking the large picture, phenomenology looks deeply into human involvements with manifold lifeworlds. Martin Heidegger's *hermeneutic* (interpretive) phenomenology speaks of allowing all things to be what they are in themselves. *Seinlassen* (letting be) was one of his themes in *Being and Time* (1962) first published in 1927 about ninety years ago. What Heidegger calls *seinlassen* enables a path of difference, even gratitude, for otherness in letting beings be what they are (Llewelyn 2003, 62). Through his background with Husserl, Heidegger's philosophy spreads toward the lifeworld in the sense of letting the natural world flourish, not using nature as a resource for consumption, not trashing nature, but touching the world with care. In movement contexts, shifting away from chronic overdrive would be a somatic way of letting be. Awareness of others and one's surroundings in an allowing frame of mind is another way of letting be. Similarly in "Letting the Difference Happen," I conceive metaphysics of difference, examining the work of mindful presence in movement arts and performance in *Dancing Identity* (2004, 136–147).

Unfortunately, Heidegger's work lives under the shadow of National Socialism through his associations with the Nazi Party, no matter how valuable his insights. *Dancing Identity* includes my extensive reading and critique of Heidegger. I substitute somatic "matching" for terms of "mastery," as these appear in his work and extensively in the arts; at the same time, I recognize how Heidegger deconstructs aesthetic terms of mastery in art, especially in critiquing dominant goal-setting and historical dexterity, understood as discipline (1999, 144–145). In a curious way, he advocates "lack of art" as a point of beginning. He published *Being and Time* (1962 [1927]) a few years before his political turn toward fascism. By now, however, it is clear that we cannot separate the man and his times from his philosophy (Farias 1987). In one of my observations on butoh and WWII, I look into Heidegger's early Catholic upbringing and the roots of his anti-Semitism (2010, 119).

We turn to Heidegger's Jewish teacher Husserl concerning eco-phenomenology and conscious engagement of the lifeworld. It is significant that Heidegger dedicated *Being and Time* to Husserl, even as their relationship became strained, and that both philosophers advanced environmental themes. I read Husserl's work as an extended journey in dedicated philosophical thinking. His ideas underline generations of phenomenologies. Yet, because he was Jewish, the infamous race laws in Germany of 1933 stripped him of his academic standing and privileges.

In today's world, we have opportunities to shift often-marginalized environmental concerns to center stage through collaborations between science and art. Ventures of art and technology are alive in the work of dancers, as we see in this volume (see Plate 3).

The ecological body has been and still remains a large part of phenomenologies of performance. Our human body relates to earth as "the living earth," not dead inert material. As in a dance, the earth is alive in a full orchestra of flowing change. Husserl first recognized "the flowing change" of the world as a matter of conscious perception (1995, 182–183).

Consciousness matters, as phenomenology holds at its source. It brings consciousness to mind in several ways and describes the contents of consciousness through related experiential themes, beginning with the body:

- Corporeality—lived body and the living of body and world
- Materiality—lived things, living things, and the living of things

- Relationality—we-life, lived self and other, intersubjectivity, intra-subjectivity, and ecology
- Temporality—lived time and the living of time
- Spatiality—lived space and the living of space
- Motility—ability, movement, growth, change, and morphology
- Kinesthesia—kinesthetic awareness as access to the lifeworld
- Aesthetics—experiential values of felt life, affective life in arts and performance, and interexperience in collaborations
- Ethics—responsibility for living justly, development of conscience and empathy
- Embodied Mind—as generated in action and delineated in performance

This limited list on experiential themes reveals central topics for dance and performance studies, as we have only begun to sketch and will become more apparent throughout our book. Studies in phenomenology are supported by an intellectual history that has branched into various bodies of knowledge, as we consider in Chapter 2.

2

Branching into Phenomenologies

SONDRA FRALEIGH

As philosophy, phenomenology has more in common with the intuitive processes and observational skills of the arts than with those of science; nevertheless, Husserl projected his philosophy as a transcendental science. He originally published *Logical Investigations*, the root text of phenomenology in 1900–1901 (English translation, 1970), but he didn't consider his philosophy complete, even in subsequent writing. In his old age, he designated his trusted assistant Eugen Fink to the task of furthering his "transcendental method." Husserl himself provided notations and additions (Fink and Husserl 1995). Despite this, Fink's attempt to explain the phenomenological method of reduction remained provisional. Fink considered his extensive work on Husserl's philosophy "a draft" (1995, xlvii–xlviii).

Unfinished Work

With its genesis in Husserl's transcendental outlook—and its later philosophical expansions in existentialism, heuristics, hermeneutics, ecology, neurology, and performativity—phenomenology emerges with concrete approaches and inspiring concepts, but not with an exact methodology. Thus, my standpoint, and that of our book: There is no single phenomenological method. Several methods have developed with adaptive frameworks to guide distinct strands of qualitative study and research, as I explore throughout this chapter. This pluralistic way of looking at phenomenology is not intended as one of closure.

In various ways, phenomenology invites artists and other scholars to examine dance performance as experience. When writers apply phenomenology in studies of the arts, the result might well be called "applied phenomenology." Artists and practitioners have unique experiential and pragmatic perspectives, but applications require study of the groundwork of phenomenology. Does phenomenology represent truth? If we can speak of experiential truth, I believe it can and does. *Truth* is not a master word in phenomenology but part of a fuller fabric of experiential understanding and knowledge.

Dance as something humans do is not abstract in application; assimilating perception and imagination in action, dance produces embodied ways of knowing—or embodied epistemologies—subject to interpretation. Dance and performance advance tests of phenomenology in application to experiences from the tangible to the nonmaterial. All forms of phenomenology are concerned with lived experience and lifeworld and as such are ripe for researching dance and performance.

Husserl's view of "the lifeworld" is foundational throughout varieties of phenomenology. His lifeworld concepts are basic to understanding intersubjectivity, as well as the more complex and less binary concept of intrasubjectivity, interexperiences shared with others, and applications of phenomenology to the more-than-human world. Husserl's views are not anthropocentric; rather, they are inclusive, anticipating the present epoch when human activities globally impact earth's ecosystems. Some propose the geological term *Anthropocene* for our time, as we see in Robert Bingham's analysis in this text. Transcendental spirit in Husserl doesn't point to normative understandings of spirituality. Instead, Husserl brings attention to habit like a somatic therapist, "inhibiting" norms (*inhibiting* is his word and also a key term in the somatics of the Alexander Technique). But his concern for individual and social habitus goes still further—toward inhibiting self-identifications of ego by bracketing ever further toward a renewal of the human person (he also uses "soul" for "person")—all this, in recognition of the "flowing change of the world" (1995, 182–186).

Forms of Phenomenology

Philosophical phenomenology is basic to all other forms. It suspends presuppositions, moving past the obvious and toward what Moshe Feldenkrais called "the elusive obvious" in his somatic movement education. As grounded in philosophy, phenomenology sometimes draws upon the history of philosophy and seeks to explain the contents and operations of conscious awareness. Regarding this, it refutes dualistic, hierarchical language, demonstrating that perception is influenced by intention and that without feeling there is no consciousness. It holds that the brain is not simply mental, but part of an entire symphony of conscious embodiment. Neurobiologists also advance philosophical themes of embodiment, as Antonio Damasio does in tracing generative concepts of self and body in *Self Comes to Mind* (2012). Thus embodiment as a phenomenological theme sustains *neurophenomenology*, which we take up at the end of this section.

Transcendental phenomenology is defined in Edmund Husserl's philosophy and provides the root of phenomenological inquiry. It accepts subjectivities of the "normal mode" of awareness, and seeks to go beyond this through awakening a state of "transcendental subjectivity." In this effort, Husserl seeks to go beyond accepted norms through a bracketing or reduction of the normal mode or "natural attitude." In thinking and writing, *bracketing* is the act of suspending judgment, also called *epoché* and phenomenological reduction. I extrapolate for dance and performance arts that bracketing can be found in conscious hesitation and waiting. In the interval lies treasure: "In the phenomenological reduction there occurs the awakening of the transcendental constitution of the world" (Fink and Husserl 1995, 13–14). This awakening is not necessarily religious, but it could be; more directly, it suggests intuition and spirituality. In pursuing the difficult questions of transcendental phenomenology, Ami Shulman and Hillel Braude develop Chapter 10 of this book.

Existential phenomenology, a philosophical and literary movement influencing the art, religion, and psychology of the latter half of the twentieth century, is still evolving aesthetic and therapeutic forms of subjective experience. As a branch of philosophy, it is founded on Husserl's ontological insights on the nature of being but develops them in a more openly expressive mien. Existentialism provides impetus to *sex and gender phenomenology* through Simone de Beauvoir's philosophy and novels, continuing in the contemporary feminism of Judith Butler and others. In the present text, Karen Barbour's Chapter 12 situates feminism historically in phenomenology, dance, and performance. Existentialist views of Maurice Merleau-Ponty, Jean Paul Sartre, and Martin Heidegger draw Husserl's transcendental phenomenology toward psychology, even its liminal and unconscious terrains. Christine Bellerose's Chapter 9 locates the Japanese concept of *ma* as a liminal space-time event at the nexus of existential phenomenology and the lived body. On Husserl's terms, initial observations are naive and full of assumptions. Thus, moving toward a pre-reflective intuitive grasp of phenomena, the "things" of consciousness, requires letting go of bias and accepted theories. This standpoint encourages descriptive accounts of lived experience, including those of dance and performance. When these include discoveries in poetry or nonverbal expression in the arts, they overlap heuristics, the mode we discuss next.

Heuristic phenomenology often has autobiographical features and employs discovery modes of inquiry by following the author's experiential narrative. This mode may also involve narratives and insights of others. Like all phenomenology, it aims to illuminate its subject and employs experiential description. It might also include photographs, drawings, video links, poetry, film, and other forms of expression. Psychologist Clark Moustakas articulates this approach well in his book, *Heuristic Research: Design, Method, and Applications* (1990). Transpersonal psychology as initiated by Carl Jung, also presents heuristic elements, particularly through Jung's discovery model of "active imagination" and the art it inspires, as we see in Amanda Williamson's Chapter 5 on language, art, and somatic process.

My Chapter 6 on living phenomenology takes heuristics in a performative direction, drawing from common tones in music and morphic relationships in dance and life. Post-intentional phenomenology incorporates elements of post-structural thinking into traditional methods, as outlined by Mark Vagle in *Crafting Phenomenological Research* (2014). Intention as quality of purposefulness is important in this view, as in all phenomenology, but here it is seen as shifting or unstable and overlapping. Such shifts emphasize the morphic quality of sense perception and consciousness. In a similar vein, Max van Manen's *Phenomenology of Practice* (2014) provides artists and practitioners an avenue toward practice as phenomenological research.

Hermeneutic phenomenology and analysis makes use of interpretation and admits the subjective position of the author involved in making and articulating meaning. Traditionally, hermeneutics is about drawing meaning from textual analysis, but meaning-making itself can become the focus, including meaning in the arts, as we see in this volume. Meaning comes through interpretation, not as objectively complete, but as ongoing. It also arrives through performativity. What we examine later as *performative phenomenology* can be understood as hermeneutic as well. There are indeed many correspondences in various kinds of phenomenology. In her previously published chapter on hermeneutic inquiry, "Dance in the Hermeneutic Circle," Joanna McNamara explains that phenomenological hermeneutics emphasizes the value of subjective understanding within various contexts (1999, 164–178). McNamara's Chapter 8 in this book delves into a sense of place, where in the current evolution of the city of Detroit, place becomes text, film, dance, and discovery. We understand a place in recovery through her on-site participation and interactions with fellow artists. The aesthetic and cultural situations of dance provide unique opportunities for hermeneutic phenomenology.

Three recent strands of phenomenology have precedent in earlier forms but take unique directions. As newer and less familiar approaches, I develop them in more detail next.

Eco-phenomenology concerns human experiences of natural and cultural environments. Because Husserl elucidates an encompassing view of lifeworlds, his work is also the root of eco-phenomenology. Seen in context of our present work, environmental issues have far-reaching implications for performative participation in the lifeworld. Beneficial experiences of environing nature and the more-than-human world are of specific import. For example, in "Towards a Posthuman Ethics," Michael Morris shines light on the ecological body through moving with others (2015, 201–217). Bioethics emerged persuasively through the work of value theorist Paul Taylor in *Respect for Nature* (1986). A recent anthology, *Eco-Phenomenology: Back to the Earth Itself*, also inspires an agentic participatory view (Brown and Toadvine 2003). From similar participatory standpoints, Robert Bingham addresses the urgencies of eco-phenomenology in Chapter 3 of this text, and Joanna McNamara's Chapter 8 looks into the revitalization of Detroit.

Like ecology in its study of living systems, phenomenology turns toward our relationship with the planet. Both ecology and phenomenology derive from a concern for our being-with-the-world as human while also being part of something larger than human. In tandem with philosophy and the arts, eco-phenomenology shows that we need to proceed with heartfelt connectivity to nature. We carry culture in our heritage and habits, but we are also animals of the natural world who share the earth with all other life forms. We all breathe the same air. Shall we be friends of air and earth? Shall we find the sacred in water? Shall we be our own best friends?

Relative to this, shall we give up *mastery* (mind over matter) in favor of *listening and discovery*? This is a phenomenological question that relates to "discovery" as a concept, and at the same time accounts for the aspect of form in dance. Soma is formless potential until it is discovered in commitment to actions and experienced as able. Dance gives us an embodied way of attending to ecological concerns. We see this in Bingham's Chapter 3 and the butoh of Atsushi Takenouchi who follows the lead of Kazuo and Yoshito Ohno, his butoh mentors and mine. Atsushi's butoh film, *Ridden by Nature*, is represented in Figure 2.1.

Embodiment remains an important theme in eco-phenomenology. David Abram's first ecological phenomenology, *Spell of the Sensuous* (1996),

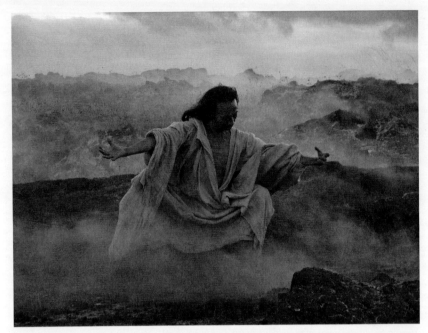

Figure 2.1. Atsushi Takenouchi in *Ridden by Nature*. Photograph of Takenouchi taken in Hawaii during the film project, "Ridden by Nature." Film by Kiah Keya, directed by Kathi von Koerber, featuring dancers Takenouchi and von Koerber. Photograph © 2007 by Hiroko Komiya.

illuminates the affective in nature, including the generative in human life. Likewise in *Wild Hunger* (1998), Bruce Wilshire's phenomenology studies addictions through his conviction that addictive dependencies stem from emotional deprivation and an inability to access the regenerative sources inherent in nature. Relaying her experiences of dance and performance in "Performing Body as Nature," Alison East writes of how performing with (and as) nature gives us the opportunity to activate the renewing sources of our own nature (2015, 164–179).

Performative phenomenology might be seen from different vantage points. I see it as a strand of phenomenology that pays attention to embodied actions (and conditions) apparent through behavior and utterance, especially movement interactions and gestures of speech. Performative "parts" of phenomenology correspond with parts in scripts, novels, plays, and performance arts, attesting that performance is a pervasive component. There are many examples of this, in the twentieth-century dramatizations of Sartre, the resonant poiesis of Maurice Merleau-Ponty, and the originative feminism of Simone de Beauvoir with its existential focus on dynamics of birth and becoming woman. Early in the history of phenomenology, her writing was full of happenings, not just ideas. Beauvoir wrote plays and novels to ground her philosophy of ambiguities. Much later, Judith Butler's contemporary phenomenology outlined "performativity" as a political/feminist concept in *Bodies that Matter* (1993). Her work might be termed feminist or gender phenomenology as well as performative. I produced a textual "Anti-Essentialist Trio" with Butler, Merleau-Ponty, and Beauvoir as performers (*Dancing Identity*, 2004, ch. 4). The presence of performativity in text might leave us wondering whether language has not co-opted the body. To be sure, language can be performative, but can it perform as dancers do? This question reminds me that writing is also an art, and language plays a part in our understandings of art. Language and art can illuminate each other. In one sense, all phenomenology is a performance; it isn't enough to explain phenomenology, ultimately, it is a *doing*.

The work of Deleuze and Guattari introduced performativity into philosophical phenomenology—explicitly—to challenge fixed meanings and the idea that the world is easily tamed by words. They have therefore been close conceptual friends of the arts. They are theorists, but their theory is lively and morphic. Morphology is for them a wide phenomenon relative to sense and the movements of thought. I am not the only one to notice this, especially in its relationship to butoh. Laura Cull connects butoh metamorphosis to metamorphic elements and themes of Deleuze and Guattari (Cull 2013, ch. 3). Deleuze also authored many solo works, writing prolifically about the arts, with cinema as a primary interest. He has influenced performance studies, musicology, anthropology, gender studies, and literary studies.

Shifting through patterns of experience and bodily states in *Kafka*, Deleuze and Guattari provide accounts of conceptual and social metamorphosis that inspire segues with morphology in performance (1986). Theirs is a philosophy immersed in changing states and circumstances, performative readings, and open-ended meanings. Their book, *A Thousand Plateaus* (1987), asks provocative questions, such as: "How do you make yourself into a body without organs?" And, "Who does the earth think it is?" Soma spills into these questions. Or it splits and striates.

Consider the question about organs discussed in *A Thousand Plateaus*, specifically in the section, "Plane of Consistency: Body without Organs" (1987, 506–508). The authors view a plane of consistency that knows nothing of substance and form. Rather, it exists in relations of speed and slowness that tie together heterogeneous elements and resist conclusions. Plane of consistency (PoC) and body without organs (BwO) are parallel and smooth, just as the power of the composed and the composer (in music and dance) are parallel. They belong to each other. PoC is connective, operating smoothly and with somatic reversibility, as a dance that moves forward can also move in retrograde and assemblages can disassemble. If my immersion in the world constructs me, I also construct my world immersions.

If I take these ideas toward the human soma, I could say that in spilling over form and into consistency, the nomadic and ongoing body of soma-psyche exceeds organic assembly; it is both-and, as alive in organic substance, but much more than organs. It is partially understood through biology, but not caught there. Soma, complex and pervasive, takes on multiple meanings, incorporating psyche as living breath and malleable essence. Soma cannot be reduced to essence, nor is it form. It maintains a deep consistency (PoC) as a both-and phenomenon, both special and ordinary in its powers. It is *special* as a topic of study and *ordinary* as a basic unsung stratum of existence. Soma as body, whether animate or sleepy, is always with us, humming along unnoticed. We can coax it to attention, however, through mindful use of motility and with sensibility and perception as partners.

I might coax my body into a slippery somatic whole, for instance, dancing smoothly without organs—spiral with snakelike consistency where ends and beginnings merge—surpass habitual assemblage, become slithery reptile and morph to my heart's content—if while roaming in nature, I chanced on a desert plateau and lay down in the sun, became consistent with it—my nomad consciousness easing as thoughts disappear—where BwO is PoC and a thousand plateaus.

Deleuze's philosophy is performative, but is he a phenomenologist? For Deleuze, the performative task of art is not to "represent" but to produce "signs" that will jolt us out of our habits of perception and into events of creation (1994, ch. 3). This is also the central task of phenomenology. Commentators like Stephan Günzel see Deleuze in light of phenomenological philosophy. From his own point of view, Deleuze writes of Sartre as his teacher, includes insights from Husserl, and critiques Heidegger, whom he resembles in many ways. Most of all, Deleuze is inspired by Merleau-Ponty's concepts of "flesh and folding," demonstrating that art pursues the same venture as phenomenology. Art practices *epoché* and shows affective phenomena as such. Deleuze shows further how phenomenology can become a phenomenology of art (Günzel 2014), suggesting how the things of art (objects, appearances, and performances) jump toward our feelings for them.

Physicist Karen Barad explains how matter and meaning are entangled in performative approaches to epistemology, ontology, and ethics. She calls into question the basic premises of representation by focusing inquiry on the practices or performances of representing. In her transdisciplinary view, subject and object are entangled intra-actively through performance (emerging through doing). She suggests intra-action as a more complex happening than interaction. Matter is never devoid of meaning or value, nor is memory a record of a fixed past (2007). As mattering, dancing materializes in bodily processes of being and becoming, arising and receding, falling and dwelling. As mattering, dance is an indicator of value. First, dancing holds experiential values that are intrinsic by definition, and intrinsic values do not serve other ends; they have value in themselves (Taylor 1961). We dance for the dancing, but cognitive purposes can also generate the dance, as explained later through Karen Barbour's Chapter 12. Theories of enaction reveal how experiential and cognitive values are joined in creative contexts, as neurophenomenology reveals.

Neurophenomenology presents a particular perspective on embodiment and enaction through the work of Chilean biologist, philosopher, and neuroscientist, Francisco Varela, and the previously mentioned work of Antonio Damasio. Varela advocates passages between experience and science through the tradition of phenomenology (1996). This model can speak to dance and performance, especially at the somatic level and in terms of image in performance. When we move and dance, we generate imagery both abstract and concrete. Embodied images are "the main currency of our minds," according to Damasio (2012, 170), and mind as embodied is more than the ability to think in words. Images are surely constructed in thoughts and ideas, but also in colors, sounds, visualizations, rhythmic movement, tastes, smells, and remembered stories. In dancing, images are affectively felt and cognitively processed. Kinesthetic and tactile images arrive somatically through movement and touch, first through sense impressions, and then, for many, in "feelings of knowing" with distinct patterns and attunements that can be described as cognitive phenomena—understandings ingrained through kinesthetic attention and awareness. Part of Damasio's project is concerned with embodied creativity—showing how "the ability to transform and combine images of actions and scenarios is the wellspring of creativity" (1999, 24). For a current example of neurophenomenology in dance studies, we look toward the work of Glena Bateson at the intersection of science, aesthetics, and movement (Bateson and Wilson 2014).

My Story in Phenomenology

In both dancing and writing, I have morphed through several strands of phenomenology. My first book, *Dance and the Lived Body* (1987), examines dance through *existential phenomenology*. It looks toward the expansive experience of dance in view of self and other, since relativity of self and other(s) is a major theme of phenomenology. It also turns attention toward *the dance itself*, defining its ontology or identifying features and bracketing and questioning taken-for-granted definitions of dance as "self expression" in the writing and accepted views of that time. This leads toward a descriptive aesthetics in delineating aesthetic models that sustain classical and modern/postmodern dance forms. As a witness, I describe many contemporary and classical works—from Balanchine's ballet to butoh, from the modernism of Martha Graham, Anna Sokolow, and Merce Cunningham to the postmodern drift of Garth Fagan and Twyla Tharp, and also taking up the athleticism and daring of Elizabeth Streb. My story reflects my experiences in modern and postmodern dance (beginning in 1958 and continuing into contemporary forms) and my early study in Germany with Mary Wigman in 1965. Wigman provides me an expressionist lens for later examinations of butoh and the contemporary Tanz Theater of Germans Pina Bausch and Susanna Linke. I describe Bausch and Linke in relation to the expressionist backgrounds of butoh in "Shibui and the Sublime" and "Liebe," two chapters of *Dancing into Darkness: Butoh, Zen, and Japan* (1999).

Dance and the Lived Body draws upon historical elements in both philosophy and dance but with a focus on existential approaches. The scope of inquiry is descriptive aesthetics and dance as theater art. The view of this book in your hands is much wider, including descriptions of phenomenological experiences in dance improvisation, dance in the lives of children, dynamics of dance in religious and spiritual frameworks, dance conceived somatically for human development, performance in light of ecology, contributions of transpersonal psychology to performativity in somatic contexts, analysis of dance through the *free fantasy variation* of transcendental phenomenology, discovery and rejuvenation of place through dance and film, liminal experiences in dance explained through Japanese cosmology, dance in relation to epistemology and feminism, and perspectives on living phenomenology through bodily attunement.

In bracketing the taken-for-granted, my early work delineates dance through the concept of "the lived body" as aesthetically constituted movement of our own doing, making, and perceiving. Merleau Ponty's *Phenom-*

enology of Perception (1962) and his work *Primacy of Perception* (1964) are central texts in *Dance and the Lived Body*. As a whole, the book points toward an existential ontology of dance, elucidating dance as experience and performance. It describes the passage of dance between dancers and audiences through the living of space and time, taking an empathic and symbiotic phenomenological position: "affirmation of bodily being is a potential value for both the dancer and the audience, because they share the dance—*as body*" (1987, 55).

Several strands from Merleau-Ponty, Beauvoir, and Butler assist my later book, *Dancing Identity: Metaphysics in Motion* (2004). I critique Heidegger's postmetaphysical phenomenology in his *Contributions to Philosophy* (1999), a deconstruction of traditional metaphysics. I also include personal life stories of body and earth—extending metaphysics toward the real and enduring ecological crises of nuclear testing near my home in Utah, with never to be undone damages to nature and people. These have been some of my sources, but there are many possible, unplumbed versions of body, earth, and dance in the potentials of ecological phenomenology.

Moving Consciously, my recent text with other contributors (2015), evolved in part out of phenomenological inquiry into teaching dance and performance somatically. If we can grasp somatic teaching approaches in *tabula rasa thinking*, then we will also be speaking about a somatic style of learning. *Moving Consciously* evolves definitions of somatics in a phenomenological way. At the same time, it acknowledges the entire field of somatic movement studies, or "somatic movement arts." Somatics enlivens movement arts when taught with affective narratives and attunements. Phenomenology keeps us curious about somatic contexts for creativity and learning, and it outlines ways of describing experiential values of dance and performance.

We might wonder whether somatics provides a model for yet another form of phenomenology. Or is somatic awareness simply an experiential thread that extends from Husserl through all phenomenologies? And how about the important questions of sex and gender relative to phenomenology and embodiment? The act of questioning is itself phenomenologically generative.

Editor's Note: Amanda Williamson, one of our authors, stimulated my interest in editing and writing for this book through her extensive interview with me, "On Dance and Phenomenology," and her publication of my article, "Phenomenologies in the Flowing Live Present." The interview and article both appear in the journal she edits, Dance, Movement & Spiritualities *2.2 (Fall 2016).*

3

Improvising Meaning
in the Age of Humans

ROBERT BINGHAM

In the introduction to *Vibrant Matter*, philosopher Jane Bennett describes noticing, while standing on a Baltimore street, a tableau of five diverse items: a dead rat, a man's glove, a bottle cap, a stick, and some scattered oak pollen. The tableau is strangely charismatic, drawing her attention in. As she lingers in its midst, Bennett begins to notice a change:

> As I encountered these items, they shimmied back and forth between debris and thing—between, on the one hand, stuff to ignore, except insofar as it betokened human activity . . . and, on the other hand, stuff that commanded attention in its own right. . . . In the second moment, stuff exhibited its thing-power: it issued a call, even if I did not understand quite what it was saying. (2011, 4)

The stuff appearing in the first instance to be inconsequential trash becomes, in the next, vibrant matter whose story exceeds meanings captured by the notion "trash." Bennett recognizes that as her view changes, so does that which she is viewing, and she begins to wonder how other things may be different than they seem. For much of the rest of the book, Bennett reflects on the nature of matter and the way humans relate to it, seeking insight into matter's meaning in a world splintering under the weight of humanity's environmental demands. As extractive economies transform earth's ecosystems to accommodate the "hyperconsumptive necessity of junking [commodities] to make room for new ones" (5), Bennett makes an appeal to rethinking matter:

> If I am right that an image of inert matter helps animate our current practice of aggressively wasteful and planet-endangering consumption, then a materi-

ality experienced as a lively force with agentic capacity could animate a more ecologically-sustainable public. (51)

Bennett appeals to rethinking matter conceptually, as something lively and creative, yet she also appeals to rethinking matter experientially. How might one do this? She does not explain, and her encounter on the Baltimore street suggests that, in that moment, the choice to view the tableau in depth emanated from the power of the things themselves, rather than her intentions alone. Still, she seems to favor an attitude of receptivity to matter, which she suggests could foster conditions suitable to change:

> The hope is that . . . [*Vibrant Matter*] will enhance receptivity to the impersonal life that surrounds us, will generate a more subtle awareness of the complicated web of dissonant connections between bodies, and will enable wiser interventions into that ecology. (4)

"Improvising Meaning in the Age of Humans" is written with a similar intention. Like Bennett, I aim to account for the vibrancy, agency, and creativity of nonhuman things and beings as a means of responding to a global environmental crisis brought on by prevailing patterns of human activity in relation to planetary "resources." As a dance improviser and phenomenologist, I approach the subject in a spirit of playful rupture of assumptions about what is human and what isn't, and where knowledge resides. Rather than attempting to formulate an "original," clear-cut theoretical position on these questions, however, my aim is to provoke further questioning into how dance can and does transform, heal, revitalize, and aestheticize human-earth relations in the context of a planet in crisis. In short, I am asking, and inviting the reader to ask, what it means to dance in the "Age of Humans" (Robin 2016).

My orientation is what Abram refers to as the "more than human world," and humanity's coexistence with nonhuman things, beings, histories, and temporalities (1996). I am asking how, as someone whose personal world view was formed in the context of anthropocentric religion, schooling, and cultural practices, I might learn afresh how to know the world and to develop the capacity to tell stories that do not, intentionally or unintentionally, reinforce humanity's positioning at the center of the universe of significance in relation to all other living beings on earth. How might this influence my sense of responsibility and citizenship? Dance is the backbone of the investigation. Through improvised, somatically guided dancing joined with the phenomenological procedure of "bracketing" assumptions about phenomena I encounter while dancing, I enter a world whose nonhuman denizens "become strange" (Sheets-Johnstone 2011, 124) in the nature of their vibrancy and in their coparticipation in my own human movement and thinking. In this world, matter matters (Barad 2007). From the perspective of this world, I confront the issue of environmental crisis as a *reason to dance*.

How might one define "environmental crisis"? With seemingly daily reports of record-breaking heat, storms, drought, wildfires, oil spills, and poisoned water, it is challenging to find an organizing principle that speaks to both specific circumstances, including human and nonhuman suffering, adaptation, and resistant action, and to the global nature of anthropogenic changes to planetary beings and systems. "Global warming" and "climate change" signal earthwide change, but, to someone like myself unschooled in the profound complexity of these phenomena and their effects, these representations can seem innocuous, particularly when their effects are not obvious to me where I reside. Moreover, from a lay perspective, the terminologies appear to be limited to the domain of "weather," which, for much of my life lived in contexts of middle-class urban American privilege, existed as a backdrop to existence, generally pleasing or irritating, the emblem of banality in the realm of human significances: *we talked about the weather*. In my experience, weather, until very recently, did not figure as a living expression of earth's nature and meaning.

The meaning of Anthropocene, the proposed and recently approved designation for our current geologic time period (Working Group 2016), extends beyond human-caused changes to weather patterns, as it includes anthropogenic changes in the chemistries and behavior of soil, water, air, plants, animals and ecosystems worldwide, including changes associated with global nuclear fallout following decades of Cold War weapons tests (Simon et al. 2006). As a pithy, unhyphenated term, *Anthropocene* signals the entanglement of human and earth history, and it puts pressure on enduring notions of earth as mere backdrop to human histories and composite of inert materials waiting to be extracted for human purposes. It is a contested term, however, because it does not, in itself, account for profound inequalities woven into the history of anthropogenic changes to the Earth system, nor to the relationship of ecological violence with colonialism, capitalism, and the theft of Indigenous land worldwide (Davis and Turpin 2015). Other terms, such as *Capitolene* and *Eurocene*, are sometimes employed outside the sciences; these effectively shift emphasis from homo sapiens as an innately ecologically destructive being to specific patterns of human *movement*, enacted asymmetrically across the globe, which push the Earth toward chaos (ibid.). Not all humans are equally implicated in the crisis, nor are all humans equally vulnerable to the effects of what Michelle Murphy, who studies the environmental and human impacts of industrial chemicals such as PCBs, calls "the aftermath" (2016). As Rob Nixon writes, those who contribute the least to the crisis tend to absorb the worst of its effects, particularly in the Global South, to which much of the crisis is "outsourced" (2011, 22).

Despite its limitations, I choose to employ Anthropocene as a term that, on its very surface, gives the lie to the fiction of a nature-culture split and, on a deeper level, integrates notions of human and earth time, even as I also recognize and acknowledge its limitations. Dance phenomenology led me to the concept, whose roots live in earth's unfolding geologic story. As I describe later in the chapter, geology represents a world that opened up to me through the act of dancing.

Dance as Methodology

Research for this writing took place in the summer of 2015, when I traveled to Southwest Utah to conduct a three-week, in-depth interview with Sondra Fraleigh. Fraleigh, whom I have known personally and professionally since studying with her as an MFA student in the early 2000s, is a dance artist, philosopher, and somatic movement educator widely known within and outside the academic dance community for her writing and teaching in the areas of phenomenology, dance aesthetics, somatics, and butoh. Her decades of inquiry into the nature and meaning of dance and human embodiment have consistently, if not always predominantly, included questioning concepts surrounding the relationship of humans and environmental nature. She mounts critiques of the nature-culture divide in Western philosophy in *Dance and the Lived Body* (1987) and *Dancing Identity* (2004), and all of her many writings on butoh discuss somatic transformation into and through phenomena such as mud, slime, rock, animal, ash, and so forth. She describes butoh's intersubjective engagement with nonhuman subjects, including chickens and pigs, and the intention in butoh to "recover the body that has not been robbed," as butoh founder Hijikata stated (Fraleigh 2010, 4). In my understanding, this refers to the recovery of the body living beyond the grasp of conceptual thought, including limiting notions of "human."

In *Dancing Identity*, Fraleigh argues from an eco-feminist perspective against both masculinist ideologies of mastery—mind over body and matter, "man" over nature—and social constructivist perspectives that, in her view, marginalize nature by consigning it to the status of "construction" (6). She proposes, as an alternative, a philosophy of *matching* that emerges conceptually from enfleshed practices of listening and response in somatics and dance. Matching is not about imitating but about attuning to subtle rhythms and qualities flowing within a given intersubjective field. In somatic partner work, such attunement might entail following and supporting a movement process with gentle touch or through nonjudgmental witnessing. By articulating a philosophy of matching while simultaneously widening the lens of inquiry to include nonhuman nature, Fraleigh suggests that practices and dispositions oriented to matching can extend beyond somatics and dance studios to include the living earth itself.

In my interview-based heuristic research with Fraleigh, I wanted to further develop this line of inquiry, which she had initiated decades earlier. In particular, I was interested in discovering what directions it might take if framed in the contemporary context of environmental crisis. While Fraleigh discusses, in *Dancing Identity* and elsewhere, her own lived experience of the specific historical crisis of Cold War nuclear testing in southern Nevada, her writing prior to "Butoh Translations" (2016) is not framed in terms of environmental crisis on a global scale. She has written that "we forget our connection to nature at our peril," which may be viewed as a warning of what is to come (*Dancing Identity* 2004, 11). Are the consequences of our break with nature ours? Are they earth's? This ambiguity was a space I wished to enter with her. Through an interview process that included extensive conversation, improvisations, choreography, and photography, we explored, through these different channels of enacting our embodiment, our individual and collective relations with the body of earth. We asked, through solo and shared processes, what meanings emerge when dance is framed in the context of environmental crisis, and, at times, we danced without a frame. What follows is a phenomenological account of this inquiry, which spirals between thick description of a particular morning of dancing and theoretical reflections on consciousness, body, matter, and time.

I

Sunday, June 14

I pick Sondra up in St. George on the way to Ivins, a small town a few miles from Snow Canyon. We are heading to Xetava Café, where we will have *al fresco* breakfast on an outdoor patio shaded by trees. At 8 a.m., it is already hot, and the interior of the car feels like an oven. As we pass the last of the strip malls and fast-food chains lining the perimeter of St. George, the heat mellows, becoming a balm that slows the tempo of time. We reach the café and, as we settle at our table, I feel the day stretching toward the cliff-lined horizon.

Several minutes pass as we browse our menus, shaded under a tree where a bird chirps brightly. I feel our descent into desert time; the conversation will begin when it is ready. Some moments glide by and then, together, we place down our menus, smiling. Sondra begins to speak. Several minutes pass before I realize I have forgotten to record, a mistake I will regret months later, as I transcribe this exchange.

> SONDRA: . . . *I wish I could put my finger on it, witnessing current neuroses of all kinds, overload. So much focus on the self, which Buddhists say ultimately doesn't exist . . . Take the notion of the self . . . I like reading Damasio,* Self Comes to Mind, *where we get to come to terms in human history with what a self can possibly be. Some people I feel so connected to . . . that I don't feel otherness, I therefore make the mistake probably of "overflow" [laughs], and too much empathy, too much connection. I don't have this with a lot of people, but some, I do think most of us have that, where there's not too much of a clear demarcation. But I've learned boundaries as a teacher. You've got to have them.*
>
> ROBERT: *When you've had that experience, that dissolve of a demarcation, has dance been the conduit or an agent in that, a somatic . . . or has it been something else?*
>
> S: *Somatic resonance. I don't get that with everybody I dance with, just sometimes, well a lot of times, and dance can really facilitate it I think. It doesn't necessarily bring it, but it does facilitate it, that dissolving of boundaries—Oh! When I go to Snow Canyon with people, students, you can call them that, but they cease to be students, we're just all there together. The environment really holds us all, and the boundaries dissolve of their own accord, because people are truly relating to something bigger than self. I think that's one of the great benefits of dancing in natural environments, and even sometimes site-specific works, though it might be a burnt-out trailer home . . . the environment, what we commonly call nature, may be gorgeous opulent interesting places, but even desolate tragic ones: they call to you of something larger than yourself.*

As we continue talking, the conversation drifts toward our diminishing desires to choreograph for indoor theatrical spaces. For me, this feels like a confession as I consider the implications for a future career in academia. In this moment, the spaces that Sondra and I inhabit seem very different, as she is retired from the academy and relishes the freedom to admit that her pursuit of dance, as aesthetic practice and basis for philosophy and healing, is motivated by love. Still, we share a common search for meaning outside institutional containers. This search will take us, after breakfast, to Snow Canyon, where we will brave the heat to dance for ourselves, each other, and the spacious red earth. We have applied no specific label to our process, though we have agreed that we will document it with photographs and video. Still, it is not clear if these images will be formalized later as art works. I am grateful for this ambiguity, because it will invite unself-conscious attention to sand and rock, and it will provide time for the land to assimilate into our dances.

Our pace picks up when we realize that it is 9:30. The line of shade has moved halfway across the table, exposing our forearms to the sun. We quickly pay up and head for the canyon.

*　*　*

Ours is the only car in the parking lot. We walk into the canyon, removing our shoes when we hit the cool pink sand, our feet benefiting from its limited absorption of heat. We are carrying two large, plastic bags of costumes I have borrowed from a friend in Moab, which I selected according to Sondra's request for "fanciful" dancewear. These include a red tutu, a futuristic form-fitting mask, a honey-colored beehive wig, creamy silk pajama bottoms, a knitted red wool shawl, and several other items. We settle on a tiered, curving section of the canyon, where a few scrubby bushes and patches of sand are scattered about. At first, we move on our own, molding our bodies to the warm stone. I have selected the edge of a terracelike formation, where flat ground begins to slope downward toward a lower terrace. I arrange my body haphazardly and close my eyes, quickly entering a dreamlike state. As I settle into the uneven ground, the world around me begins to breathe, the sky, ground, and cells in my body merging into a common medium of slow, wavelike patterns of heat and energy. I remain for a long time, feeling tissues responding to the horizontal plane and soft undulation of stone beneath my body. Soon these undulations grow into a rippling dance that spreads through my back and out into limbs; I picture pebbles dropping into a lake, one by one, from the perspective of the water. The waves shift direction, as if a wind were forcing the liquid surface to bend toward shore. The rippling transforms into roll, and I become a snake sidewinding along the red earth. Several feet away, I pause and allow limbs to grow, finding myself on all fours.

Briefly, I back up onto two legs and rear upward before melting back down to the ground, rolling to my back with arms splayed. The intensity of the sun against my lids causes my eyes to water; my cheeks burn. I partially open my eyes and roll my head, now a leaden weight against the stone. Sondra, a few yards away, is trying on the shawl. How long have I been dancing? I pull my body off the ground, staggering slightly as I make my way down the slope. Minutes later, we are laughing and mugging for each other's cameras. I end up wearing the tutu over a billowing yellow taffeta skirt, which inspires me to begin another extended sequence of dancing. Sondra switches her camera to video mode, following my movement while offering periodic prompts and affirmations. When I watch an excerpt of the video months later, I see that I have discarded the skirt and tutu, which lie in a pile several feet from my dancing body. In the video, I appear on all fours, clad in the mask and black underwear, sliding my hand forward and backward along the sandstone. I am absorbed in the movement, but suddenly pause to ask, "Do you want me to come to standing"? I recollect my quickening awareness of being filmed and of the possibility that my dancing may become a composition for other eyes; this moment of self-consciousness visibly rigidifies my body. Sondra replies gently, "Just keep going, you're doing great. And find a way to lose the mask at a certain point. Go where you want to go; let your body do what it wants to do. Feel the essence of . . . that petrified sandstone, the butterfly of it, the softness of it. Let it guide you. The place will do it." Slowly, I peel off the mask, my elbow reaching upward toward the fathomless dome of sky.

*   *   *

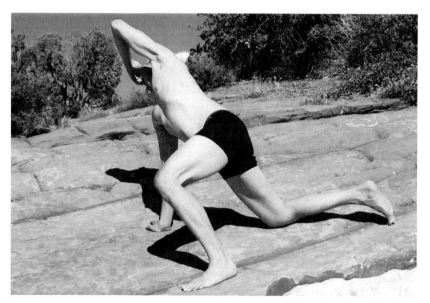

Figure 3.1. Robert Bingham dancing in Snow Canyon, Utah. Photograph © 2015 by Sondra Fraleigh.

Fifteen minutes later, our roles are reversed. Sondra, wearing the shawl and copper wig, is ambling slowly across an expanse of petrified dune. While I photograph, I observe her concentration and the detailed rhythm of her walk. She appears to be in conversation with the stone, feeling it out and responding to its curves and crevices through her feet. Where the ground slopes more steeply downward, her walk becomes unsteady, shedding any trace of the kind of grounded, heroic gait I associate with modern dance techniques. I recall Eiko Otake's statement that "Sometimes it is not only about the human" (Lepecki 2011, 51), feeling certain that Sondra's dance, too, is not only about a human self but about the ground and earth; perhaps it is a prayer or offering. Several uneven steps later, she pauses and lowers herself slowly to the stone. She settles on her side, and my eyes water as I see her body forming a perfect echo of the dunes running along the horizon behind her; inexplicably, I think: *I am home.* Behind me, a woman with two children pass by, carrying the sound of a heated argument that fades quickly as they disappear over the next hillock. Sondra continues to move incrementally, her glacial pace not affected by their passage. I see that her hands are shaping themselves to the wig, which she gradually removes and presses away from her. Suddenly, I become aware that she is grimacing. A whole-bodied expression of grief amplifies as she drops the wig onto the ground, and then it quickly fades as she settles onto her back. I am reminded of the astonishing speed of the desert squalls I have witnessed, which rear up under miles-high stacks of dark clouds before vanishing into blue sky. Sondra becomes still. I lower myself to the ground to see her profile etched against the sky.

II

Sondra and I are in Snow Canyon to feel the world in its immediacy. The immediate, worlding world, which embodies what Edmund Husserl referred to as the "the flowing live present," is available to direct experience only through the particularities of place (Bruzina 2004, 30). Improvised dancing is our method for sensitizing ourselves to these particularities, as we assimilate fragments and textures of place into the pathways and rhythms of our movement. A light gust of wind might ripple through an arm, or a stretch of sandstone might be the anchor from which to reach toward the sky. As patterns of movement unfold, panoplies of further movement possibilities arise (LaMothe 2015). Our "task" as dancers is to remain present to this process and to engage, or allow to pass by, emerging movement possibilities and impulses. The reward for our committed attention is the change in the canyon, which becomes vivid and participatory, as if it, too, has chosen to join the dance. The delineations of body and ego become fuzzy, if not fully dissolved, in the presence of something larger, as Sondra remarked at breakfast. As I danced, I felt the local assemblage of things, including my own body, melt into an underlying field of energy—an apparently boundless continuum permeating this body and environment. Clearly a shift in consciousness occurred through the act of dancing. Philosopher Shigenori Nagatomo describes how somatic attunement through the body may yield a transformation from the "provisional dualistic tendency" characteristic of everyday consciousness to a holistic state of consciousness experienced as oneness of perceiver and perceived (1992, xxv). Earlier, as we pulled into the parking lot, I perceived the rocks, sky, and junipers as things external to my body, and the landscape, while beautiful, appeared as a somewhat generic "southern Utah desert" scene, only moderately distinct from other locations in red rock country. Yet as my dancing began, the environment vivified and particularized, clarifying its participation in the physical movements of the dance and awakening my senses and imagination. Through the gross kinesthetic give-and-take of yielding and pushing into the ground, as well as a subtler, felt inter-resonance with the energy of the environment (1992), I verified my interdependent relationship with the vibrant matter constituting this environment; a deep sense of care awakened. Perhaps my attunement to finer layers of energy elicited the feeling that "I am home," or the sense of home arose from exploring, with Sondra, the fragile contingency of our dancing bodies held by the dizzyingly vast landscape. Sondra has mentioned many times the feeling of being held by the canyon, including in an article she wrote some months after this morning of dancing together. In the article, she describes her dance as a process of surrendering to the pain, beauty, and impermanence of the canyon:

> Through this dance, I feel more about what happens in and around me. I listen to a mother cuss her child as they pass by our quiet dance in the canyon. Forgetting why they came in the first place, they completely miss the incredible landscape given them by nature. Meanwhile, the canyon suffers their neglect, while I morph and try my best to attune to the beauty that holds me. . . . Tell me what to do to make this moment last. I know this canyon was dusted with nuclear fallout from the Nevada testing site at Frenchman's Flat about sixty-five years ago. And yet, I lie here in the suffering, consenting to have nothing but love in my life. (2016, 71)

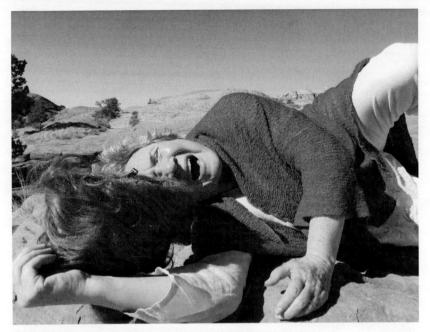

Figure 3.2. Sondra Fraleigh dancing in Snow Canyon, Utah. Photograph © 2015 by Robert Bingham.

III

For several minutes, I have been sitting downslope from Sondra, observing her profile against the unbroken blue of sky. It is so peaceful to be here in stillness on the soft warm stone. Time dances in the ripples of heat emanating from the canyon floor. With an exhale, Sondra stirs into action, rolling over to her side and up to sitting. We face each other for a long while, smiling, our eyes soft. There is an unspoken agreement not to speak and, instead, to allow the energy of this moment to play within our tissues. Something in the tenor of the day has changed, downshifting to a slower temporal gear. I decide to ride the changed rhythm, keeping it alive in movement. I lie down and begin to roll unevenly across the terrace, eventually ending up on a bed of fine pink sand. My body spills outward, legs and head spiraling away from each other. I scan internally, feeling various pressures and torques across the landscape of tissue. Where does suffering reside in a body? I imagine it as a hot ball of energy pushed and rolled into different corners of my body, like a pinball in slow motion. In some places, the ball gets hotter and denser; in others it dissipates. I allow it to settle within the gnarled thicket of my solar plexus. For over two years, I have sensed that something is not right here.

The feeling changes continually, morphing into qualities of density and bloat, like a restless creature that has made a home just below my heart. Six months ago, I sought medical attention, but nothing showed up in the X-rays and stress test. Sprawled out in the sand, I choose to assume a friendly attitude toward this mystery, meeting it on its own terms, without attachment or aversion (Chödrön 1994). My dance, centered within the perimeter of lower ribs, becomes ever more subtle and internal, distilling down to a feeling of long, even waves flowing through my cells, which somehow reminds me of meat falling off a bone: the freedom of it. I feel myself become matter in the first person: particle and wave, solid and not solid at once. The subtler my attunement, the more wavelike I imagine myself to be, an apparition floating in emptiness sculpted into the shape of canyon and sky.

According to quantum physics, as a material body, I am, just as this environment is, both particle and wave (Barad 2007; Bohm 1980). This presents an intellectual riddle. A particle occupies a defined position in space, while a wave is movement itself, unavailable to such definition. Matter is, mysteriously, both. Not only did physics reveal, a century ago, matter's irreducibility at the quantum level, it demonstrated that the apparati used for observation influenced the behavior of observed quanta, suggesting that the apparatus and observer—the entire context—must be considered part of the observed phenomenon. These and subsequent discoveries would lead physicist David Bohm (1980) to theorize, many decades later, the universe as Undivided Whole in Flowing Movement: all is related to all else in a web of interconnectedness, with the web itself irreducible and ceaselessly changing; the web is the world's worlding. Surface appearances, which suggest independent being, thus deceive. While distinctions clearly exist among phenomena, which are identifiable in perception and representable in language and thought, underneath these distinctions there is an integrative dance of change from which differentiated phenomena emerge and back into which they dissolve. Physicist Karen Barad refers to the coparticipation of distinct phenomena in the world's worlding as intra-action—*intra* indicating that, at the quantum level, phenomena are already aspects of a larger, interconnected field or whole. In this view, there is not a preexisting world within which interactions occur, but an unfixed, relational dance of ongoing "intra-action produc[ing] new worlds" (2007, 170).

The implication of a holistic, interdependent—or, perhaps better, "intra-dependent"—universe that emerged from quantum physics flew in the face of the view in classic physics of a mechanical, knowable world "composed of individual objects with individually determinate boundaries and properties" (107), and its companion, Cartesian dualism, which viewed mind, associated only with humans, as existing on an abstract plane independent of the mechanical operations of body and universe (according to ecologist Carl Safina, Descartes performed live dissections of dogs apparently without regard for their suffering: as nonhumans, they were mechanisms driven by instinct, devoid of mind or soul (Mowe 2016, 4)). Despite the onto-epistemological interventions of quantum physics and relativity (Bohm 1980), the laws of classic physics were not invalidated, as they remained highly accurate in describing and predicting the behavior of gross objects; classic physics is useful for building bridges (Gilman 1993, 11). Yet the latter misrepresented subtle being, the quantum level of reality at which dualistic notions of independent subject (such as observer) and object (such as observed) fall apart. Perhaps the coexistence of gross (classic) and subtle (quantum) reality might be understood through analogy with matter itself, given its dual nature as particle and wave. Since the revolution of quantum physics, several physicists have drawn ethical conclusions from the behavior and nature of matter's quantum dimension, which implies a lively, interconnected whole. Some contemporary physicists argue that the thinking and practices of present-day science (Laszlo 2007) and of Western civilization *writ large* have yet to catch up with the discoveries of quantum physics, even after 100 years:

> Since most of the distinctive institutions of western civilization—materialistic science, market economics, our legal system, the Bill of Rights—are based on the assumption that the world is composed of discrete units, the idea of interconnectedness rattles the foundations of our whole society. (Gilman 1993, 11)

Drawing metaphorically on the wave-particle duality of matter, he continues:

> Might we humans also, in some mysterious way, have both particle-like individuality and a wave-like shared beingness and interconnectedness? . . . those of us from the West . . . need to stretch our ability to understand our more wave-like, interconnected qualities. (11)

Perhaps attuning to subtle energies within and external to the body can elicit a deeper sense of intra-connection and enhanced commitment to living more reciprocally with this beleaguered planet, recognizing that humans are not the only beings to whom earth's "resources" matter. Philosopher Yuasa (1993) hints at this in his theory of body, which integrates gross body (physiology) and subtle body (ki energy). According to this theory, which is grounded in a combination of Daoist and Buddhist philosophy and Western philosophy, psychology, and medicine, the body is irreducible to a bounded, determinate biological system as conceived in Western medicine. Instead, it is an open system whose life-energy, ki, intermingles with the ki energy permeating the environment. Body-mind-environment and, ultimately, universe are unified within the "invigorating activities of *ki*" (Nagatomo 1992, 202). This conception of a human-environment continuum enlivened with ki is associated with an ecological view of homo sapiens that is, according to Yuasa, distinct from that which predominates in the West:

> The view of human being espoused by . . . [East Asian] philosophy maintains that the human being is not a *homo faber* who conquers nature, but is an ecological, receptive being made alive by the invisible power working from beyond nature, for the human being is originally a being born out of nature. (1993, 188)

While ki permeates human and nonhuman phenomena, it operates, Yuasa argues, at a deep, subtle level within the body, and perception of its activity is not available within everyday "provisionally dualistic" consciousness. Perceiving ki requires the kind of finely tuned somatic awareness cultivated through integrative mindbody practices such as meditation and martial arts. Yuasa makes no mention of dance as a means of cultivating such perceptual acuity, nor does Nagatomo, who translates Yuasa's work from the original Japanese. However, Nagatomo's theory of attunement (1992), which draws substantially on Yuasa's work, extends the domain of somatic engagement beyond the specific self-cultivation activities identified by Yuasa toward a more expansive potential field of practices that may or may not be Asian in origin. Nagatomo thereby suggests that a broad range of attunement practices are capable of eliciting experiences of oneness beyond subject-object dualism, experiences which he describes variously as oneness of perceiver and perceived and felt inter-resonance between body and living ambiance.

Nagatomo's frequent use of the term "living ambiance" implies that any given environment possesses an inherent vitality, regardless of the nature of its constitutive parts and of Western, biologically based definitions of living and nonliving. The quality of consciousness elicited by attuning the body can reveal the intra-resonance of body's and environment's vitality, in distinction from everyday consciousness, or natural attitude, that splits body and environment into two. What might be called body listening in dance and somatics practices can, similarly, deepen a sense of felt intra-connection with environment through attention to subtle, changing qualities in the total field of matter-energy constituting self-and-environment. Sondra's description, at breakfast, of dancing with students in Snow Canyon references a dissolution of dualistic consciousness: *the environment really holds us all and the boundaries just dissolve of their own accord, because people are truly relating to something bigger than self.* This reference bears a resemblance to Nagatomo's description of the phenomenon of attunement, whereby the emanation of an energy from the personal body . . . calls for a recognition of its pervasive presence in the living ambiance which embraces the personal body as a contingent being, for it shares the same "natural" elements which comprise the totality of physical nature. (1992, 203)

By shared "natural" elements, he refers to traditional Buddhist philosophy, which holds that all phenomena, including the human body, are comprised of the same constitutive elements of wind, water, fire, and earth. Perceiving the personal body's subtle energy elicits recognition of its continuity with the energy permeating the ambiance. Such recognition may call forth vivid affective qualities. In Sondra's description of somatic attunement to the canyon, including its suffering, she spoke to the capacity of dancing with earth to elicit an earth-centered love transcending the metaphysical privileging of a human self. From what source or direction does that feeling flow? In his philosophy of direct experience, Kitaro Nishida writes: "It is not that experience exists because there is an individual, but that an individual exists because there is an experience" (1990, xv). Could this also be said of love?

IV

I am mid-dance, and suddenly my mind is scrambling to capture the moment. I am thinking: trying, in vain, to formulate a clear thought around this moment's meaning. Yet as I continue falling into the thrum of land, body, and sky, the possibility of intellectual capture evaporates into the blue. *There is only change.* All of a sudden, a hawk cuts across the otherwise unbroken blue of sky; the field of being uniting the sky and my body immediately shifts. I begin to roll again along the hot canyon floor, a physical recognition of the relationality of all to all else. Around me, the rocks continue their slow dissolve into sand, which, in time, will grow into soil feeding the sweet-acrid–scented junipers.

The roll ends in stillness. I begin to snake my arms outward, feeling the sand's soft caress with my fingertips. The desert's hot, slow ontology urges me to pass beyond human temporality into a geologic history that vibrates in the molecules of sand and bones. Accounting for such a passage requires a shift from "the language of epistemology to that of ontology" (Bennett 2011, 3), to things in themselves, infused with the evolutionary story of earth. Bone itself is an emergent phenomenon within the unfolding dance of earth, whose history, according to Manuel De Landa, can be traced to a specific moment in geologic time:

Soft tissue (gels and aerosols, muscle and nerve) reigned supreme until 500 million years ago. At that point, some of the conglomerations of fleshy matter-energy that made up life underwent a sudden *mineralization*, and a new material for constructing living creatures emerged: bone. It is almost as if the mineral world that had served as a substratum for the emergence of biological creatures was reasserting itself. (11)

Here in the desert, the mineral world's assertiveness is nakedly displayed in the monoclines, those huge, diagonal slabs of earth that look like frozen ocean breakers, and in the laccolithic mountains that ripped through the earth's surface millions of years ago. These cousins of my bones. Through opening fingertips, I try to harmonize with the slow desert ontology, whose solid appearance belies the land's liquidlike morphology spanning multiple geologic epochs. My leg turns inward, initiating a meandering sequence of movement that passes across the topography of my ribs and spine. My head lands on its side, a heavy boulder coming to rest. Suddenly, I recall another boulder I saw recently, a chunk of rock that had fallen from the midsection of a three-hundred-foot cliff just south of Moab. The gash in the cliff wall looked fresh, perhaps the loosening of cracked sandstone following a recent downpour. Desert squalls, though infrequent, can be ferocious, very different from storms where I live back east. Numerous times, I have been warned by locals to steer clear of dry river beds whenever there is the threat of a downpour; when these occur, water rapidly accumulates in the multiply merging channels, sometimes carrying boulders and other debris, and an innocent-looking dry bed can become a raging river in minutes. Noticing that bit of collapsed wall, I walked closer to get a better look. As I drew near, I began to see elaborate patterns in the boulder, which, like many of the red cliff walls in the area, was partially covered by a charcoal-colored patina. Moments later, the patterns clarified into a dense, multilayered display of thousand-year-old petroglyphs interspersed with scratched-out names and dates from the early 1900s. For a split second, I experienced a dizzying temporal dysphoria—a physical sense of human history from the perspective of geologic time. The seemingly fresh collapse of the wall must have occurred thousands, maybe tens of thousands, of years ago. There was an intimacy to the well-preserved marks, as if they, too, were recent, perhaps chiseled into the wall just days or weeks earlier. To the right, a large, bone-dry length of wood was propped up against the eight-foot-tall boulder. I followed the beam with my gaze, noticing more petroglyphs above. It was now clear that this was a makeshift ladder of indeterminate age. I climbed to the top of the boulder.

The dizzy feeling returned as I saw an even larger display of snakes, horned animals, geometric patterns, and early-twentieth-century graffiti. Different dimensions of time and history competed with each other on and around this massive stone, which was, itself, an expression of agency issued forth by "recent" geologic processes. I felt my *species* infancy, an uncanny, bodily recognition that humanity's entire 200,000-year history on earth is little more than a geologic blink of an eye. Yet, within a fraction of this blink—a minute tremor in space-time—this species fuses with earth's geology, transforming itself into a geophysical force as it transforms earth's awesome vibrancy into a commodity-generating *resource*.

V

Two hours after our arrival at Snow Canyon, it is time to leave. I peel myself away from the rock and brush the pink sand off my skin. We stuff the costumes into the bags and head toward the car. Halfway there, I pause and turn around. I need to see the canyon one more time, to have a final moment of resolution and thanks.

Once in the car, Sondra and I talk about marionettes and Grecian statues.

> SONDRA: *In his story, Heinrich von Kleist asks why human beings can't be as graceful as marionettes. He believes it is because the marionette has no consciousness, and the human is conscious, or more to the point, "self-conscious." Do we, then, fall out of grace, when we're aware of ourselves? Well, even in awareness, humans might be beautiful. Where does beauty and consciousness lie, and what does it mean to be conscious of "self"? This is a really good story for dancers because we're asked to be interesting, expressive, beautiful, ugly, all those things. And darned if we don't work at it! . . . So there is this little vignette in the story about a statue—where the young man is plucking a thorn from his foot. He's just doing that, and in that moment he's so beautiful and somebody notices it and tells him. Then suddenly he's trying, admiring himself in the mirror, and he can't "get it" back ever again. It's an interesting story about spontaneous grace and consciousness, especially self-consciousness and reflexivity.*

Sondra has referenced von Kleist's essay "On the Marionette Theater," with which I am not familiar. As she talks, I take the narrative at face value, as a cautionary tale about self-consciousness and the tension between the pre-reflectively lived body (self) and the body (self) objectified in thought and language, which can produce the familiarly distressing feeling of self-consciousness. This may be experienced as phenomenological dualism, with conceptualizing mind seemingly distinct from living body, a feeling that perhaps reinforces Cartesian dualism, if my thoughts *about* my body lead me to believe the thinking "I" is something or somewhere other than a whole body thinking. Perhaps "falling from grace" might be viewed not from the perspective of an audience but from the first-person experience of falling out of oneness.

Dancing, with or without an audience, furnishes an opportunity to play across a horizon from a pre-reflectively lived bodily self to a self projected in thinking, where both dancing and thinking about dance are rhythms of bodily becoming in which one can participate consciously (LaMothe 2015). When I transcribe my exchange with Sondra months later, new more-than-human meanings emerge related to vibrant matter beyond human consciousness and semiotics, including a consideration of the marionette and statue prior to their status as stand-ins for human concerns; these new meanings quickly morph into thoughts about thingness and *becoming thing* in dance. Lepecki (2016) writes about thingness in *Singularities*, highlighting a range of contemporary performing artists who interrogate objecthood by shifting the source of their movement from self to thing, allowing things to be agents of change. Like Bennett, he differentiates object and thing: "The relationship to subordination is what turns things into objects. An object is self-willing manipulative humanity" (2016, 33).

The work of the artists he cites offers reflections on thing-agency, whether the things in question are exploding bubbles or sleeping pills, and they challenge the subordination of things at the hands of humans, a subordination that is, at the same time, a superordination of human subjecthood: "The more we let things be things, the less heroic we need to be, stepping out of cliché that is humanity" (36). By allowing things to be things and to show themselves as themselves, in Heideggerian terms (Moran 2000, 218), these artists topple the cliché of self-assured, masterful humans who control themselves and the things around them, including their meanings. In these performances, focus shifts to the agency of things in the performers' midst or, in the case of the sleeping pills, within their tissues. For Lepecki, the foregrounding of thing-agency represents a "modesty [that] goes against the cliché of narcissistic presence in western theatrical dance" (2016, 36), and it represents, further, a critique of the pressure, in contemporary neoliberal capitalism, to perform a confident, successful self who is in control: "Who would bet on . . . an insecure Self?!" (13).

Lepecki's use of the word "cliché" is significant because it indicates that he does not equate Western theatrical dance categorically with narcissistic presence, but instead acknowledges that exceptionalist expectations—beauty, talent, charisma—hang in the midst of its studios and theaters. I know this firsthand, and I relate Lepecki's references to narcissism and heroism to Sondra's comment about the kinds of expectations placed on dancers. Yet dancers mount challenges to these, as Lepecki describes, and as I witnessed during our morning at Snow Canyon. Sondra's traversal of the canyon floor was a poignant antidote to dancerly exceptionalism, as she allowed the stone's idiosyncratic shape to ripple through her body and flower into a stumbling walk. If, as Lepecki writes, the contemporary reality of neoliberal capitalism demands a relentlessly striving, confident, and ever-improving self, a performance practice of letting things be things or, as Ishmael Houston-Jones once said during an improvisation class, "trying to not try," is a significant challenge to this ethos. And it may also be a relief, if, as Eiko states, "it is a relief sometimes not to be confined to the human" (Lepecki 2011, 51). Collectively, these artists seem to say: try laying down the mantle of human exceptionalism and allowing oneself to be a living thing among things. If human exceptionalism, as a stance or habit, enables nonreciprocal relations with a planet reduced to a composite of "resources," might it also enable nonreciprocal relations with one's own body as it strives to live up to the cliché of exceptionalism? Is not dance, as a method for collaborating with—rather than forcing or ignoring—body and earth's rhythms of becoming, an especially potent site for challenging the burden of the exceptional human?

As we drive down the windy road out of the canyon, I think: *knowledge lives in flesh and things*, and in this moment my body surrenders into the whirring of the car's engine and our gentle descent toward the valley below. It is a mistake to believe that knowledge is contained within a human brain, or even a body. This flesh is entangled with the world's. Matter and meaning are entangled (Barad 2007), and knowledge is woven through the world's ontological dance of becoming. Human thinking, and human brain, are not the bank vaults of knowledge. Husserl's call to "return to the things themselves" continues to offer a particular alternative to privileging humans as the center of the universe of knowledge and significance, because it requires setting aside (human) representations *of* things long enough to touch things, with open senses, and to feel the nature of their power. This basic tenet of phenomenology impels me to take time to listen to the world, transforming the way I relate to it, and this, in turn, casts blissful doubt on my assumptions about where power and knowledge reside. In this moment of forgetting what I think I know, the world emerges as a *dancing* world. Now forgetting becomes remembering, and this is a moment of great relief.

Performing Life and Language

4

Improvisation as Paradigm for Phenomenologies

VIDA L. MIDGELOW

"When phenomenology is true to its intent, it never knows where it is going." These words open Sondra Fraleigh's seminal essay, "A Vulnerable Glance: Seeing Dance through Phenomenology" (1991), in reference to Maurice Merleau-Ponty (1962, xxi). Fraleigh goes on to describe how phenomenology "develops unpredictably according to the contents of consciousness" (1991, 11). She notes how the present-centered approach and descriptive aims of phenomenology means that it is open to temporal change and shifts in focus for it has no inherently appropriate, or inappropriate, topics.

I want to start here, not only to direct you to the writing by Fraleigh and Merleau-Ponty but also to note how easily in this opening sentence it is to replace the word *phenomenology* with that of *improvisation*. It is the intersection between these two practices, when they are understood as methodologies that offer ways of revealing and constructing the world, which I explore here. Later in the chapter, I focus on improvisation based in Skinner Releasing Techniques that are broadly somatic in approach, thus grounding my discussion within a particular improvisatory form. The ways in which somatics can be understood in terms of phenomenology has been richly illuminated by Fraleigh (2015). She notes how both somatics and phenomenology operate at a level of embodied reflexivity and share concerns with consciousness and intentionality. Indeed, she has proposed "somatic movement practices might even be called phenomenology in action" (19). Similarly, I seek to go beyond illuminating dance improvisation through a phenomenological lens to turn instead to a consideration of improvisation as methodological paradigm for phenomenologies. I propose various somatically informed improvisation

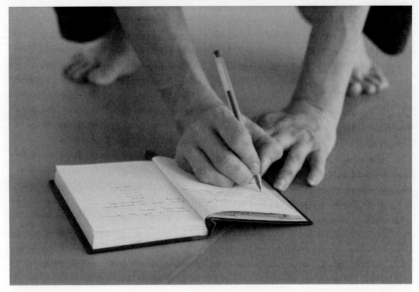

Figure 4.1. Vida L. Midgelow. *Writing Following Improvisation*. Photograph © 2011 by Tim Halliday.

strategies through which the phenomenologist may approach the casting of phenomena and articulation of experience differently.

Making this assertion I am, of course, making a link to the insights of Thomas Csordas, who wrote the insightful essay, "Embodiment as a Paradigm for Anthropology" (1990). In this essay, Csordas distinguishes the body—a biological, material entity—and embodiment. Embodiment "has as a principle characteristic the collapse of dualities between body and mind, subject and object" (7). Further as a paradigm, embodiment is considered as an indeterminate methodological field defined by perceptual experience and the mode of presence and engagement in the world. In this proposal he draws on the work of Merleau-Ponty and Bourdieu, such that the dialectic between perceptual experience and cultural practice is harmonized. As such, he writes: "Embodiment begins from the methodological postulate that the body is not an object to be studied in relation to culture, but it is considered as the subject of culture, or in other words as the existential ground of culture" (5).

Foreshadowing his work, "Somatic Modes of Attention" (1993), Csordas attends to sensory modalities, social interactions, and how we make meaning in these modes. Describing the ways of attending to and with one's body in surroundings that include the embodied presence of others, our bodies, "are not objects to us. Quite the contrary, they are an integral part of the perceiving subject" (Csordas 1990, 36). Elaborating examples of people's embodied experiences in healing and spiritual contexts, he foregrounds the particular concepts of the pre-objective and habitus, wherein the pre-objective rest in how we experience "manifestations as spontaneous and without preordained content." He continues saying that the "manifestations are original acts of communication which nevertheless take a limited number of common forms because they emerge from a shared habitus" (15). Thereby, Csordas notes how the pre-objective is not pre-cultural; rather, he invokes the bond between the material, corporeal, cultural, spiritual, and psychological to describe what we might call a mindful embodiment.

In these writings, Csordas includes extended phenomenological descriptions and demonstrates how phenomena are understood in the interconnection between people—world relations. He also implicitly attends to the relationship between the research and the researched. This is an intersubjective connection. It requires of the researcher a particular kind of "openness" in order to attend to what is present such that I propose that the phenomenologist, like the improviser, needs to enter her (research) practice open to that which is present and ready to follow that which emerges as it arises, swells, and takes shape, without predetermination, without knowing where things are going. Thereby, I suggest a phenomenological methodology is not just an approach to be applied to dance improvisation, but that the doing of a phenomenological study is itself improvisational. Or more specifically (and more modestly), the tools and insights of the improviser can augment the work of the phenomenologist.

There is no one way of going about a phenomenological study. My own understanding of phenomenological research is that it can be understood as phenomenological when it involves the researcher adopting a special open phenomenological attitude that is highly embodied and responsive to change. Paying particular attention to the interconnectedness and situatedness of the researcher/researched, the aim of such an approach is to assist in making manifest a rich articulation of the lifeworld or lived experience as it is in the making. This process is inherently improvisational and involves a different way of knowing the world. For, as Van Manen notes, "whereas theory 'thinks' the world, practice 'grasps' the world—it grasps the world pathically" (2007, 20).

Improvisational knowledge is pathic to the extent that the act of practice depends on somatic sensibilities and relational perceptiveness, alongside other aspects of knowledge, that are rigorously pursued and that are in part pre-theoretic and pre-linguistic (2007). Thereby, the improviser, like the phenomenologist, operates in attuned and intuitive modes, recognizing how as an embodied agent she is acting with a level of responsiveness to the thingness of the changing world. But, unlike traditional phenomenology, this practice arises through somaesthetic means to give rise to attitudinal, sensate, and creative insights to inform artistic and other experientially generated research enquiries.

Practice that "grasps" might be best considered a form of "process phenomenology" (Kozel 2015). This process orientation is significant for it enables us to understand and celebrate the midflow, the never to be complete, the messy and amorphous. Such difficult-to-grasp forms, processes, and changes are an inherent feature of life. As Mesle writes: "Whatever people may dream or speculate regarding timeless, changeless, becomingless eternity, it is clear to me that nothing in our actual life's fits this category." Stated directly: "Life is simply change—becoming and perishing. The joy of life is the journey" (2008, x).

"Process philosophy is an effort to think clearly and deeply about the obvious truth that our world and our lives are dynamic, interrelated processes and to challenge the apparently obvious, but fundamentally mistaken, idea that the world (including ourselves) is made of things that exist independently of such relationships and that seem to endure unchanged through all the processes of change" (8).

Mesle's emphasis on process offers an approach that might aid us in overcoming the problems and limitations of conventional phenomenological orientations. A pathically generated process phenomenology focuses on the practice of researching through/in change and asserts an ongoing dynamic process. As Van Manen writes: "Phenomenology formatively informs, reforms, transforms, performs, and performs the relation between being and practice" (2007, 26).

Merleau-Ponty points us in this direction, too, without fully elaborating the means through which it might be done. Although he doesn't explicitly write about improvisation (or indeed dance), his thinking does bring to the fore the incomplete, inexhaustible, spontaneous, and indeterminate. He makes it clear that the phenomenal realm is often ambiguous, subject to transformation and experienced in flux. This being so, a proper phenomenology he writes "must plunge into the world instead of surveying it, it must descend toward it such as it is instead of working its way back up toward a prior possibility of thinking it—which would impose upon the world in advance the conditions of our control over it" (1968, 38–39). This urgency of process and this "plunging" encounter is inherent within improvisation, for improvisations are processes in an essential sense that require the improviser to fully commit to being open and vulnerable to the situation. Being and becoming simultaneously, improvisers, as I discuss in what follows, operate in convergent and processual modes—foregrounding change and responsiveness.

Dance Improvisation and Phenomenology

Insistent, driving, repetitive the music pulses through me.
Bah ba, bah ba, bah ba.
Knees bounce to the pulse and feet step.
Bah ba bah ba, bah ba.
A bouncing skip propelling me on a clear diagonal trajectory.
Then I hear it, a low tone, long and continuous—it is there, in the
  background. My arms open releasing the previous rhythm to extend
  out—fingertips reaching out on the horizontal, shoulders wide,
  like a bird of prey. I begin to take long sweeping curving rotations.
  Diagonal lines become arching curves.
Smooth. Swooping.
Embracing.
I look out and I smile, my curving rotations meet the pounding feet of my
fellow dancers. And then. And then another arm glides open, the smooth
motion echoing my own and I see my body in hers and her body in mine
  and
we are flying.

*   *   *

Improvisation is always and already an operating feature of our lives—it is already everywhere, for our lives are unscripted and unscriptable (Hallam and Ingold 2007). This said, and given the seeming obvious truth that life is change (after Mesle 2008), the ideas I discuss here could be seen as redundant, for these processes are occurring all the time and without need of any intervention. Yet, just as we often don't pay attention to our bodies, because bodies are often absent to us (Leder 1990), our improvisations too go unnoted. It is to counter such disappearances that I draw our attentions to these processes.

In order to understand the significance of improvisation, we need to understand its nature. Just as Csordas writes, "There is a sense in which corporeality is integral to every domain of existence, but if embodiment is to be useful as a methodological field it must (like textuality) have a definable scope" (2011, 14). We could similarly speak of the need to define the scope of improvisation.

First, it is important to note that improvisation in art practice is not an unplanned, unpracticed, make-do activity as is perhaps a common misconception. While it might be useful to be able to adapt quickly in unforeseen circumstances, the notion of "pure" improvisational spontaneity and "freedom" as an improvisational consequence is a myth, and, as Daniel Goldman (2010) has shown, a dangerously unhelpful one. Indeed, it might well be that our unfettered improvisations, our spontaneous actions, tend toward the ill considered, leading as often as not to culturally affirmative, unreflective ways of being.

So rather than a false sense of "freedom," I emphasize in line with Csordas, ways that improvisation can be understood as grounded in shared practices of the body that are carried out through common understandings within a given community. These practices are experienced largely in the pre-objective realm but often give rise to shared perceptual articulations. As such, improvisation in performance, as discussed here, rarely leaves us to our own unfettered devices and is generally productively and consciously undertaken in communal settings. In these modes, improvisation is generally a rigorous, focused, and purposefully pursued way of going about things. And for our purposes here, it is significant that this "thingness" in somatically informed improvisation is focused toward attitudes of attending and processes of opening. But I get ahead of myself, and we will return to these specifics.

In my own writing, I elaborate improvisation as a wide field of practices and argue that improvisation may be considered "as a way of going about things for it has no inherent content" (Midgelow forthcoming). As a "way of going about things," we can think through the scope of improvisation as it entails entering a convergent space in which creative process and performance are one and the same generative occurrence, and in which the work evolves as a process. In other words, in improvisation, thinking and doing, planning and executing, become blurred through processes of, at times, compositional, but always in-the-moment decision making.

Often structured by various frameworks, be these shared movement techniques, compositional practices, tasks, scores, or the like, in-the-moment nature of improvisation foregrounds irreversibility. This is a risky thing, for improvisation involves entering a space, often with others and believing something (even if that something is "nothing") will happen. This something, in somatically based forms, is commonly developed through (inner) listening, initiating, responding, and redirecting within more-or-less open terrains of possibility. This entails a willingness to be vulnerable and assailable, enabling the improviser to follow routes and note emerging pathways—to catch and respond to that which becomes apparent and sparks the imagination. This happens in real time and foregrounds how and what we (can) perceive is fluid. Open to each context, the improviser seeks to let go of fixity through a deeply seated receptivity to self, others, and the world.

Improvisation is "always in the making," for as a process-driven mode of operating, improvisation is embedded in "the ways we work" (Hallam and Ingold 2007, 1, 3). Building upon such reflections, improvisation is articulated here as a practice that is sharable with others (but in forms that challenge the norm of the research "artifact") and as methodology for phenomenology (but in a way that sits in distinction to the more language-directed methods of conventional approaches). Understanding how improvisation is an always present but often hidden part of the ways we work enables us not only to acknowledge but also celebrate the mobility of our interceptive and intercorporeal connectivities that shape our lived worlds. For, to use Merleau-Ponty's terminology, we are part of the world and coextensive with it, constituting but also constituted.

Thus, the improviser and phenomenologist operate through (ever-changing) immediate experience and social interactions, while simultaneously co-forming specific materially and structurally embodied insights. Both entail intuitive and in-the-midst (as Merleau-Ponty might say) reflection. Further, they move, at times, toward reflective description or various languaging and/or scribing systems as a way of making immediate experience more explicitly available to ourselves and to others.

Some Practical Concepts: Skinner Releasing Technique and Open Source Forms

Inhaling, chest rising. The air is mist, thick with water its palpable texture touching my inside and my outside. Like the flow of a running droplet, the upward lift of my skull and chest, ripples downward— shimmering from skull, through shoulders and into my pelvis.
The watery mist, connecting me to the world.
Transforming.
The light of the world entering my lungs and spreading until I am aglow with
soft warm yellow hews. Moving as light my back opens and I explore the space behind me—illuminating that which I cannot see.

The shoulder blade opens, reaching out—so the space across my back
impossibly expands—reaching as if I could touch those about me from
*   where I*
sit with the tip of my scapula.

*   *   *

Stepping onto more specific grounds, I want us to consider the concepts, practice, and improvisatory explorations in Skinner Releasing Technique (SRT). I do this in part in order to avoid the generalized use of "improvisation" and "somatics" (as though these were singular practices). Doran George (2014) and Susan Foster (2011) have argued that, in somatics or at least "somatic dance training," distinctions between bodies and between movement traditions are lost because the anatomical basis of these approaches seems to provide a universal basis for movement. Further, in his critical reappraisal of "nature" and somatics, George proposes that the conceit of nature as a somatic premise has cultivated "a canonical body as an invisible category of nature, which purportedly accounted for ontology, yet marked difference and enacted exclusion from its supposedly universal purview" (2014, iv).

These positions are certainly worth noting, even if we might want to challenge some of the limitations in the account of somatic practices that these writers offer. That said, Csordas has shown somatic attending doesn't have to be undifferentiated. Rather, he suggests a movement toward particularities of specific lived corporealities, and as such, here I draw on my own corporeality as embedded within a movement practice. While SRT has received very little academic attention, it is a form that I have practiced for many years and it is for this reason that I look to locate myself here.[1] Reaching to the known offers me rich experiential materials developed through kinaesthetic immersion to consider. At the same time, it also carries inculcated modes of habituation—coloring (perhaps limiting) the perceptual openness I might desire. Yet such observations are part of my creative and reflective process. This improvisationally focused approach requires an experienced self and repeated engagement. Not in the sense of a static set of exercises, knowledge, or competencies, but in the dynamic sense of experiences as a dialectic interplay between being and becoming sensitive to the qualities and intensities of situations. In this way, possibilities of improvisation are "born of habit" (Merleau-Ponty 1962, 238), while at the same time repeated engagement illuminates and potentially alters habitual responses in creative and insightful ways.

SRT sessions, developed by American dancer and teacher Joan Skinner,[2] move between image actions and movement studies. The image actions involve tactile activities (in the form of hands-on partner work called "partner-graphics") to ease or release holding patterns and "blocked" energy, while the movement studies (often traveling) give the imagery an immediate kin-aesthetic effect and promote an integrated alignment of the whole self. These movement studies are improvised and evoked by guided poetic imagery. The classes seek to enable creative and accessible explorations of Skinner's move-ment principles, such as multidirectional alignment, suppleness, suspension, economy, and autonomy.

Skinner's work has been developed into improvised performance by artists such as American dancer Stephanie Skura,[3] alongside the increasing partici-pation of SRT internationally, including in Britain where the long-standing practice of Gaby Agis, and more recently Joe Moran, Florence Peake, Alex Crowe, and Sally Dean, among others, have shown the potential of SRT for performance.[4] Here, I expand upon Skura's work in particular. As a member of Joan Skinner's teaching faculty for many years, Skura has explicitly carried this deep knowledge into her own improvisation practice. She describes her approach, called Open Source Forms (OSF), in the following way: "Fluidly expanded from Skinner Releasing Technique (SRT), Open Source Forms is about cross-fertilizations and deep commonalities of SRT and creative pro-cess: shedding outer layers, finding primal energy, agility navigating subcon-scious realms, and imagery as powerful tools for transformation" (Skura).

The improvisatory body evoked in SRT and OSF is best understood not in terms of representation but as system. For in these practices, as in other somatically focused movement forms, there is an emphasis on assisting bodily change—via the creation of bodily circumstance, imaginal worlds, and the evocation of particular modes of attention. SRT inherently seeks to facilitate change and enable the refiguration of the body as a site of differing and in-dividually differentiated qualities—such that there is no desire to codify or unify bodies, and we can both note and "release" habits, creating scope for transformation. In the following, I go more deeply into the improvisational aspects of these movement forms foregrounding "releasing" and "autonomy" (from Skinner) and "score-making" (from Skura). These ideas are considered here as practical concepts and as metaphors that illuminate our consideration of improvisation as a paradigm for phenomenologies.

RELEASING

My legs feel light and weighted at the same time. I rest upon on my back and hands support me. Guided—my legs fall, skim and rise, folding in the hips,

*knees and ankles. Floating away—dislocated, disoriented—my legs are no
longer my own, my legs are becoming anew.
Starting to move with this touch, my legs seek to embody looseness—hips
sockets opening, legs are falling, rotating, jiggling jangling legs.*
. . .

*In baggy trousers and top hat, I am a jaunty traveler coming home.
Tumbling and unsteady, I am a baby taking my first steps.
Treading in deep water, I am fishing in a warm sea.*

*   *   *

Releasing is a complex notion to define that incorporates "letting go" in physical, emotional, and perceptual terms. Skinner says: "One releases immediate fixed states of being to become available to the aligning process. In turn, the aligning process releases psychophysical energy" (Skinner et al. 1979, 11). The release of tension is, in effect, a release of perceptions, of preconceived ideas, which are manifested in habits. In order to participate in responsive, adaptable processes, one releases habitual control in order to (re)experience the physical principles of human movement. Skinner might argue that when one becomes more harmoniously aligned with these principles, a new well-being and freedom are realized.

In the performative writing that started this section on releasing, I am drawing on an arch of SRT that goes from a partner graphic to extended improvisation. Beginning resting supine, my lower limbs are supported and facilitated into movement by my partner. I then enter an experiential improvised study in which I carry the residual sensations from my partner's touch as a basis from which to explore an ease and looseness of movement in the legs. Skinner calls this the "loose leg dance."

In these processes we find practical ways through which a phenomenological research process might begin, as we move away from what Husserl calls the natural attitude toward a phenomenological one. I ask, as if for the first time, what are legs? What do they do and how can they move? How does this movement feel? What is this sensation? How do I understand by body anew? This is akin to the process of phenomenological reduction whereby, just for a moment, I seek to put aside my habitual body and what I think I know, feel, and experience it as and consider the experience as if afresh. In this process, I have allowed myself the space to suspend my judgments about my legs (for example) and to try moving them in less known ways.

This particular attitude doesn't happen of its own accord and goes beyond an attitude of defamiliarization. Here, I am not only considering and imagining phenomena newly, but am using particular strategies that bring about a reexperiencing and a sense of "'wonder' in the face of the world" (Merleau-Ponty 1962, xv). The hands-on partner-graphic and follow on movement study have given space for me to "let go" of my familiar perceptions and accustomed usage. As I improvise, I attend to the possibilities of these "releasing" legs. My improvisation task is to stay with the proposed image in conjunction with the tactile sensation. There is no intent to form another, fixing, way of doing things, but rather to work on how I continually experience in "nonnaturalized," nonhabitual, ways. I am, as Merleau-Ponty after Husserl describes, attempting to bring forward the attitude of the perceptual beginner. So while these legs propel me daily and I have returned to this improvisational image many times, my task is to consider it an "ever-renewed experiment" and perennial investigation (Merleau-Ponty 1962, xv).

Importantly, the processes from partner-graphic to movement study guide us into a way of being in which I can be vulnerable and open to all that is occurring or might occur. This takes trust. Trust and risk. This combination is important, for phenomenology requires us to move through landscapes that are new to us. Allowing ourselves to be vulnerable to the complexity of or own embodiment and intercorporeally porous to the live worlds of those with whom we move (and research). This interconnectedness is important to the way we might exceed the representational or projected image and how the perceived and perceiver become intertwined and always in motion. Little can be assumed in advance, and in each revisiting, we are invited to undo and relearn in a perpetually improvised repositioning of limb to torso, center to periphery, my body to your body, and as Merleau-Ponty would have it the visible to the invisible (1968).

Another way that SRT supports risk and release is through the notion of "suppleness." Skinner teachers commonly bring a natural sponge into their classes in order to help dancers understand suppleness. Holding a dry sponge, I might notice its hard, crisp edges. It is light, almost insubstantial, but also stiff, unyielding, and easy to crack and break. On soaking the sponge, I might note that it is heavier but also soft in my hand. Squeezing the sponge it moves, contracts, and expands easily, easing into different shapes. It feels full. In suppleness—like the water-filled sponge—the ability to soften into change is the quality that is sought. Moving with a sense of this "sponginess" we are able ease into change, remaining in an open dynamic state. In this state the dancer is able to avoid physical jarring and be responsive to changing circumstance. Skura describes a similar sense: "travelling through

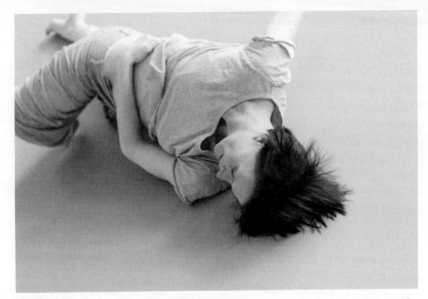

Figure 4.2. Vida L. Midgelow, Improvisation: *Becoming Animal*. Photograph © 2011 by Tim Halliday.

my porousness, softening me even more. I am suspended in water, softening through space, moving in many directions at once" (in Hamp 2013, 20).

Engaging a supple "sponginess" as a phenomenologist allows us to note things that may arise unexpectedly, without being jolted or thrown "off balance." It might be in this state we can respond more effectively to these situations, avoiding what might be initial sensations of resistance or rejection. This malleable state allows the improvising phenomenologist to navigate with a quality of ease, readiness, and openness. In doing so, it is also important to recognize that such qualities are not easy to achieve and require practice.

AUTONOMY AND CONNECTIVITY

Fingers brush across the back of my knees and then trace lines, like a wide toothed comb, up from my ears and out above my head.
Knees softening and head floating—suspending on imaginary "strings" my
skull opening upward. My spinal column lengthens. The skull weight starts to dissipate from the rest of my body.
Moving into the room I lean off balance—my head lengthening away from me. Rocking, I tip into space.

*Head dropping toward the floor, my neck hangs loose, head leading the way
to the floor and body flowing through.*
Supine.
Tip of head and tail of spine curl toward each other.
Opening the left side of the body and concaving in the right.
Reversing side to side. I slide and slither, becoming snake.

* * *

Skinner, informed by the work of F. M. Alexander,[5] proposes that no one
part of the body presses on another and that any one part of the body can
work autonomously from the rest. Here, there is an emphasis, for example,
on allowing the shoulder blades to slide easily across the back ribcage while
moving independently from the movement of the ribs and spine. Or, encouraging the head, as in the description earlier, to balance lightly on the spine,
releasing the neck and shoulders from its weight.

This autonomy of movement evokes a spacious body in which different
parts of the body can be considered in detail as the potentialities of each are
independently explored. Exploring the movement potentialities of the arm,
for example, might arise from one of Skinner's images wherein an imaginary
gossamer thread extends out from the middle figure. Using this image, a
movement quality of lightness and floating often arises and an ease of motion
occurs. Or perhaps, to extend Skinner's work, we might explore the image
of the folding such that many connectivities are experienced. Here, if we
still focus on the arm, we might experience many articulations—the action
of the phalanges, the intersection of rotation and flexion in the wrist, or the
nexus of motion to which the elbow and shoulder joints give rise. Through
the process of dancing with the image of folding, this nexus may give rise
to movement akin to a marionette wherein the arm can hang loosely, jiggle,
or shudder, as if each part were able to move independently from the rest.
These improvisational explorations provide opportunities for seeing what is
there, and they may indicate, or even change, habitual usage and release unnecessary holding patterns. Thereby, SRT as a system seeks to progressively
encourage, cultivate, and refine sensory proprioceptive skills—preparing the
individual to be more open and receptive to bodily motion.

The spaciousness described here is not only focused toward skeletal relations
but also reflects out, multidirectionally, to the space immediately around us and
beyond. Attending to the mutability of the balance, for example, Joan Skinner
writes: "Balancing on two feet becomes a multidirectional, multidimensional

experience in space. There is not, as found in traditional methods, a singular reference point for balancing, such as a set of muscles, a particular center of the body, or a concept of upness and downness" (Skinner et al. 1979, 10).

By extending out in multiple directions the idea of autonomy also has within it the important correlates of connectivity and bodily (re)orientations. For through the experience of the body in dynamic change—in finding its ground through ever-shifting balance—we don't look for hard or fixed properties but a softness and fluidity in which we are able to note, but not be held by, our position at any moment. I see this as evoking a productive state of flux. This offers a spaciousness wherein all elements have equal potential rather than one part, or one thing, or indeed one person, being emphasized over an/the other.

When taken as metaphor—the notions that no one part of the body presses on another alongside its correlate of connectivity—is akin to the Merleau-Pontian notion that human experience is not reducible to a sum of parts but is rather a weave of consciousness, body, and environment. Teaching us to notice how we touch and are touched, such a phenomenological synthesis maintains and asserts integrity precisely insofar as it emphasizes our being-toward-the-world.

SCORE-MAKING

The use of language-based guidance in the form of poetic imagery is core to SRT and OSF. Skinner has related her use of images to Suzanne Langer, saying "the image is a gestalt: you experience it as a totality, not as parts leading to a whole, and you absorb it that way all at once" (in Hobson 1997, 37). In her work, the images, arranged into what she calls "image clusters," are at times indirect and oblique, at times related to nature or a quality. Here is an example of an image cluster:

> The whole body becomes one cellular, like an amoeba—one pulsing, breathing, expanding, contracting, liquid unity. Bones and muscles spread out on the floor like spilled water. With every inward breath I seem to take in the whole atmosphere and then breath it out again, taking it in and letting out the whole sky. The whole body becomes a breathing organism like an enormous bellows—breathing in space and energy, breathing out a release of tension in a rush of air. . . . Definitions get lost: me-body-mind-atmosphere-room-up-down-moving-static . . . Rather than trying to perceive things you become perception and it releases you into a vast realm of experience." (Skinner et al. 1979, 10)

In offering such image clusters to a class, Skinner proposes them in a drifting series of suggestions that may remind, deepen, or extend the idea that the dancer is working with. They are allowed to resonate intuitively, stimulating movement or sometimes just being present without defining how the image might be manifest. As clusters, they are designed to lead the dancer into deeper feeling states, or what Skinner calls "totalities." As metaphors, the images give rise to kinesthetic knowledge, weaving together the interior and exterior of the body and connecting each dancer to the group.

In OSF, images are formed more clearly into scores for performance wherein a score might be seen as a guide to initiate movement or provide a shape and structure for improvisation. A score might be formed of words, images, or drawings. Scores for improvisations, unlike music or dance notation scores, are not intended to codify or capture the performed movement. Rather, they offer invitations or impulses from which to dance. The process of forming and performing a score can act as a tool for accessing, developing, and clarifying awareness and for honing and nuancing materials.

For Skura they offer a way to integrate intuitive and analytical faculties and find forms from and for improvisation. Developing a score from improvising, the scores offer a way of asking: What happened? What seemed resonant or potent? Using an alternating structure of dancing, scoring, dancing, and scoring, the movement, words, and drawings resonate with and build on each other. Skura's scores might attend to the physicalities, sensation and energies, spatiality, interconnections, or arising associations. Her strategies suggest structures through which improvisations can be performed, the scores giving us something to work with in an increasingly focused or refined ways. So rather than continually searching for the new, or the next thing, a score keeps bringing us back to the same, such that we can explore it again but each time differently. Through the repeated asking of: "what is the *thingness* of this thing," and phenomenologically, "how do I experience this thing," we deepen our knowledge of what the "thing" is—its shape, texture, tonality, or associations. At the same time, even while focusing on the experience, the experience itself is changing, because, as we move with an image, the image is also transforming. Further, when working with scores there is always the possibility of resistance or even a creative rejection of the boundaries of the predetermined structure. Pushing against the score allows us to find its edges, to sense its limitations; this process similarly enhances our knowing.

> I am moving sideways, smoothing the rough edges and sliding around
> to find another way. Crossing right over left while traversing sideways,
> arms flicking out in multiple directions.
> My hands flicker; fingers splay—flying open stretching my tendons to the
>   end

of my fingertips. Then, softening, I being to dissolve.
Like plastic under heat my edges are starting to curl in and up, molding
    and morphing, by body bends, ripples and bubbles.

Score: Folding and Melting, Forming and Reforming

Running, legs extending at full reach, I circle the studio. Round and
round. Falling—I fall into the floor, my body collapses. All effort
    dissipates and I lay crumpled, heavy, chest rising and falling—my lungs
        burning, my body radiating, pulsing, tingling.
Rest.
Shifting across the floor I roll. Folding and curling I am in a continual
    motion.
The momentum of one roll, tumbling into the next
—a ball running over shifting surfaces.
Arriving.
I hold myself into the wall as if it were a transient surface.
Becoming water, glass, rock.

Score: Moving in/on/as Transmuting Surfaces

A solid crumbling
A folding melt

It is clear then that for Skura score-making is not about closing options, but rather a process through which dynamic flux and process is emphasized. It offers frameworks from the practice as a way to reenter the practice. This is a feedback-loop process in which, as Kozel notes, "the performative moment is initiated by the intention to enact a reflective chiasmic loop" (2011, 208).

This strategy gives us a practical reframing of Merleau-Ponty's core philosophical notion that "my body simultaneously sees and is seen" (1968a, 162), an awareness that he uses to describe a self-reflexivity (in seeing myself I am also being seen by myself) that then ripples out into layers of chiasmic meaning. Proceeding through complex weavings, shifting through and circulating around in an ongoing series of intersecting ideas, scoring offers a tangible way to note, track, respond, and feel our way through. The iterative, but never complete, process enables the "composition" of ideas to emerge from and remain embedded within the process, rather than the phenomena being unnaturally forced and molded.

During these improvisatory practices, connectivity and variation is openly to the fore—to space, to sound, to sensation, to the dynamic and bodies of others. Receptivity to these materialities and intercorporealities enacts the lifeworld in intuitive and at times novel ways. We might see this as a practical way through which we can refine our insights of intuiting or seeing essences via ongoing imaginative and physical variation such that phenomenological description and practice actively circulate. The ongoing process implicitly reminds us that we can never fully imagine all variations, yet through the emergent processes of improvisation (see Midgelow, forthcoming) at least some variations that we could not have pre-thought or pre-imagined can become evident.

PHENOMENOLOGY AS AN IMPROVISED RESEARCH INQUIRY

In activating an improvisationally attuned phenomenology, I have proposed that through somatic modes, improvisation can become as significant to phenomenology as embodiment is to anthropology. More specifically, I have indicated some core ways in which the movement forms of Skinner and Skura might offer us insights into how phenomenological explorations might be enabled and pursued.

Retooling the phenomenologist as an embodied improviser, I have pointed us to: the requirement for letting go, vulnerability, and suppleness as ways of being that enable us to experience as if anew; the ability to attend to in-dividual elements within a context of integrated wholeness via the notion of autonomy; and a process of scoring as a phenomenological method that attends to variation and change and can move us toward a sense of (transi-tory) essence. Through these in-motion strategies, the phenomenologist may be able to sense, embody, and describe the complexity of the ever-changing lifeworld. These practical concepts offer attitudinal, physical, strategic, and creative "tools" through which the phenomenologist may approach the cast-ing of phenomena and articulation of experience. Importantly, these are activated through the use of one's body as a locus of sensory appreciation and critical engagement.

Best understood as forms of process phenomenologies (after Kozel 2015 and Mesle 2008) that arise from and elaborate the pathic (Van Manen 2007), the emerging phenomenologies remain, as is the nature of improvisation, in process, unfixed, and unresolved. They reflect Merleau-Ponty's insight that pure impressions are not only imperceptible but also undiscoverable (1962, 4) for, as Van Manen observes, we don't hear a pure sound sensation or "sense impression" but the barking of the dog or the ringing of the phone (2007, 17). This being the case, I focus here on catching experience in the act of making the world available, offering a counter modality from abstraction and logic to provide ways through which that which is in flux and otherwise unseen can be touched and experienced, leading to greater possibilities and the ability to sense more of how we are present in an ever-changing world.

While phenomenology seeks to open the pre-reflective experience and to distill and illuminate the essence of embodied experience, this retooling moves us away from the conventional procedures of phenomenology that have focused on writing and language-based description as the process for both research and representation (Van Manen 1989, 31–32). Instead, through dance improvisation as based in somatic practice, research is undertaken through touch, bodily awareness, and physical action. These are processes that move beyond description phenomenologies for SRT and OSF and are not only descriptive but also transforming and transformative practices. Deeply embedded in inter/corporeal listening, release, and imaginal worlds, they may at times be quiet, small, and still in tone and quality, but these methods are not passive. They may invite us to enter image-based worlds yet they do not (only) describe; they seek instead to create experience and deepen our somaesthetic being. Here, meaning is lively in the body and can effect change. This expansion of phenomenologies finds resonance with Van Manen's notion that a "phenomenology of practice operates in the space of the formative relations between who we are and who we may become, between how we think or feel and how we act" (Van Manen 2007, 26). Reforming and transforming (to use Van Manen's terms), these practices cultivate an awareness of how to become attuned to inner and outer sensations. Expanding this sensibility improvisationally, we learn to understand how perception is in constant flow and how to research in, through, and about that which is in motion. They ask us to open a space of possibility, making us more critically and somatically aware such that the "how" of being able to notice is transformed and our bodily knowing becomes more acute.

> *Quiet, non-rushed and gentle—I dwell here. Waiting for you to join me.*
> *Listening I hear my blood—I hear the swoosh of wind—I feel/hear the*
>   *rumble*
> *of laughter gurgle from me.*
> *As your hand touches my skull, and I rest into your hand—we begin, each*
>   *transformed by the other.*

Notes

1. I am grateful to Stephanie Skura and SRT teachers Gaby Agis, Rebecca Skelton, and Usha Mahenthiralingam for the training they have given me through workshop intensives and the Skinner introductory and ongoing class series.

2. After graduating from Bennington College in 1946, Joan Skinner performed with the Martha Graham Company and taught in the Graham school until 1951 when she began to work with Merce Cunningham. Sustaining a serious injury led her to the Alexander Technique and, from 1957 onward, she focused on her teaching. She developed her individual approach from the mid-1960s until in the 1980s when the SRT teaching program was launched. This program has codified the practice and enabled the method to spread internationally. For a fuller biography, see http://www.skinnerreleasingnetwork.org/about-joan-skinner (accessed October 12, 2016).

3. Stephanie Skura directed a New York–based performance company for fifteen years. Now based in the Pacific Northwest, Skura works independently with several companies, artists, and institutions. She was one of four core faculty and teacher trainers at the Skinner Releasing Institute 1994–2006, working closely with Joan Skinner to help shape the SRT Teacher Certification Program. Skura's current performance work, including *Surreptitious Preparations for an Impossible Total Act* (2015, 16), *Two Huts* (2012), and *Noir Noir Noir* (2013) integrates improvisation and a visceral approach to language with dance and theater. See http://www.stephanieskura.com/bio.shtml (accessed October 12, 2016).

4. In the U.K., the Skinner Releasing Network has been a significant catalyst for the development and wider recognition of SRT. Introductory biographies and further web links for each of the artists mentioned here can be found on the network's webpages. See http://www.skinnerreleasingnetwork.org/teachers (accessed January 15, 2018.

5. The Alexander Technique, as developed by Frederick Matthias Alexander, is a hands-on educational process that seeks to refine posture and address unnecessary muscular and mental tension. See Alexander 2001.

5

Falling in Love with Language

AMANDA WILLIAMSON

babbling

In somatic movement dance studies, participants are often encouraged to write, speak, mark-make, or paint from the felt sense—sometimes prior to, or after moving, or both. A felt sense may refer "to a way of knowing that is not just logical 'but responsive,' that is, awake to the bodily evocative dimensions that makes words personally relevant and workable" (Todres 2007, 31). Likewise, the embodied, poetic, and aesthetic hermeneutics established in movement-based somatics also listens into bodily experience, preceding the language-formulation process. Captured so neatly by Les Todres quoting Eugene T. Gendlin—"language cannot work alone"—language "needs the body and 'the more'"—and "even though language and experience are implicated in one another, they cannot be reduced to one another nor replace one another in the ongoing aliveness that is understanding" (Todres, 23). The heart-tended, exceptionally detailed, focused, and aesthetic appreciation of language enacted in somatic movement processes has enchanted me over a number of years and, in particular, how language can carefully unfold from sensory feeling.

In somatic explorations, the journey from prereflective or preseparated moving experience to writing, dialogical exchange, and image making often moves back and forth between deep body sensing and language formulation. This process invites participants into the intimacies of embodied language and image making. As in Gendlin's work (1996, 1997, 2003), participants contact and track subtle sensory perceptual flows that stir and feel meaningful at a bodily level, and call for further expression in language. Dance developed within philosophies of somatic awareness cares for the constancy of moving body in one's life journey, but also, and perhaps less obviously, to follow Thomas Cheetham's ideas—to the sea of language in which we live (2015). Reflecting a concern to attend to language with intentional care, James Hillman urges readers in an age of body therapies not to forget the healing power of words (Hillman 1996). In somatically guided movement, embodied language is brought into being through a number of approaches, engaging with a far wider phenomenological and therapeutic concern to not hold words at a distance. From Jung through Hillman, I observe a love for the somatic, alchemical, and imaginal articulating through language, where the "subtle bodies of language, soul and image are required to counteract the abstractions of conceptual thought and of spirit" (Cheetham 2015, 69). Additionally, I observe how Gendlin's phenomenological approach of *focusing* (2003) draws upon his concept of the "responsive order" and how "flow and embodied understanding" ensue from there. Gendlin in kinship with Hillman, "provides a healthy counterpoint to a 'logical order' that tends to produce 'abstract principles'" (Todres 2007, 35).

For Hillman, language is an extension of the biological world from which we evolved (Cheetham 2015, 50). It rises from the same matter. "Language is utterly ubiquitous, and as natural as earth, air, fire, and water" (2015, 61). These quotes emphasise the alchemical somatic basis of language exquisitely developed by Hillman through his alchemical hermeneutics (the materials, substances, and imaginal forms through which the world is ensouled) (1975); but equally, these quotes reflect Gendlin's somatic process, and his experiential technique of moving between a felt sense into language formulation (2003). While not the same, both Gendlin and Hillman share common ground in critiquing the nominalism of language and conceptual rationalism, and they draw attention to the healing power of words in the embodied therapeutic process.

The meeting points and cross-fertilizations that continuously shape and spiral together within the fields of somatic movement and dance, archetypal psychology, somatic psychology, and phenomenology are beautifully witnessed when Hillman writes an endorsement in David Abram's book (1996), and equally where Don Hanlon Johnson writes an endorsement in Gendlin's book (2003). Perhaps it is Johnson's lifetime work where the merging and interlacing of phenomenology, somatic movement practices, and somatic psychology shine most (1987, 1992, 1994, 1995, 1997, 2006, 2014). Overlaps between phenomenology, archetypal psychology, and somatic formulations of language are witnessed in many places. A further example is through Les Todres, a psychotherapist, who acknowledges James Hillman's contribution not only to archetypal psychology, but also to phenomenology (2007, 11–12). In light of this, it is notable that Hillman was inspired by Edmund Husserl (1989). All fields noted earlier find ways to sensually entwine the somatic and the linguistic, critiquing how disjunctive language abandons us in our sensual and fleshy living.

Gendlin's phenomenological ideas of bodily interaction in language and his notion of the "responsive order" are quietly present in somatic movement and dance (1996, 1997, 2003). In the first part of this chapter, his ideas help me unfold an aesthetic embodied appreciation of language akin to the processes enjoyed by many somatic movement and dance participants worldwide. Equally, and of no less importance, in the second part of this chapter, I unfold Hillman's alchemical and imaginal understanding of language and how he provides a profoundly heart-tending experiential approach. Hillman's idea that words have soul substance; words are emissaries, metaphors, and carriers of meaning; and words are rooted in flesh and in the alchemical/imaginal materials of soul are enacted in the second half of this chapter (1975). With further references to Les Todres (2007), Don Hanlon Johnson (2014), David Abram (1996), Thomas Cheetham (2015), and Martin Buber (1970), I travel in this chapter closely with both Gendlin and Hillman, attending to what I see as two vital approaches to language formulation infiltrating somatic movement practices. Of note, they are not exact theoretical applications, but rather are varyingly modulated and often developed in the somatic studio. Here I am interested in Gendlin's and Hillman's infiltrations and meanderings into somatic movement and dance: how they merge, and may overlap, and are part of a far wider paradigm of embodied scholarship critiquing conceptual rationalism.

Weaving through these theoretical and experiential paths, I offer three practice-based enactments in this chapter. Sondra Fraleigh shares her experience of tracing embodiment to language during a somatic movement session. Mary Abrams enacts her somatic process, unfolding language from sensing and moving. I offer an imaginal dance to language process at the end of this chapter. In an early chapter hop: Participants in somatic movement and dance sessions are often invited into "a bodily inclusive hermeneutic cycle in which one's bodily-sensed-situation-in-relation-to-words gives words a new life" (Todres 2007, 24).

trickling

Van Manen neatly writes: "It is best to think of the basic method of phenom-enology as the taking up of a certain attitude and practicing a certain attentive awareness to the things of the world as we live them rather than as we con-ceptualize or theorize them" (2000, 460). Somatically informed movement and dance reflects and enacts phenomenology's broader ethical call—to live phenomena closely, rather than conceptualize phenomena and hold the world at a distance. Bringing awareness to living body, closely attuning to our life-full body of flesh, and not holding body apart as an "it" is central to somatic movement philosophy. Bringing awareness to how we live in language, and how language lives us, is equally central to somatic perspectives, but not so commonly written about. In somatic movement dance processes, one does not want to overprioritize language viewed in postmodern trajectories or indeed endlessly critique language as disjunctive and therefore deceptive; rather, a delicate and subtle flow between body and language is embedded in somatic movement philosophy.

fleshing

> When we think of "body" we may traditionally think of something solidly there. In the Cartesian sense, there is the body and the world, the body and the mind, inner and outer. But approaching embodying more naively, we find a living body that inhabits situations intimately; it interweaves the realms as a matter of being, and is often "lost" out there in the textures, the senses, the flesh, the histories, and the meanings that come from the flowing excess of the lifeworld. (Todres 2007, 20)

Todres, in his extensive writings on embodiment, highlights how "em-bodying is where being and knowing meet" (ibid.). Following Gendlin's ideas closely, he accentuates "how the body knows its situation directly" and prior to language formulation (ibid.). He writes: "Faithful to the depth of bodily relational understandings, we could say that the way we are bodily in situations exceeds any precise formulation or patterning of it" (21). Preceding language, bodily experiencing is thus full of meaning, knowing and intelligence (Gendlin 2003). "The body is an intentional body, primordially relational, and co-arising with its situation that is not just fleshly perceptual but also full of implicit meanings and relational understanding" (Todres 2007, 21). Crucially and following Gendlin, bodily experiencing is not passive:

The role of the lived body becomes crucial as a double realm that both textually experiences the prereflective "more" of a world that it is part of, and at the same time, gives perspective and reflection (shared or alone to this experience). (2)

deepening

Gendlin (1996, 1997, 2003), a philosopher and psychotherapist (influenced by Husserl, Merleau-Ponty, and Heidegger), originated the therapeutic approach "focusing," and creative similarities and modulations of Gendlin's focusing method appear in language formulation processes in somatic movement and dance (although similarities with Gendlin's methods may not always be made explicit to participants). One of the main similarities found across somatic movement and dance studies and Gendlin's approach is what he terms *preseparated multiplicity* (Todres 2007). Sometimes referred to as the *prereflective* in somatic movement sessions, Gendlin refers to *preseparated multiplicity* as an experiential bodily realm prior to the separation language uniquely requires. Noted by Todres, for Gendlin, "body is the intimate medium of 'the more'" (2007, 22). The "more" of the body precedes the distinctions and separations language requires. The "more" is our body's excess and a pregnancy of meaning. Thus, for Gendlin: "perception is not primary, as perception is already based on a distinction between 'over there' from 'over here'—something important is happening before this spatial distinction in the way that meaning unfolds" (21). The "more" is both fertile (expansive), and yet specific (expressing through directional bodily animations). In Todres's words, learning to language from "the more" is

> not reflectively already achieved before us; one needs to go into a kind of "murky" or a kind of "down there" or "in there," a "not quite that but something else." This involves an aesthetic experience and process of finding the words or differentiating movements, or symbolizing something in such a way that does some of this "more" a degree of justice. The more is "very fertile. Many strands or specific meanings can come from it—but it is itself an 'unseparated multiplicity.'" The more is "very specific even though it is unseparated in direct experiencing. It is specific in that it implies particular directions, actions, and speech." (22)

In somatic movement studies, participants are often encouraged to listen into "the more" and to the directions, subtle pulses, and movements that babble, ache, skate across, and rumble in flesh—animated movements that call us to find words or images (Johnson 2014). In Gendlin's experiential model, "'closeness' refers to bodily-participant-knowing, while 'distance' refers to the language-formulating process'" (Todres 2007, 34). Rhythms of closeness and distance are both required in the act of knowing.

His experiential technique shifts back and forth between closeness and distance, and one listens into pre-separated multiplicity waiting quietly for a felt sense to form. In Gendlin's words:

> A felt sense is not an emotion. We recognise emotions. We know when we are angry or sad or glad—it is vague and murky. It feels meaningful, but not known. It is a body-sense of meaning. When you learn how to focus, you will discover that the body finding its own way provides its own answers to many of your problems. (2003, 10)

For Gendlin, the felt sense is not just there; it forms as you learn how to let it form through tending to your body (ibid.). His model has profound implications because he is calling for body experience to presence intimately in language, and such intimate participation with nonverbal intelligence has the potential to shape human actions. He explains:

> Your body is not a machine, rather a wonderfully intricate interaction with everything around you, which is why it "knows" so much just in being. The animals live intricately with each other without culture and language. The different cultures don't create us. They only add elaboration. The living body is always going beyond what evolution, culture and language have already built. The body is always sketching and probing a few steps further. Your ongoing living makes evolution and history happen—now. (viii)

merging

Gendlin offers six phases to his focusing method:

- Clearing a space: silent sensing and sensing into body or body parts.
- A felt sense: tending to, or allowing a felt-sense to form.
- Handling: allowing words and phrases to emerge from a felt sense.
- Resonating: moving between a felt sense and words or images.
- Asking: asking into this felt sense and its quality, and noticing subtle shifts and releases.
- Receiving: the somatic reception of meaning about one's life and body while noticing ongoing shifts, releases, and responses (43–45).

Gendlin's focusing techniques are found in somatically informed movement studies and notably across a range of somatic practices where participants are encouraged to explore processes such as the below, and in many variations and modulations.

SILENT-SENSING

Participants are invited to sense into the body before or after moving. Sensing into preseparated multiplicity and "the more" needs silence, or moments of silence; a deepening into the textures, expanse and tentative formings of a felt sense.

TENDING TO AND LISTENING FOR A FELT SENSE

Participants are encouraged to listen for a felt sense beginning to differentiate from preseparated multiplicity and "the more" (a felt-sense, not yet articulated in language, but pregnant with bodily feeling).

MOVING FROM A FELT SENSE

Participants are invited to move or dance a felt sense, listening to the qualities of a felt sense and motoring out its imaginal intelligence.

OPENING TO LANGUAGE AND IMAGE

After moving, participants are invited to open to words and images emerging from a felt sense and moving time, incarnating a felt sense in words or images, then crossing back and forth between a felt sense and the differentiations of language and image.

RESONATING WITH LANGUAGE

Participants are invited to dwell with words or images that have immerged from a felt sense, moving back and forth between a felt sense and its flesh-full words and images, and to see if the words and images are aesthetically satisfying.

RECEIVING AND NOTICING

Participants are encouraged to receive words or images back into a felt sense, noticing how the words or images create subtle shifts and effect change at a bodily level.

SHARING, SOUNDING AND DIGESTING

Participants are invited to share and sound their embodied language or images in dyadic or group dialogue, digesting and toning experience with others.

* * *

In these somatic movement sessions, language and image are encouraged to incarnate with bodily intimacy and, through an ongoing invitation for the human body, to be intimately present when languaging or imaging. As in Gendlin's focusing sessions, participants in somatic movement sessions are encouraged to dwell in closeness, allowing the intimacy of the felt sense to express outwardly through movement and in language. This back and forth between "the more" of experiencing, an emergent felt sense, and the differentiations of language forming from a felt sense is central to languaging somatic experience in the studio. Gendlin reflects a similar ethical approach to languaging found in somatic movement and dance studies, providing a healthy counterpoint to abstract principles. The flow he advocates puts body and language in a flowing responsive relationship.

Gendlin's responsive order teaches that knowledge cannot be separated from interpretation and "bodily-contextual-intimacy" (35). The type of language Gendlin and Todres write of is rooted and entwined in bodily feeling. Here, we find a phenomenal practice aiming to heal disjunctive ways of knowing and certainly swimming against the tide of postmodernism, and equally we find an alternative to conceptual rationalism, where words are either "bloated in importance or dried in content" (Hillman 1996, 8).

Gendlin's practice and languaging in somatic movement processes seek to heal the split between the knower and the known, between meaning and things, between the image and word. Many somatic movement facilitators work within modulations of these processes or reflect aspects of Gendlin's work. For example, Sondra Fraleigh and Mary Abrams share their approaches. Sondra says:

> I have several ways of tuning into words, sometimes cerebrally, and sometimes through felt life, which would signal poetry. My use of imagery as the basis for language and dance comes out of stillness, as in Gendlin's Focusing process. I sit still or move without expectation and see what comes into consciousness. Sometimes a picture forms. Sometimes, it's a felt sensation in a part of my body that calls to me. An entire short story might arrive, something of fantasy or daydream, or something I would rather not own about my life. In any case, I let it ruminate until enough of it forms that I can actually dance it, or say something about it. The minute I speak, write or dance, the image melts or it rises to language. But I can usually recall the affective source. Language and dance enrich the image. This process takes fascinating directions when I focus with a partner while sitting or in movement, and we speak to each other and dance out of the imagistic, experiential states. The images morph as we share. In our approach to somatic bodywork at Eastwest, we often focus images in sitting or moving as a way to begin the process. The focused images and their morphology become the

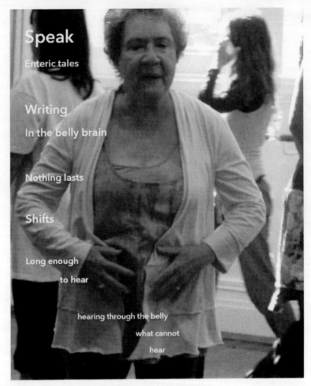

Figure 5.1. Sondra Fraleigh. Photograph © 2014 by Kelly Ferris.

basis for verbal communication in the course of bodywork. (Sondra Fraleigh, personal communication, September 2016)

Mary Abrams in her language formulation asks a question about her life before moving and sensing. She asks: "How can I feel more creatively engaged in the health and well-being of my life and work to create and facilitate a brilliantly abundant safe, loving, peaceful, and sustainably supportive future for the rest of my life?" She first asks and answers her question verbally before sensing and moving. She calls this first response in language—"narrative thinking" and "cultural flow." She then senses—tending to her question with breath, heart, skin, folds, twists, and reaches. Mary moves the same question kinaesthetically and nonverbally. After moving time, she writes again, retaining relationship to the flesh and heart of her moving experience—she finds words "awake with flow, feeling, vibration, and curiosity." Mary reflects:

> I enter the process with myself, a witness and a photographer witness. My first writing flows through with clear intention. I write my dream for life to come. I

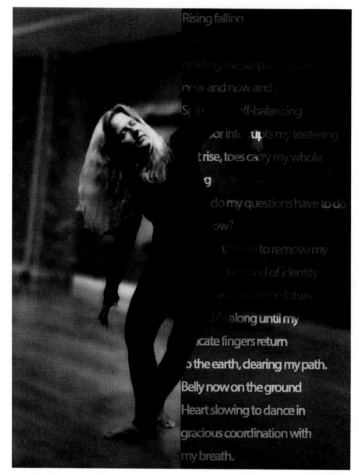

Figure 5.2. Mary Abrams. Photograph by Eric R. Hansen.

feel for the words as they stream through as narrative thinking, telling a story as I feel, see myself in the future. The words flow in sentences, proper sequence of grammatical structure and punctuation. I am moving a cultural flow.

I set the paper down, roll to the middle of the floor, end in a squatted position and begin to move. For 10 minutes in silence, my whole body-minding process shakes, shivers, teeters, spins, falls, pauses, breathes, reaches, eyes opening, eyes closing, softens, twists, folds, unfurls, and gently comes to a rest.

I reach for my pen and paper. Feeling my heart pulsing, my breath slowing, I write again. Words fall onto the page—one, two, three at a time. New line. No punctuation, no grammar, a feeling, an image, no linear progression, just word-space-word-space-word-space. My silent dance has ended yet flows through me

*in a new way as words begin to form describing now, describing then, awake
with flow, feeling, vibration, and curiosity.*

*Writing-moving-writing again, I experience the presentness of my body-being
dreaming a future. I can see more clearly what it will take to be what I am, and
be what I am becoming.* (Mary Abrams, personal communication, October 7,
2016)

gathering

Gendlin is only one of many phenomenologists seeking to heal disjunctive
models of knowing that find resonance and enactment in formulations of
somatic movement language. Merleau-Ponty, David Abram, and Don Hanlon
Johnson are commonly cited and integrated in practice and research with
a surge and passion (Williamson 2015a, b). Other theorists such as Buber,
likewise, call us to find language (and thus knowledge) that encourages balance within the subjective "I" in the deeply absorptive "thou" relationship
(1970). These theorists call for knowledge that admits vulnerability and does
not recklessly control the world. All these theorists noted above could equally
provide insightful ways of reflecting on studio practice. Abram, for example,
reflects a sensual somatic understanding of language expression central to
somatic movement pedagogies:

> Linguistic meaning is not some ideal and bodiless essence that we arbitrarily
> assign to a physical sound or word and then toss it out into the "external"
> world. Rather, meaning sprouts in the very depths of the sensory world, in
> the heat of meeting, encounter, participation. (1996, 75)

Johnson also reflects a poetic textured sensuality that seeks language beyond banal descriptions:

> It is not words that betray our deeper experiences, but banal words, ready-
> made words, truisms, slogans, ethereal generalized words. The poet, liter-
> ary novelist, songwriter, spoken word hip-hopper: words for them are juicy,
> powerful, moving, earthy, leading us to an even more complex experience of
> reality rather than washing out its colours. (2014, xiv)

shifting

In the second part of this chapter, I turn to Hillman and imaginal somatic
movement studies, specifically to heighten Gendlin's ideas of seeking language that is not dried in content, but rather fleshy and plump, entwined with,
moving, and pulsing in the materials and flesh of the world. I also choose

Hillman because he reflects phenomenology's ability to loosen a fixed sense of self—a self that is often colonized by objectification and conceptualization (Fraleigh 2016; Williamson 2015a). Hillman, inspired by Husserl, calls for us to allow "phenomena to show themselves for our contemplation" (1989, 4). In doing so, he indeed loosens, frees up, and melts conceptual rationalization. In this way, I regard him as deeply phenomenological. Equally, Hillman's experiential theories resonate strongly with David Abram's ecological phenomenology; Abram also highlights the moving materials, substances, and temperatures of language (1996).

In a second chapter hop:

Following Jung and Hillman, I move into an "illuminist epistemology" that seeks "conjunctive knowing," where the imagination is offered as a healing and remedial agent, an experiential realm that supports movers in healing the split between the knower and the known (Cheetham 2015, 43). Therefore, I get down and soulful with Hillman's soul—neither physical nor spiritual, but rather bound to both through the alchemical and imaginal—the materials, substances, and imaginal forms through which we are alchemically worked.

diving

Jungian and post-Jungian somatic movement studies, sometimes called "active-imagination" in movement, or "transpersonal" approaches, are a well-researched and deeply considered strand of somatic movement practice (Hayes 2013, 2014; Halprin 2003, 2014; Stromsted 2014; Hartley 2014). I will call this strand of practice "imaginal somatic movement approaches," which form a spiraling branch, blossoming within the broader paradigm of somatic movement education and therapy. Imaginal somatic movement approaches are rooted in, warmed and cooked by Jungian and post-Jungian lenses, and are polytheistic in their image making and repersonifying the world. Images scribbled, lovingly painted, quickly dotted or striking out boldly across the page, disclose a polytheistic appreciation of imaginal form. Image making moves away from idolatry and static religious forms that solidify and cripple the imagination; "hard facts, fixed truths, and blind certainties of compulsion and fanaticism are melted by *solutio*" (Cheetham 2015, 99).

Sounds sounding, words toning, poems inscribed and emblazoned in notepads, or words and phrases scattered on canvases are melted by *solution*. By this, I mean words are encouraged to retain their relationship with the imaginal and metaphorical, evoking anima and *solutio*—she who melts hardened concepts. When movement is stirring in cellular waters, firing in belly, settling in bones, yielding into earth's gravity, meandering and streaming through veins, it is encouraged to flow with imaginal and metaphorical sensibility (Hayes 2014). Thus, when one encounters somatic movement and dance forms lovingly warmed by Jungian and post-Jungian experiential discourses, one is entering what Henry Corbin calls, *Ta'wil*—"the mainspring of every spirituality" (Corbin, in Cheetham 2015, 98). *Ta'wil* is a mode of being and perceiving beyond idolatry and literalism. *Ta'wil* is metaphorical and imaginal; "It is a way of seeing and a way of living that refuses the literal" (ibid.). Like phenomenological approaches of suspension (although certainly not identical), in imaginal somatic movement approaches, a pre-reflective experience of imaginal phenomena is lived. One is dancing, writing, languaging, sounding, and image making on the middle path (in the imaginal and with the metaphorical).

Somatic movement and dance underpinned by imaginal studies are different from somatic practices underpinned by, for example, ontogenetic, phylogenetic, and biomorphic somatic movement exploration (Williamson 2015b). It is never entirely wise to draw sharp and unbending distinctions between different somatic movement approaches because many explore the interdependencies between the living body and living earth, and all offer a nondualistic vision of existence. Ontogenetic and phylogenetic movement practices, for example, aim to explore through "sensuous moving cellular participation, the protoplasmic unity and interdependencies of body and earth" (Williamson 2015b, 335; Bainbridge Cohen 1993; Olsen and McHose 1998; Hartley 1995; McHose and Frank 2006; Olsen 2002). Likewise, imaginal somatic movement studies are also deeply rooted in the protoplasmic, organic, and primordial, but there is a keen focus on sensing into and listening for imaginal forms that arise from somatic engagement with body and environmental nature (Hayes 2014). Here we witness the keen integration of Jungian and post-Jungian discourse into somatic movement, and therefore the approach tends to lens through ideas of the archetypal and alchemical. All approaches to somatic movement are rooted in "reverence," "awe," and the "mysteries of creativity" (Hayes 2013, 67), and of note, many practitioners mix it up, working across the two, or indeed many somatic movement approaches.

However, there are differences that are delightful to study; the main characteristic I draw attention to in the second part of this chapter is how imaginal somatic movement seeks to re-enchant and re-personify language through a theory of the redemption of matter. This is a theory that "embraces a world view in which language has body, images have body, soul has body—and these bodies, subtle though they be, are required if the world we think of as material is to have any body at all" (Cheetham 2015, 69). Noted above, this approach is illuminist and conjunctive, where the imagination is enacted to heal the split between the knower and the known (Hayes 2013).

One certainly encounters an openly spiritual and soulful pedagogical approach through the use of imagination in movement. In Jill Hayes's words: imaginal somatic movement "is a kind of dancing that listens to and appreciates the imaginal presences arising inside the physical forms of the natural world" (2014, 66). Participants are encouraged, through "sensuous engagement with body and nature" to "listen for images that arise from such a relationship" (ibid.). Imaginal form, enacted within this Jungian and post-Jungian frame "indicates something other than an image produced by a self-contained mechanical imaginative faculty in a human brain; it suggests a spiritual image-presence arising from the heart of living form" (70). Through this lens, the collective unconscious is "accessed through the process of active imagination through which the person welcomes and learns from the image as living presence" (ibid.). Participants are supported in exploring the "material/spiritual and temporal/eternal" continuum (dancing between the visible and invisible) (ibid.), and embodied imagination carries participants "into the eternal or archetypal stream of life." Body is explored as an alchemical vessel, and soul has both alchemical and imaginal sensibility. Participants are encouraged to enact the metaphorical and the symbolic and not the literal; and of note, the cultivation of somatic awareness and an imaginal sensibility are equally valued (65).

expanding

Hillman's work, following Jung, circumnavigates the hero archetype of the ego in Western monotheistic consciousness, and he roots soul making and repersonifying images and language in the multiplicity and polytheism of the anima (1975). For Hillman, words are living entities, living souls, with alchemical, sensate, and archetypal power. In short, he encourages images and language to emerge from the alchemical and the imaginal beyond the dry and conceptual. His work opens readers and practitioners to the multiplicity of the polytheistic imaginal. The larger spiritual call, when applied to somatic studies, is to move, dance, write, paint, and imagine, not from the I and God but from the we and many. Hillman writes, "What we learn from dreams is what psychic nature really is—the nature of psychic reality: not I, but we; not one, but many. Not monotheistic consciousness looking down from its mountain, but polytheistic consciousness wandering all over the place, in the vales and along rivers, in the woods, the sky, and under earth" (33) (see Plate 4).

For Hillman, the soul's first freedom is to imagine (39), and he highlights, the soul person anima; her multiplicity and polytheistic nature has long been controlled by "our anti-imaginal, anti-personifying" monotheistic traditions, which continue to keep her under control—so afraid of the nonliteral and the "spontaneity and natural polytheism of soul." (45). Preceding David Abram's ecological phenomenology (Fraleigh 2016), Hillman extensively critiques the shadow of Christian and Cartesian values, noting how our modern world view "vigorously combated an animistic, personified view of nature and "polytheistic antiquity" (1975, 3–4). He writes: "Personifying has always been fundamental to the religious and poetic imagination," but the Christian idea of the human person "as the true focus of the divine and the only carrier of soul is basic" to our modern worldview (1). Hillman writes at length about how the modern worldview restricts understanding of subjectivity to human persons: "Only they are permitted to be agents and doers, to have consciousness and soul" (ibid.). He writes that Descartes "imagines a universe divided into living subjects and dead objects. There is no space for anything intermediate, ambiguous, and metaphorical" (ibid.). The metaphorical and deliteralized realm that Hillman explored is the foci of imaginal somatic movement processes.

Ensouling and re-personifying language in the wake of monotheism and the literalistic nominalism of language in Western consciousness is Hillman's outspoken gift to us, and this gift, deeply Jungian and developed by Hillman, is the lifeblood of somatic movement practices that view imagination in movement as the "ontological continuity between the human soul, the *anima humana*, and the soul of the world, the *anima mundi*" (Cheetham 2015, 43). Akin with Gendlin, and many other phenomenologists, the split between the knower and the known, between meaning and things, and between the image and word, seeks union; but, within Hillman's approach, union is keenly developed through the alchemical and imaginal. Such a path, while very much adaptable to more secular sensibilities, particularly given its emphasis on the plurality and multiplicity of psyche/soul, is an "illuminist epistemology" based on "conjunctive knowing," where the intelligence of the imagination unfolds a conjunctive relationship between "the human soul, and the soul of the world" (2015, 43–44).

multiplying

Underpinning imaginal somatic movement processes are the alchemical archetypes understood as the *"deepest patterns of psychic functioning,"* the roots of the soul governing the perspectives we have of ourselves and the world (Hillman 1975, xix). For Hillman, one way to begin to see metaphoric archetypes is through the Greek pantheon of the Gods and Goddesses, who remind us "that there are lots of emotional atmospheres and styles of experience, mirroring the diversity of organisms and ecosystems in the biological world" (Cheetham 2015, 115). The application of Hillman's archetypal psychology opens movers to the polytheistic expressive dimensions of the human psyche: no longer "I and God" (and alone), movers enter the transpersonal—"we and many" (and together). For Hillman "the soul's inherent multiplicity demands a theological fantasy." As he observes, "polytheistic thinking shifts all our habitual categories and divisions" (1975, 168). He notes his work is theistic, but not religious—and writes that, in religions,

> Gods are believed in and approached with religious methods. In archetypal psychology, Gods are imagined. They are formulated ambiguously, as metaphors for modes of experience and as numinous borderline persons. They are cosmic perspectives in which soul participates. (169)

melting

Entries "into the imaginal signals not change of place, but change in your mode of being. Just as finding one's soul is not the discovery of a thing but a deepening of experience, so entering the imaginal involves a fundamental transformation in the condition of the world" (Cheetham 2015, 80).

Both Hillman and Cheetham critique literalism as based in a monotheistic consciousness "that is grounded in a lack of imagination"—rigidity, fixation, concretization (Cheetham 2015, 82). Cheetham says that fundamentalist religion becomes pathological when it cripples our capacities to feel and move in response to "a manifold and changing surround" (78). Entry into the imaginal in somatic movement processes thus requires *solution*—melting hardened concepts, such as the hard crack supposed between spirit and matter. Melting signals a love for metaphor, the imaginal and the nonliteral. Such dissolution of our habits, beliefs, and ways of thinking is the beginning of healing. Thus, in imaginal somatic movement processes, water as a metaphor and carrier of meaning indicates dissolution, freeing inertia in both our imaging and languaging process.

freeing

Central to Jung and Hillman's alchemical hermeneutics and their contribution to the development of imaginal somatic movement studies is "soul." Soul making, soul seeking, and soul seeing may sound lofty, and to some old-fashioned, but following Hillman, in imaginal somatic movement studies, soul is offered and experienced metaphorically. The word *soul* is a carrier of meaning (anima *solutio*); soul is not a solid thing (Hillman 1975). Trying to fix and classify soul is seductive and attractive because our modern worldview wants everything boxed, conceptualized, or dismissed by science as fallacy. For Hillman, finding one's soul is not the discovery of a thing but a deepening of experience:

> By *soul* I mean, first of all, a perspective rather than a substance, a viewpoint toward things rather than the thing itself. This perspective is reflective; it mediates events and makes differences between ourselves and everything that happens. Between us and events, between the doer and everything that happens. Between us and events, between the doer and the deed, there is a reflective moment—and soul-making means differentiating this middle ground. (1975, xvi)

He continues:

> First, "soul" refers to the *deepening* of events into experiences; second the significance soul makes possible, whether in love or in religious concern, derives from its *special relation to death*. And third, by soul I mean experiencing through reflective speculation, dream, image, and *fantasy*—that mode which recognizes all realities as primarily symbolic or metaphorical. (xvi)

And furthermore, for Hillman, soul is paradoxical: soul senses independence and interdependence. Soul lives in paradox, intermediating a feeling of personality (of me, my depth, my suffering, my life journey). Yet I can never grasp my soul, apart from the other things of which I am part. The soul "is like a reflection in a flowing river, or like the moon which mediates only borrowed light" (xvi). For Hillman, soul "is neither physical and material on the one hand, nor spiritual and abstract on the other, yet bound to them both" (68).

watering

Etymologically, soul, often colonized in monotheistic religion and its conceptual language, takes us back to the sea (*saiwaz*), back to our watery beginnings and into *solutio*. Hillman's call to ensoul the world beyond the limiting images of monotheism and literal language depends upon our ability to personify, which in turn depends upon anima. Anima means both psyche and soul and "we meet her in her numerous embodiments as soul of waters without whom we dry" (Hillman 1975, 42). For Hillman, "she is both bridge to the imaginal and also the other side, personifying the imagination of the soul," and she is "the movement through the constructed world of concepts and dead things into an animistic, subjective, mythical consciousness, where fantasy is alive" (43). Sensing soul through anima and her *solutio* is a vital archetypal experience in imaginal somatic movement modalities. Somatic movers may meet anima in the waters and fluids of body, or they may encounter her as they activate imaginal movement and language processes, where the conceptual is encouraged to shift to the metaphorical, and where we move from dry concepts and empty images into heart-tending image making and languaging.

materializing

Hillman's post-Jungian work with alchemical language and image making (following Jung) attends to the unification of psyche and logos and the re-balancing of directed conceptual thinking. Hillman highlights how "we are trapped in the literalism of language." And the therapeutic function of al-chemical language is to shift the way we think about the psyche, the soul, and the world beyond the human (Cheetham 2015, 66). For Hillman, our daily language often at best "accounts for the world in concept words rather than images or thing words. Concepts are based on established identities— what something is rather than what it is *like*" (1975, 65). While, for Hillman, concepts may be traces or husk of things, he further writes:

> And to say what something is we have to treat it schematically, abstractly, since the real thing itself is far too complex, individual and immediate to be anything but itself. So we take this being away from it, and rather than describing it metaphorically, we categorize it with a concept and say what it is. (Cheetham 2015, 65)

Language formulation in imaginal somatic movement approaches requires describing experience beyond daily concepts easily reached. Instead, coming to language involves finding words of temperatures and movements, speaking from the bodied alchemical and imaginal. Hillman writes that we must speak "dreamingly, imagistically, and materially" (69). We need

> a new angelology of words . . . so that we may once again have faith in them. Without the inherence of the angel in the word—and angel means originally

"emissary," "message-bearer"—how can we utter anything but personal opin-
ions, things made up in our subjective minds? How can anything of worth
and soul be conveyed from one psyche to another, as in a conversation, a letter, or a book, if archetypal significances are not carried in the depths of our
words? (Hillman 1996, 9)

Hillman provides a phenomenology of practice within the depths of alchemical language. Placing "the imagination at the center of reality, alchemical
language moves right to the heart of the *prima materia* of emotional life in
all its pain, confusion, density, and complexity. It provides a language and
a method for an intense struggle with perception and emotion" (Cheetham
2015, 70, 63). The "beauty of alchemical language" is for Hillman a "mate-
rialized language which we can never take literally" (Hillman 2015, 1). He
writes: "we are carried by [alchemical language] into an as-if, into both the
materialization of the psyche and the psychization of matter" (1). For Jung,
too, alchemy is "intensely somatic", and of note, "his development of the
technique of active imagination is based fundamentally on working with
images in matter—in stone and in paint . . . in dance . . . in sandplay . . . and
crucially, the embodied, material forms of language" (Cheetham 2015, 122).
Active imagination through sound, movement, mark making, painting, and
dancing is central to imaginal somatic movement approaches, but equally
one may attend to imaginal form in words. For Hillman, conceptual language
lacks substance, whereas alchemical language is a parched heart bespattered
and kicked and blackening—a drying kiss, curling and crisping in firing
sunlight—in short, alchemical language has substance, depth, and weight
and retains a relationship with the soul's alchemical materials. Of important
note, Hillman does not want us to abandon conceptual language altogether
or take alchemical language as a literal expression. Rather, he encourages us
to speak with alchemical imagination by treating "materials as ensouled"
(1989, 3)—in short, find speech rooted in the vessels, variables, transitions,
and titrating substances in which we are embodied:

> The basic stuffs of personality—salt, sulphur, mercury, and lead—are concrete
> materials; the description of soul, *aqua pinguis* or *aqua ardens*, as well as words
> for states of soul, such as *albedo* and *nigredo*. . . . The work of soulmaking
> requires corrosive acids, heavy earths, ascending birds; there are sweating
> kings, dogs and bitches, stenches, urine and blood. . . . How like the language
> of dreams and unlike the language into which we interpret dreams. When
> alchemy speaks of degrees of heat, it does not use numbers. Rather it refers
> to the heat of horse dung, the heat of sand, the heat of metal touching fire.

These heats differ, moreover, not only in degree but also in quality: heat can be slow and gentle, or moist and heavy, or sudden or sharp. (Hillman 2015, 1)

blackbirding

While not an exact application of Hillman's ideas, alchemical language is present in imaginal somatic movement studies. A redemptive theory of matter pours forth, and passions practice through a theory noted earlier: this theory in which language, images, and soul have a body, subtle perhaps, but required, if the material world is "to have any body at all" (Cheetham 2015, 69). Attending to alchemical substances worked in the vessel of body, while giving these experiences words and images, undergirds many forms of somatic movement practice. For example, in ontogenetic and biomorphic movement exploration established in Body-Mind Centering® (Bainbridge Cohen 1993; Hartley 1995; Williamson 2015b) and Continuum Movement (Conrad 2007), the materials of the body in which we are worked, watered, warmed, bubbled, poured, and cooked are of salt, saline, electricity, and mineral. We are moving substances and temperatures—sensing into our pulsating fluids, sticky substances, fluctuating temperatures, pooling and puddling emotions,

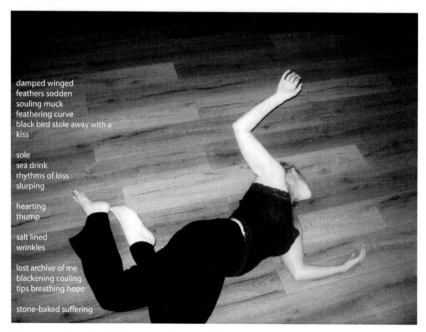

Figure 5.3. Amanda Williamson. Photograph by Scott Closson.

atmospheric bones, and sinuous firing muscles—enlivening our somas across many somatic practices. In imaginal somatic movement studies, one may attend to temperatures of loss felt in teeth and cheekbones; a blackbird landing on lips and stealing the corner of a sunlit kiss; the warming tingles of love daring to move up the spine; a subzero graying heart held in emotionless hands; a solid greening dampness of chest; or a heavy thumping muck of veins longing for a fresh river to wash out its thickness and blackness. To repersonify language, we listen to our material bodies and alchemy, sensing our unique movements, temperatures, and emotional qualities imbuing these ensouled substances with imaginal form.

6

Living Phenomenology

SONDRA FRALEIGH

When it is true to its original purpose of illuminating experience, all phenomenology is unpredictable and life changing. This chapter invites such potential through *performative phenomenology*, witnessing how change in the unfinished body occurs through life itself as a performance. Dance is the essay's performative ground and music its means. Reaching from dance toward music composition through timespace linkages of somatic life, the text progresses through a metamorphic process of common tone somatic attunements that will become increasingly apparent.

Our subtle step from existential phenomenology toward "living phenomenology" implicates "being" and "becoming" as both presence and survival. It suggests active "doings" and calls for being real in admitting life's disappointments and constraints. Daily attention to human needs is never over, and issues of survival persist, particularly in preservation of the world we live in together. If early existentialism asserted the lonely man against the crowd, living phenomenology invokes networks that bind life together. It asserts that we are responsible for each other as for ourselves. Existentially, this is what being free is about. "Being-with" takes a front seat. We are not alone in difficulty and suffering, and life need not be lonely. Living phenomenology appears in the simple pleasures of companionship and perhaps more dramatically in attention to dancing beyond illusions of control.

Existentialism was never a philosophy of closure. From the beginning, it described fluctuations of everyday life in situational uncertainties and ambiguous states of being, as Simone de Beauvoir elucidated in her work, *The Ethics of Ambiguity* (1994). Early in its history, phenomenology was forever changed in the hands of existentialists Beauvoir (1994), Merleau-Ponty (1962), Sartre (1947), Heidegger (1962), and Levinas (1974). All of them were indebted to Husserl. Expanding his method of *bracketing* (setting aside) naturalized life and worldviews, their work admitted the psychological tests and ethics of *living* a life. This chapter veers toward life as performance, hesitating briefly at this point to go back to Husserl's constitutive phenomenology: *back to the dance itself*, to ask what makes a *thing* what it is? What is performance?

To Perform on Purpose

To perform is to finish something, to know how to orient actions and to complete them, or else to play with incompletion. Performance is a way of doing. To perform is to know how to do something, and to be in "the how" of the doing. Thus performance is movement, and it is more than movement; it is comprised of intentional actions that have express purposes. If we look behind action toward *motility* (the ability to move), we can appreciate movement as the change and process that powers intentional actions.

Sense perception informed by attention and the oriented acts of intentionality is a major theme of phenomenology (Husserl 1989, 60–93, 291). Attentive perception is not passive but alive with intentionality, motility, and receptive phases. To grasp this is to understand how intentionality springs from affective sensate life. Intentionality (orientation) can be obvious as forethought for action but is tacit as attunement of attention and purpose, even as purpose dissolves in motile symbiotic processes. In the dissolve, we can be in the flow of doing and dancing, not seeming to intend anything when our attention is present-centered. We carry aims lightly in what we have learned how to do well; these are the learned abilities and individual habitus that transform how we move into life.

In life, then, a performance might be a task like giving a public speech, for instance, or consciously undertaking an interpersonal process like forgiveness. *Performances exist in the actions we take on purpose.* They arise and recede in oriented chunks of time that draw particular notice. To bring consciousness to a process or event, to live and perform as one intends, is not that unusual. We make choices daily that have effects on those around us and ripple out into the world. It isn't always easy to see the extent of our performances, but when we are aware of our chosen actions, sometimes we can see with distance, and in seeing recognize ourselves, even in transition. The major narrative of this chapter suggests tenuous exchanges in performance, noticing how perceptual qualities overlap and mix affectively.

We have said that performances have limits and are partly defined by a sense of completion or accomplishment; they are also presentational acts, including ways of functioning effectively. My thesis that life and embodiment are ongoing and in transition may seem quite apart from performative aspects of completion and accomplishment. Part of the definition of a performance is that it does finish. When I pick up one of the books I have written, I'm not tempted to read it. Rather I'm just glad to know that it is finished. The book no longer belongs to me but will be read and interpreted by others. I understand writing as a performance, but the ongoing and changing flow of my life is another matter—or is it? We court cliché in calling life a dance; in view of process, however, we might extract life's performative, dancelike elements.

Dance is, among other things, a somatic movement art. We activate somatic potentials when we move with awareness of self in relation to others and the surrounding world. I can become more aware of my surroundings through dance, and I don't need a stage to do this. Like music, dance involves acts of somatic attunement: listening (taking in) and voicing (moving out). Speaking and breathing, seeing, even dying are bodily events sited in music and dance, and we could also call them "somatic existentials," as crucial, embodied activities that shape existence.

Attuning through Common Tones

Reflecting on performative existentials gives me a chance to attune my senses. I can pause, linger, and look at a painting I like, or take time to listen to music, even as each time I revisit them, I see and hear again because I change. In the *process performances* discussed in the next section, I employ common tones akin to music composition, as when selected tones of chords in play are carried forward into new chords, and the future is suggested. The textual morphic overlaps of the performances shift and renew somatically. I am curious how somatic ties (as common feeling tones) might challenge my habits of thought, and what role tonal bonds play in metamorphosis, the intimate activity of "becoming other" that dancers practice in *butoh*, a form of dance that originated in post–WWII Japan. I have written about butoh in other contexts (1999, 2004, 2006, 2010, 2016), and once again find it relevant here. I want to say more, however, about how metamorphosis operates in experience. Describing conditions for becoming other through micro-adjustments on planes of consistency (PoC) is a major motif in the process philosophy of Deleuze and Guattari (1986, 1987). Similarly, common tones (of soma, sense, and feeling) move osmotically across boundaries in the following process performances.

Process Performances

LISTENING AND DISTANCE

Why listening as a first performance? Because, I understand when I listen well and am aware of space in the distances between sonorities. I think better and feel better when I listen: whether to someone speaking, to music, or to rain and wind. I love music and have studied it, which doesn't make me a better listener. One doesn't study listening, but it definitely helps to give attention, and one can practice attention. In deepening concentration, leveling tones of meditation help with this. Buddhist ethics lie in the present-centered attention of meditation, and also in aesthetic activities or work at hand. Listening is an art.

> I slow toward kindness when I listen,
> Or speed toward joy if a rhythm bolds me.
> I stamp if the pulse suggests it, as do Indian ragas
> Out of *spiritus mundi*—
> Or my gravity lowers to let African
> Drumming shake in my belly.
> While moving in slow figures,
> Lyrical music lifts my arms.

Jean-Luc Nancy has written a phenomenology of listening that speaks to the importance of distance in music, particularly its distance from words in not forcing meanings. Being aural and intangible, music resists solid form. Listening to music is an intimate evocative experience (Nancy 2009). Music, never quite finished in sound and time, creates forms of sound from formlessness. Music makes time for being in the moment of attending without expectations. I gather from Nancy that the distance music has from meaning is important in the spacious politics of waiting. In conjuring distance and surrendering an immediate need to know, I breathe better. Unlike visual landscapes, soundscapes remain abstract, invisible, malleable, and mysterious. In seeing, I see forms—while hearing music, I am carried through time. After the music is gone, I often still hear it. Music makes me want to move, sway, zigzag, and dance. It surrounds and powers me, but not in words. I want to hear the music in color and rhythm, to feel its twang and glow. Like evasions of dance, its ephemeral sounds will disappear in time and fade into space. And this is enough. Dance and music suffer when we try too hard to squeeze language from them or ask them to conform to analysis.

> Without troubling reason,
> We can say that
> Every non-discursive perception
> Not tamed by language
> Is held questionable by language.

SPEAKING AND BREATHING

From the previous performance, we carry *Listening and Distance* forward as common tones. Distance evokes neutrality in speech and breath. Not needing to take a breath, we can; not needing to speak, the words come fluently. Need and distance disturb each other. Neutrality is central in somatic bodywork; not needing to fix others, we can listen. Listening engenders a neutral touch and easy breath. The waiting in breath and distance appears in listening. Stillness lies in waiting. Not knowing lies in waiting. Deeper knowing is possible through the non-doing of neutral waiting.

> The voice comes mixed with distant colors
> and singing sounds,
> circling my ears.
> Freedom prepares a stony noise,
> then rides a harsh breath out.

SEEING AND UNDERSTANDING

> *Waiting* is now the common air.
> In dancing alone, I practice waiting,
> the inverse of starting or catching up.
> In waiting as in not expecting, being unwritten,
> in hope as in hope for the future,
> I see and am seen,
> and in being seen,
> am understood,
> am silently glad.

TOUCH AND MATTER

When we harm the earth, we harm our human natures. Increasingly, humans are evolving a living choreography of material touch entwined with earth. Shall we dance with earth, then, and in concert with each other? Throughout her book *Vibrant Matter: A Political Ecology of Things*, Jane Bennett advances the view that matter is alive with meaning and is not inert. She asks why one would advocate the vitality of matter? Her "hunch" is "that the image of dead or thoroughly instrumentalized matter feeds human hubris and our earth-destroying fantasies of conquest and consumption" (ix).

I extend her hunch through the material choreography of touch, using touch in somatic bodywork as an example, meanwhile drawing four common tones from previous performances: *distance, waiting, listening,* and *seeing*. In somatic bodywork, touch is deliberate and not taken for granted. It is careful, neutral, and listening. In respect of ethical boundaries, gentle touch provides somatic distance from nearness and personal involvement. In this sense, it is objective as it seeks vital material connectivity. We trust the vibrant matter of the human body under the influence of touch and aliveness of matter, and we touch with care.

Through neutral touch (akin to tabula rasa clearings of phenomenology), somatic practitioners encourage movement gently, listening for paths of least resistance inherent in the body-responsiveness of the recipient to guide the process toward ease. Persistent blocks and biases, slackness, or weakness might be evident, but the somatic practitioner trusts the bodily intelligence of the other that seeks the best for itself. She attunes to this. Somatic touch is not attuned to flesh as inert matter; flesh participates in vital life itself. When I touch, I listen to organizations of bodily structure through the resonance in bones and find structural uniqueness through the weight of bone. Finally, I experience how the marvel of movement through the grace of joints and expressions of the flesh move the body. For me, being in touch with another person through movement is a dance of inter-experience. The flow of being unified in a movement that I perform with the other is enlivening, even elegant at times. We are not depleted as we move together. Over time, we see what changes in our body-sense and common understanding, and we often share this in words.

Somatic perspectives in dance and performance are about being in sync and listening and thus less about performing for an audience. Touch is part of this embodied listening, also relating us to the world in its tactile kinesthetics. In fathoming the radiant life of the world, we touch it lightly, not through need or forcing a meaning. We find a listening distance to let the world be what it is in its nature. Likewise, can more of our own nature appear to us? Not in needing to know, but in the awareness and patience of waiting, can we see and be seen as we would like to be? Can we touch with care and attention?

Some time ago I made a request at large. On February 18, 2011, I sent an email to a group of friends and associates of my Eastwest Somatics Institute:

Dear Students and Friends of Eastwest Somatics,

I invite your thoughts on something—the inspirations that seem to arrive unbidden and take on a creative life of their own. When we prepare to hear these in the "yes" of our bodies, I think we can learn to live consciously in our chosen work and relationships. As we practice being present daily, and listen with love to others in their individuality and special beauty, the way we move and touch the world stimulates creativeness. At least this is my reflection on deep listening through movement and touch as we develop these at Eastwest Somatics. I invite you to share your thoughts on this. Take a few moments. I will bring them to our Santa Barbara retreat on moving consciously and creating the life you want.

Sincerely, Sondra Fraleigh

Dancer and phenomenologist Susan Kozel answered me On March 1, 2011:

Dear Sondra,

Thank you for letting me drop inward, to my old friend, my body in the midst of my day. I notice the voice my body chooses to get my attention, when not resorting to pain, is often simply vibration. A tingling of skin, a rippling

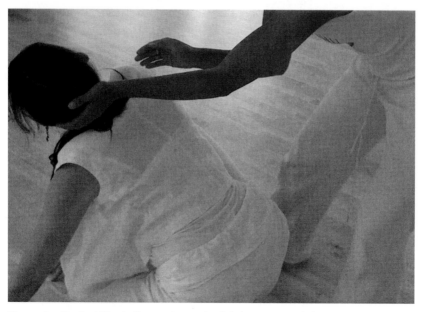

Figure 6.1. *Contact Unwinding*, an improvised dance-game and therapeutic practice at Eastwest Somatics Institute that speaks and listens through movement and touch. Partners practice roles of moving freely (moving as speaking) and supporting through touch (supporting as listening). They change roles by saying "switch," or indicating this with a single clap. Photograph © 2012 by Sondra Fraleigh.

up and down limbs or sometimes more localized. This can be a response to another's words (usually a personal story that contains some shared resonance or deeper truth) or to a situation. We can choose to listen to a toddler or not, we can choose to listen to the quiet vibrations in our bodies or not, but they always offer their own wisdom.

With all warm wishes, Susan

Her response is an example of *living phenomenology*, accounting for process through the unfinished body and the intrinsic wisdom in listening. Listening is a sensory part of music, dance, and touch. Kozel's message also reminds me that life is a performance in tactile styles of listening (2007). It has affective contours and timings that we can pay attention to or not. Performance is often considered to be something done on stage for an audience, but the stage can be anywhere. As Shakespeare famously said: "All the world's a stage, And all the men and women merely players" (*As You Like It*, Act 2, Scene 7).

LOVE AND AMBITION

Love is not a constant feeling for me, but I trust it to appear often. It has a warm approach, gentle as moonlight, and a sure way of linking my hands with others in the dance. It banishes depressive heaviness in my chest. Like many, I thrive on the daily work and play of dance, a matter of doing and application, and a risky matter of love. The matters of dancing are circumstantial and contextual; they can inspire, or they might turn bleak and ambitious. Here, I introduce *matter* as a common tone, which could break like a wave in several directions.

We don't usually think of dance or any of the arts for that matter as fraught with ambition. Are they not about expression, communication, and empathy? Dance, like most activities, is what we make of it and how we make it matter in the countless doings of our lives. Having lived a long life has given me pause to consider the consequences of my varied affections and choices. I want to dance in the light of love, not ambition, but I still have ambitions.

This much I know, love is more important than ambition, is generous in its acts, and says, "yes," whenever it can. Love also forgives; its invisible threads extend beyond the present. The love in forgiveness may be the saving dance of grace on the other side of death. I believe that love is a performance. We show up for it, and give up to it, or else it doesn't matter. Love carries us into grief and gets us out of it. We love those we care for, and the extent of our love is our measure. Love moves flesh and animates matter.

WORLDING AND SUFFERING

Worlding is a favored word in phenomenology, a floating signifier popularized by Heidegger, usually indicating something ongoing and generative. Turning toward the "environing world," Husserl's use of worlding preceded Heidegger's. Worlding may sound odd, but it works. "To world" is to actively belong to the world as a whole—referencing origins, perhaps ethnicities and governance, and most surely expanding consciousness beyond confining racial boundaries.

To weigh worlding with belonging, I ask how the experiential tone of *ambition* from the previous performance might overlap and texture tones of *belonging*? To wait without ambition is one way of worlding, as when I walk outside my door in early morning to greet the horizon. In loosening a dance, I'm alive to the world's sunrise, and in my gaze and breath, I belong to the golden distance. Worlding as belonging is an experience of love without boundaries. This spread beyond ambition in world familiarity is comforting.

Husserl and Heidegger both spoke of worlding as a wide and present phenomenon—of consciousness spreading toward nature and spirit while encompassing culture and sociality. We invoke the world to expand the affective flow of life beyond rooms and reach. As inclusive, the world is welcoming and also full of suffering. In seeming, it may not seem welcoming for minorities pushed aside or people who feel they don't belong. Novels and human narratives tell us that the world has been experienced as unfriendly, unstable, unfair, and in upheaval as far back as recorded history. And today's world has unique threats and joys. We travel fast, and live longer. We are globally and interculturally connected through technology. Terrorists can strike anywhere, and they are both locally and globally connected. Warfare can be conducted through the internet. Performances can be rendered digitally for aesthetic purposes or politically without scruple through contagions of technology. Performative ghost images arise in media. The possibilities are multiplying as I write.

We are concerned as never before that humanity is accountable to the more-than-human world, and that we share a common fate with all life. Minds are required to be more nimble. Technology is vastly expanding the reach of human existence in a vivid lifeworld of nature. Husserl's term *lifeworld*, connecting world to life, and nature to world, is still relevant—and maybe even more so today in a world driven by ambition where human desires of many kinds run amuck. We have a lot to learn about nonattachment from Buddhism, and from phenomenology, to learn about letting go of ego-driven goals.

World is womb and container; all that exists is held by the natural world and animated by it. In his *Sixth Cartesian Meditation* written with Eugen Fink, Husserl taught that "human subjects are only in the world by the fact that, as bearers of world-consciousness, they produce the sense, world, for themselves at every moment" (1995, 166). This doesn't mean that nature is not tangible, just that humans come to know the world in relation to their own perceptions and direction of intention. We leave body prints in sand, and we can lie down in the grass to feel its soft and bristly textures. Where I live in Utah, our spectacular canyons have vast, twisting zigzags and grainy slopes that carry and fascinate those who pay attention. Their sandstone ridges spring to life for barefoot dancers navigating soft folds and sharp crests of smooth rock, a reminder of how adaptive the foot is, and how the whole body moves in response to changes in the foot and a sense of place (see Plate 5).

"I am a child of the universe, I belong here." When I practice this yoga mantra, the world becomes my friend wherever I am, and I can empathize with those who struggle to belong. In being world-friendly as an activist, I can advocate for the belonging of everyone. The natural world in its profundity makes room for variety and reminds me to be inclusive. As a teacher, I have many opportunities to practice this.

Writing of "place worlds," contemporary phenomenologist Edward Casey speaks of world and nature in the plural (1993, 194). Similarly, the place worlds of our experience are also many, as we see throughout this book. Wilderness places are environments that produce atmospheres, specific in mood and affect. When I dance with others in Utah's canyons, we meld with the audible tempos and vivid colors. The ebb and flow of the weather moves through us as boundaries disappear. Site-specific dances in nature allow us the freedom of *disappearing in place*. We can practice self-forgetting in such disappearances. In appearing and disappearing, we dance as we world beyond prejudice and difference.

I have come to appreciate butoh as an art that pays attention to environment as place—in its radical shift toward performing nature—linking the human body to all that is not human. Moreover, butoh takes the suffering of nature as thematic, as I explain in "Butoh Translations and the Suffering of Nature" (2016). The suffering of the world and nature are common tones between butoh and Buddhism. Butoh is not Buddhist, but it shares a common ethos and aesthetic in touch with suffering and evanescence. A hybrid dance of Eastern and Western elements, butoh worlds with enigma and morphology. Its many place dances and theatrical performances embody varieties of material nature, morphing into the more-than-human world. As in Buddhism, butoh dancers do not push away awkwardness, pathos, or paradox. Weeds are fine in butoh. They allow a play of nature within (see Plate 6).

SHOW ME BUTOH

Perform as you like.
Show humors distant,
Fair your eerie gaze.

Tread on riverbanks—
Nowhere out there.
Be visible limitless miles.
Show heaps I cannot see—
Detachments of snow,
Empty footprints behind.

Show faces glancing back—
Old as the East
And first in every dawn
Before my face was born.

FREEDOM AND GRAVITY

Husserl teaches that the way we direct our intentions toward the natural world produces, or "enworlds" it, in consciousness. "Enworlding" is his correlative term for individual and community striving "in a cultural world constantly in motion, in motion as to the way it already is and in motion with the horizon of future forms." In relation to nature, cultural striving continues its motion toward "the creation of a new environing world" (1995, 190–192). Can we promote, then, in sight of current ecological crises, human strivings that improve the world and do not exploit it? For phenomenology, nature has ontic being, which on first glance is as fragile as our own. Nature changes in our subjective perceptions, but this doesn't alter nature itself. "Subjectivity . . . alters nothing of the unity of nature as core in its own ontological form" (1995, 189). Husserl's philosophy points phenomenology away from ephemeral ego and toward the existence of nature and spirit, even as this includes creative striving.

Gravity pertains to all things earthly, and thus to *suffering* and *worlding*, the somatic tones we carry forward from the previous performance. Gravity inflects these tones with striving and moral grounding. As a natural force, gravity is weighty and relates to the seriousness of suffering; it keeps things bound to the earth. Dance, we are sometimes taught, should defy gravity. The ballet as aspiring upward is an aerial aristocratic form that seeks to escape the bounds of gravity, at least in its illusions. In any case, all dance grounds in a gravitational field that holds bodies on earth. Diaphanous visions of ethereal dance may seem effortless, but this is only in the seeming, like classical ballets maintaining their ageless fluidity in the face of extreme challenges.

Grace is not the opposite of gravity; rather, grace is a quality of action in easy rapport with movement and effort. Grace doesn't waste effort and is not about ornamentation or grandiosity. Being graceful, the dancer has learned how to bring the right amount of effort to performance. I enjoy teaching novices who are exploring dance for the first time, especially as they learn how to do a new movement, repeating variations until it becomes second nature. We commonly use the term *second nature* to describe something that has become easy, natural, and doable. This assumes that nature is easy in its worlding actions, even in storms. Strife is part of its dance. Second nature has its blind spots, however, especially through keeping dominant behaviors and powers in place—thus, the tenets of phenomenology that require us to question what is (or seems) natural.

In my dance, I can use gravity as a friend, not fighting it, but allowing its flow through me and experiencing the ground as support and springboard for flight. Freedom is a quality of affect that grows from gravity, especially in spirit. If I dance in the spirit of gravity, not denying my weight but moving with it, I can be generous in my movement, finding freedom in balance, center, and ground; in finding ground, I can admit suffering as part of life. This has moral implications for how I treat others. In both practical and moral matters, people can find generosity if they are centered in being present, balanced in feeling plentiful, and have the ground beneath them as support. I can support others only in my ability to support myself. I can wish them well if I am well, even when I don't feel well. It doesn't stretch the bounds of plausibility to see spirituality in wellness and generosity, and also in relativities of suffering and disease as we live them.

Japanese phenomenology does not separate body and spirit from the vastness of nature; it moves past the material body we are so attached to in the West, voicing the immaterial energy body, ki or chi, permeating and connecting all beings, and operating in humans through bodily self-cultivation techniques such as meditation and martial arts. Shigenori Nagatomo's work, *Attunement through the Body* (1992), introduces this perspective. Likewise through attuning, Japanese butoh, also called "ancient dance," engenders a morphic philosophy of becoming. As a contemporary genre, butoh is nevertheless ancient in moving consciousness back toward the liminal primitive brain and in shedding cultural norms. It is not about being weird, even if some performances seem so. It often plies edges of liminal awareness, letting beings be, and not soliciting appreciation or commanding control.

Grounding originally in Tatsumi Hijikata's identification with mud, butoh yields to the earth. I like performing the basic butoh walk, *hokotai*, because it is slow, neutral and intimate with gravity. I can relax into it, even when I'm conjuring animal awareness. Improvisational dances of butoh occur through movement most people can perform, if not through the lens of highly produced theater that motivates many professional butoh performances. Shaking, shivering, falling, floating, gliding, waiting, trembling, and changing: these are just some of the morphic movement states explored. Because butoh's exploratory, therapeutic modes move with gravity and accept pain rather than hiding it, dancers can allow pain to be and to change in the movement at hand. From the first time I encountered this dance form, I experienced myself as part of something bigger than self or locale, dancing into darkness and the energetic lines of ki, light, and spirit. For this, I have Japan to thank, especially my friends and teachers there.

Show me butoh—
Dark and weightless.
Hand me butoh's light.

DREAM AND STRANGENESS

In the dead of night and hollowness of my chest, I met my father in a dream. His look was wild, and his eyes wide with gravity. He couldn't wholly unbend his knees, as he hopped about strangely and looked up under the faces of a group of people inhabiting a large vacant room. I don't know where it was. But I remember he was wearing his everyday muddy workclothes that he wore to the meadows early in the mornings. Who were these people, and why were they there? I had no idea. They seemed phantoms. He went from one bland face to another trying to see something, and I was trying to figure out what it meant.

The dream started to unfold questions I had about my father (or about myself through him). Did he want approval? He looked up in a beseeching way that made no sense. Why did he persist in looking up from under faces while turning his head in a neck-wrenching torque? Might he be trying to get attention in this peculiar way? Or was he trying to connect through facings, to find the hobbling, churning stuff of really facing something above? (Am I trying to face something, no matter how unyielding or unpleasant?)

I thought about the phenomenology of Emmanuel Levinas—about the face and facing others—and its ethical basis (1974). More than his teachers, Husserl or Heidegger, Levinas underlines our subjective responsiveness to others. Subjectivity, Levinas holds, is an ethical matter, not theoretical. Responsibility orients consciousness away from self and in a meaningful direction (ibid., ch. 4). Levinas maintains that *empathy* develops consciousness in human responsiveness and constancy to others. And he makes me wonder, could it be that the strangeness in dreams keeps us honest, on our toes, and looking askance in unexpected facings? Dreams are the stuff of alternative selves and wild otherness, time travel, and flight.

I awoke to books, light, and coffee, to my own sleep-ridden face passing in the mirror. Dreams are like that. They fade quickly, but sometimes they leave traces of odd terrain. The dream about my father is not one I need to solve. It left enough queasiness in me and a common tone of gravity's pull. It morphs as I write, however. Right now, I remember it as a contingent tableau and opportunity to be surprised. I'm grateful that I can look, see, remember, and be surprised. I am still here. My father is gone, standing up, and fading fast. Now in my lucid daydream, he is sitting on a log by a river, facing it while releasing the agony of his brother's death in World War II.

I have friends who say they don't remember their dreams. To me, the importance of dreaming is in the moment of having, not in remembering. Nothing lasts long enough to remember truly, and experiences can't be reconstituted as they were, but dreaming does its odd healing work, nevertheless.

Strangeness is important in life and in art. Strangeness exists in the courageous choice to move on a hunch. Artists and performers don't like to repeat themselves. Rather, they seek to find the hidden potentials in their materials and performances. In dance, this material can arrive in various guises: as body, idea, or living magma. The substance of dance and performance lives in the glues and suspensions of our material bodies, flowing with the same life and habitus that animate all gravitations.

SIDLING AND METAMORPHOSIS

In this section, I invite the reader to join me in a somatic exploration. Drawing on common tones of *strangeness* while courting difficulties of *gravity* and *weightlessness*, a problem-solving study in lateral movement might suffice. In the following one, I invite you to lie down on the floor, on sand, on soft sandstone, or on grass, and without the use of your arms or legs, move your body slowly and smoothly from one side to the other as a whole. At first it may seem impossible, and then, bit by bit, a way may open up, partly because you understand more about what you are doing, and how you might find more flair laterally. Maybe you concentrate a little on the shoulders and find more translation to the side there? The neck and head might become an issue. Do you slide the head on the ground, lift it up, or let it roll? Try sliding it softly, slowly and gently, while leaving the neck relatively relaxed.

Can you translate the pelvis to one side in slow gentle motion? Think of guiding the movement through the hips. To scoot (or glide) one hip sideways, the waist might side-bend slightly, tilting the opposite hip toward the head a bit, but not by lifting it off the floor. This is all about sidling or translating sideways, keeping as much contact with the floor as you can. Side-bending at the waist (side-folding) causes the ribs to fold. This makes one leg seem longer than the other, not anatomically, but functionally. Rest a minute on the long side. Don't worry if you don't get this right away. You will find a way that works for you. Be satisfied with the exploration. That is enough. Find ease.

This movement study can bring an illusion of lateral motion through the pelvis, but it is actually modulated with up and down through slight side bending at the waist. (Something has to give.) Finally, with the shoulders and pelvis involved and the head traveling slowly along the floor or ground, you might land in a C curve. What joy! You will probably favor your habitual C. I move left to land with my head on the right and right ribs folded, which is a left C curve. (No one has a perfectly straight spine.) Then I rest, reset, and try again on the other side to land in a right C curve. This helps to balance the sides of the body through the spine. In this way, the body moves laterally through space, but a bit snakelike in itself. (You might be finding out something else about how you move. Great!)

For me, this is a phenomenological exploration because it teaches me about my bodily held bias toward the left C curve of my spine, and I find out other things about myself along the way, how I always try too hard in the beginning, for instance, and need to work mindfully at letting things go. We all have spinal biases, also tempo and stress biases, just as we have biases in seeing, smelling, and hearing. Some of these go back to the womb, and some are acquired tastes. They play out in our relationships. How could they not, unless we become aware of them and learn how to temper the curves, the tempos, and the stresses?

Discovering about ingrained bias and how to work with it is a big part of the work of the Feldenkrais Method of somatic education, which intersects with my work in Shin Somatics regarding the unfinished nature of embodiment and mindfulness. Every time I take myself through some matter of lateral motion, I learn something new about my bodily held biases and mind in movement, and I'm not finished with the learning. I learn most of all that my movement is malleable as is my body. It doesn't matter how old I get, I'm different every day. Learning about my habits helps me observe embodied dispositions in others, opening an attentive way to practice hands-on somatic therapy.

Today was super-special because my puppy jumped up on the couch where I was resting and crawled into my arms. Not needing any lateral motion, I just rested with her while we synchronized our breath.

> These are the times I don't aspire to grow, or to change, or to be
>   empowered,
> or to learn anything new.
> These are dancing sparks of time that allow me to rest into the
> beauty of now, now, and now. These are the times I feel complete,
>   even weightless.
> In time, I will find an upright relationship to gravity,
> sense a desired direction, and go there, tweaking
> steps inevitably along the way.
> Something will call my attention,
> even if I don't aim to rise and move.
> The intentions have already been deeply embodied and practiced—the
>   relationship to gravity and sense of direction.
> If some discarded shoe or costume appears in my way, or someone calls
>   to me, I can adjust.

INTENTIONALITY, OTHERNESS, AND GLOBAL BECOMING

Each new day offers naked potential for renewal, and every lateral glance its strangeness. Failure as lack or breakdown can be dissolved in living life on purpose. The past follows along, or we drag it, but when we realize that we can live consciously, we have choices in how we intend our lives. We gain more possibilities for purposeful use of the past, calling it up in memory, or letting it disappear in dance. *Intention is the direction of attention* and key to living life on purpose. In creative activities and performances, we get to practice uses of attention.

I know I'm directing my attention in specific ways when I dance and when I move laterally. In dancing, I let go, especially when I improvise and let my intentions roam. In moving laterally, I can also let go, but only after considerable experimentation and patience. Or else, I can morph into a scaly lizard, not through imitation, but through finding common tones sidling between lizards, the small dinosaurs, and me.

> Lazy ... and listening,
> squamata scaling,
> watching, waiting
> and withholding.
> Dreaming ...
> reforming and leaving.
> Light ... and belonging.
> Hushing ...
> drying.
> Flipping, surprising, quadrating.
> Mating, worlding and suffering.
> Dying ... slackening, conforming,
> ruling and drifting.
> Waiting ...
> Fading ... distancing.
> Envisioning ... levitating,
> slipping, resting ... and remaining still.
> Tailing.

Hijikata founded bodily processes of becoming other in butoh (Fraleigh and Nakamura 2006, 11–13), which is a matter of directing intentionality. Tones of butoh *metamorphosis* thrive on intentional states of becoming other where all arrivals fade, unlike many Western forms of dance that hold final balances and posed silhouettes, perhaps for camera endings. Butoh echoes with common tones across dissimilarities (human, animal, mineral, insect, earth, plant, object, material, weather, water, ice, ash, season), and with uncertainties appreciated in Buddhism. The morphings of butoh link it performatively to reactions in organic chemistry through emphases on substance and substitution, elimination and escape. Likewise, the popular inheritors of phenomenology, Gilles Deleuze and Felix Guattari, argue for their concept of becoming—that metamorphic becoming is not a metaphor:

> Metamorphosis is the contrary of metaphor. There is no longer any proper sense or figurative sense, but only a distribution of states that is part of the range of the word. The thing and other things are no longer anything but intensities overrun by deterritorialized sound or words that are following their line of escape. (1986, 22)

But where they speak of "the range of the word," I seek lines of escape in unsettling performance.

I am cautious, however. Distribution of states, words, and movements can be challenging in terms of cultural attribution. Butoh is a global phenomenon, but it originates in Japan, which should not be lost or forgotten. Its extensive practices broach the question of ethics in performance. Is everything game for global development? There must be some rules or we should create them. I am aware of being on foreign land in Japan, but also mindful of my reasons for being there and the radical accord and solubility embodied in all that I share with Japan. On falling in love with butoh through the performance of Nakajima Natsu in *Niwa* (The Garden, 1985), I studied Japanese and went to Japan to learn. Gratefully, I was welcomed, and in generous ways I will never forget, since America and Europe have had complicated histories with Japan. I write of these in three cultural contexts: migrations of American and German modern dance to Japan, American colonialism in Japan since 1857, and World War II and globalism of butoh (2004, 2006, 2010). Through experiential studies of butoh and Zen, and by way of my travels in Japan, I have repeatedly sounded out common tones, first through *Dancing into Darkness: Butoh, Zen and Japan* (1999).

I write in the belief that ethical praxis lies in the art of paying attention with aims toward listening and reciprocity. Differences make the world fascinating and also violent; they require respectful engagement. Phenomenology offers a pragmatic, experiential path toward cultural inquiry. In the case of Japan, one honors the teacher; thus, I continue to learn from my butoh mentors in Japan, even though butoh is more an imagistic process art than a traditional form. Its morphology moves globally and transcends culture while recalling it. Butoh teaches me about my human continuities with seeming otherness. To morph is to become—to change, magically, and yet to cohere.

STORY AND WEIGHTLESSNESS

We begin this story with a common tone of *morphology*, and once more with Husserl, who produced a rich variety of influential manuscripts on topics of human life and history, intersubjectivity, and "the flowing live present." This phrase is a fundamental of Husserl's phenomenology (Bruzina 1995, xiv), describing his temporal concept of present, primordial time-consciousness, an idea almost impossible to grasp, yet actualized concretely through dance and the lived body: in every changing motion of "the now." Dance is a time-conscious transformational art, ripe for ontological concerns of philosophy from Husserl through Sartre to Deleuze and Guattari.

The latter create scenarios where individuals overcome repressive forms of identity and stasis in a constant process of becoming and transformation, not so distant from striving toward renewal in "the flowing live present" of Husserl (1995, 192), or recalling Sartre's philosophy of freedom and becoming in *Being and Nothingness* (1965).

Unexpected common tones of *intentional mindfulness and metamorphosis* enter my personal story through these philosophies, blending with *touch*, another common tone lingering from a previous performance. Before I studied matters of touch in the Feldenkrais work, I had no idea I would someday become a dedicated somatic teacher and evolve my own style of hands-on bodywork related to dance and developmental yoga. Now when I use contact and touch in somatic therapy with others, I mind my body, breathe easily, and feel my feet on the ground. At first I use gentle micro-movements that invite and listen for developmental paths in the body of the other to become available. When they arrive, I can expand upon them. I let go of doing and enter the space between the other and myself as thought and sense impression blend in the flowing life of the present. I don't consider that I have any special healing powers, but as a performer and yogini, I have developed keen attention.

People can learn how to be with others in a beneficial way. Healing begins with feelings of trust and ease rather than dis-ease. Those who have a desire to assist others in healing can learn how. It isn't a special talent, but maybe it is a special calling—in the desire to assist and the patience to learn. One of the fascinating parts of this calling is the personal growth one undergoes. The body itself changes, accruing consciousness through movement and image. Inviting metaphysics of gesture and generosity, mindfulness expands, and the heart finds freedom and purpose in the weight of bone.

Somatic bodywork—intrinsic and responsive—converses without words. It invites trust, and in this interval, connective partnering flows between the practitioner (as a guide) and the active-recipient. Eventually, words come, particularly in contexts of listening and not advising. As participants find their own solutions, the exercise of choice and thus freedom in movement can become a source of knowledge and healing; while listening together from deep states of awareness, partners can excavate pain and body memories. Admitting pain in somatic processes, acknowledging it, allows hurt a way out.

Somatic transformations call for trust in positive ontologies of embodiment relative to agency, action, and freedom. Philosophies of change and morphology teach us that we can change at any time of life. Now we have a chance to write the story of our human oneness with other life in proximity, likeness, and kindness. Kindness derives from kind: In kindness, we strike common tones with others. In choosing to be kind, we live in light of our *freedom*, a common tone this essay shares with Jean-Paul Sartre.

Friends sometimes ask me why I write so much about "dead white guys." Actually, I send them love letters for providing me a springboard to write about experience and freedom in movement. My goal has been to describe *freedom as experienced* in dance and somatic modalities, while finding my own voice in the current century. I composed a work of electronic music, *Tidal Space, Elemental Time*, as a love letter to Sartre—for his writing of *Being and Nothingness*—sending phenomenology toward experiential matters of freedom. *Tidal Space, Elemental Time* progresses improvisationally from nothing toward being in profuse common tones, linking synthesizer sounds with piano and orchestral instruments. Michelle Ikle and Amy Bush perform a version of this music in site-specific dance near waterfalls and on railroad tracks near Geneva, New York (Fraleigh, Youtube Music Video, June 11, 2017).

I gain from Sartre that the body subject is lived and not known (1965, 300), and freedom as lived is a subjective experience that roots in responsibility. For me, subjectivity is danced, and I can be authentically free in my dance only when I am responsible for my own freedom and I value the freedom of others as I value my own. This perspective can be chanted in a Buddhist mantra: "May all beings be happy, may all beings be free."

But I promised a story: I think I'll choose one slightly askew with lateral nostalgia and hints of global becoming. Recently, I visited my hometown of Circleville, Utah, nestled in a verdant valley that time forgot. At the Butch Cassidy Café, I chanced across my friend of sixty years ago and asked her how she was.

"I'm crazy, Sondra," she said.
I laughed.
"No I'm really crazy," she underlined. "I mean it."

I knew she had suffered two strokes, so I hesitated.
Then I asked her about another high school friend of ours.
"Oh, she's dying," was the swift reply.

I was alarmed, and said I wanted to visit her.
"Oh no, she won't see anyone," my friend said—"Never leaves the house, and her husband waits on her hand and foot."

So I inquired what was the matter.
"She's dying of self-pity," came her answer.

This conversation took place as she was passing beside my table on her way out. People in Circleville figure things out quickly and seldom mince words. As the door was closing, my friend shot back:

"I googled you, and know you teach around the world.
Do you still read a lot, and do you dance?"
"Yes," I said I did, as I took care not to be "uppity."
(That would never fly in Circleville.)

Then she asked me if I remembered what I wrote in her high school year-book.
"No," I said, preparing for something really stupid.
She said I had written, "I don't come to your house just to eat. I really like you."

As our eyes met in hilarity and sadness, I could see she was thin and tired of everything. Then she smiled from across the years, and I felt her warmth and pain.

I wanted to live my life in that sweet town, to have children and grow old with my family and friends. But life had other plans for me. My friendships are worlding more all the time. I say I don't give advice, but here is a little. Don't try to control life; that's when it really starts, and you get more than you asked for. I'm happy with whatever comes to me now, and I love to visit Circleville. Like Japanese butoh and Butch Cassidy's weathered cabin in the meadow, its pace is slow and peaceful amid the suffering. At night, you can see the heavens glittering with stars and, in the day, silver oak, weightless with euphoria, dropping every heavy memory.

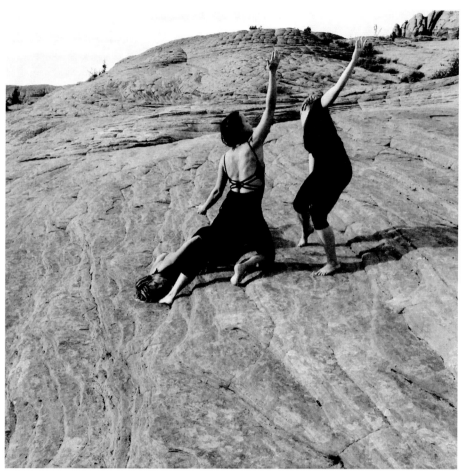

Plate 1. Ecological Bodies. Dancing at Snow Canyon in Utah: Denise Purvis, Megan Brunsvold, and Sara Gallo. Photograph © 2015 by Tom Gallo.

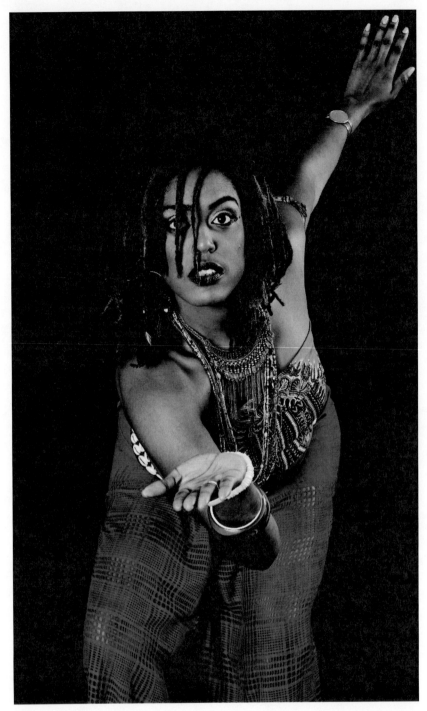

Plate 2. In *Dancing with the Wind*, Nathalie Guillaume dances across time and cultures, as she quotes Buddhism: "if you want to know your past life, look at your present condition. If you want to know your future life, look at your present actions." Padmasambhava. Photograph © 2017, at Little Haiti Culture Complex in Miami, by Woosler Delisfort.

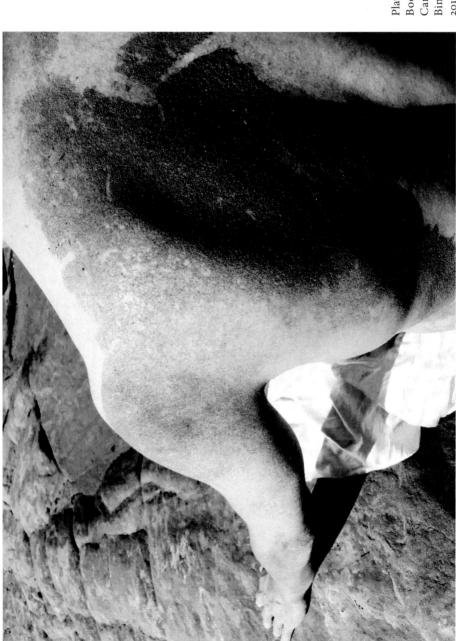

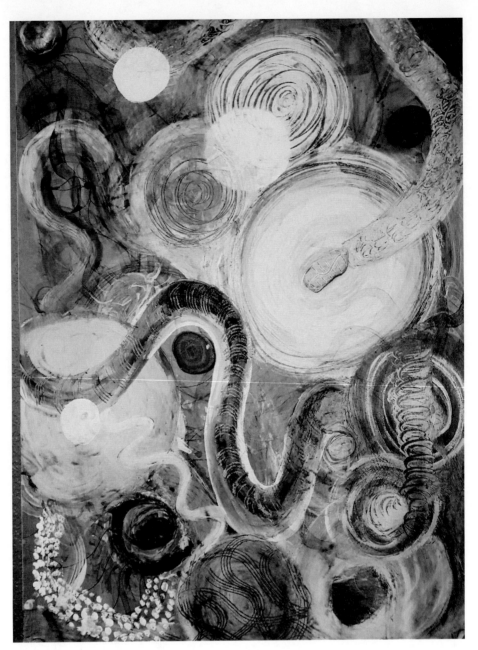

Plate 4. Painting by Amanda Williamson.

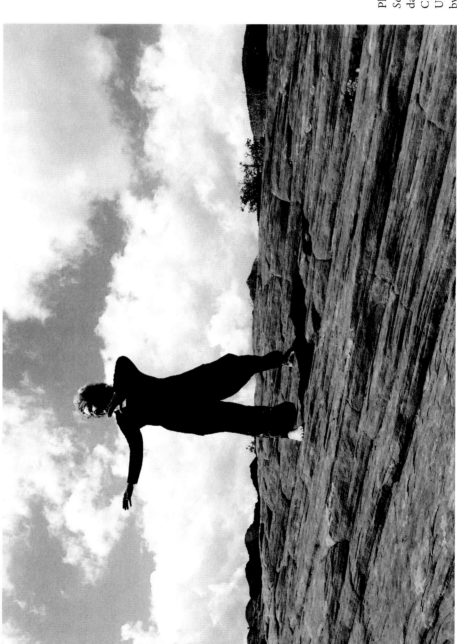

Plate 5. *Footing Seventy-Seven.* Sondra Fraleigh dancing barefoot in Snow Canyon in Southwest Utah. Photograph © 2016 by Alicia Bright Holland.

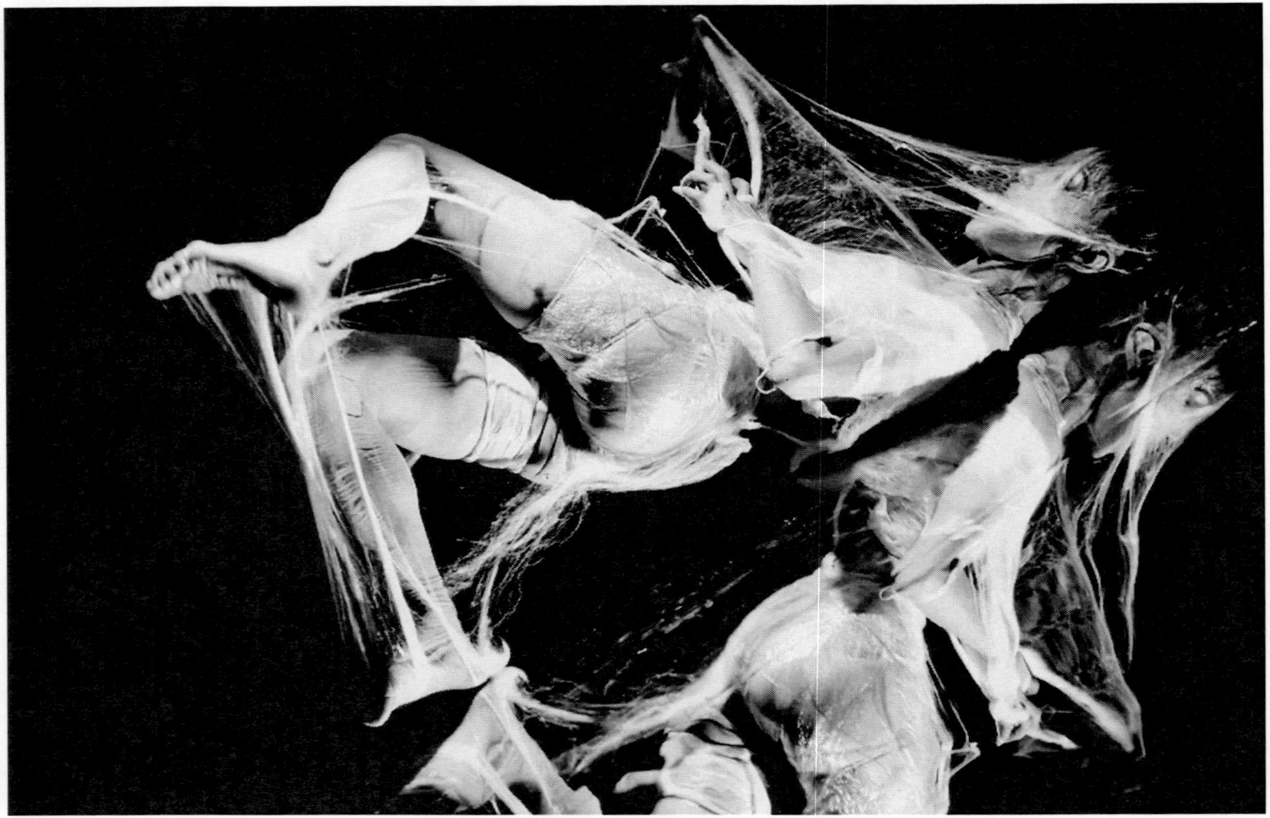

Plate 6. Butoh dancer Yumiko Yoshioka in *Birth of a Creature*.

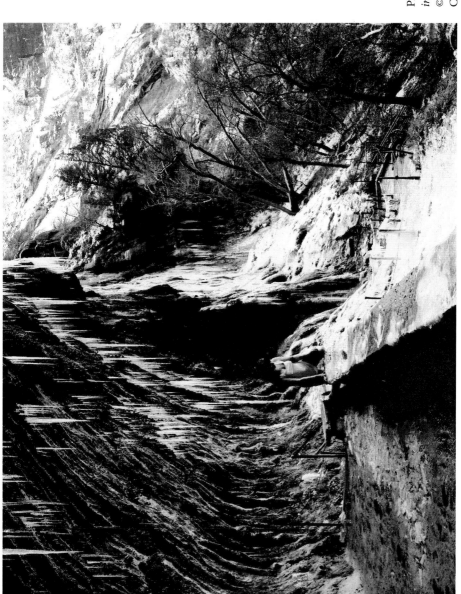

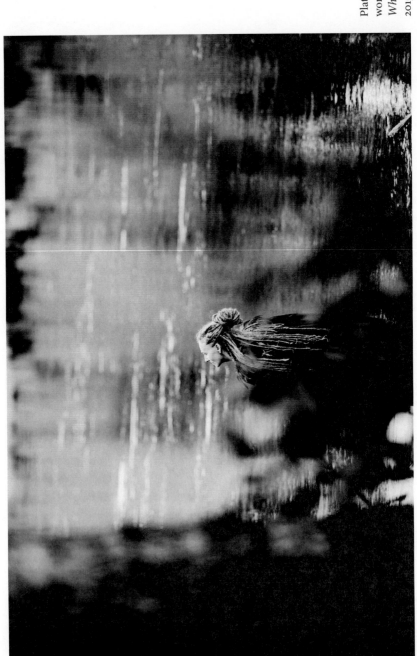

III

Body and Place

7

As the Earth Dances
A Philosophy of Bodily Becoming

KIMERER L. LAMOTHE

In 2005, when I moved with my family from a compact bungalow in a Boston suburb to a sprawling, retired dairy farm in rural New York, I carried with me a sense of what I knew and a stack of questions I wanted my new life to help me answer. Our move was a grand experiment. My partner and I were determined to discover whether we could create a sustainable life for ourselves and our children, while living as artists in close proximity to nature. Could we create a world in which the love that dared to dream it possible remained the most important thing?

In eleven and a half years since, life on the farm has radically altered what I thought I knew and what I intended to pursue. In the space between then and now, a philosophy of bodily becoming has taken shape in me, pulled into presence by the movements I have made and been moved to make by the challenges of rural living. This philosophy has emerged as a gift and a responsibility: a perspective on humanity in which dance appears as vital to the ability of humans, individually and collectively, to sustain the health and well-being of the earth matrix of which we are one moment. This philosophy might just as easily be named an ecokinetic phenomenology. The task of this chapter is to describe it.

I

WHAT I THOUGHT I KNEW

At the time of our move, I thought I knew what dance was. I had been dancing seriously for at least twenty years. While studying modern, ballet, Haitian, and Kathak techniques; making dances to perform in theaters, classrooms, and churches; or performing solo and with various companies, I had learned that dancing opened in me the kind of experiences described by others as "religious"—experiences with names like connection, flow, transcendence, and overpowering love. Dance was my core. My passion. My connection to the divine. I also knew that more than anything else, time spent in the natural world inspired me to dance. It catalyzed in me a sensory shift in which impulses to move come alive.

This experience shift happened the first time our real estate agent pointed us to the high point of the farm property—Moon Rock. As I crested the hill, I felt the familiar surge, the joyful quickening that bubbles into a deep need to lift and leap, reach and bend, twisting round in a happy, hopeless effort to take it all in and let it all out, both at once. It was why we moved: I knew I could dance here.

I knew as well that, as much as I had enjoyed teaching and writing at Harvard for seven years, I felt stuck. I had reached an impasse in my research in dance, philosophy, and religious studies. Dance, I had come to believe, is revolutionary. As American dancer Ruth St. Denis averred, dance contains the "seeds of a new order" (1950–1959). As Isadora Duncan affirmed, danc-

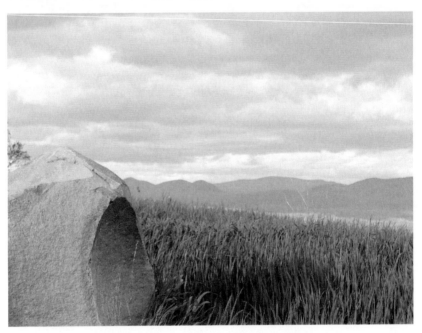

Figure 7.1. *Moon Rock*. Photograph © 2017 by Kimerer LaMothe.

ing gives rise to a "new conception of life" (1928, 101). Both of these dancers, moreover, found support in the writings of Friedrich Nietzsche, for whom "dance" represented an affirming alternative to the Christian values he perceived as both permeating Western culture and hostile to human life (1954; LaMothe 2006, ch. 1–3).

Nevertheless, in academic conversations that I observed, dance, while rising in status, was also being boxed in by theories and methods that treated "it" as one more acceptable object of cultural or historical study whose meaning and function could be parsed by various rational explanations.[1] Dance was useful, functional, symbolically relevant, even religious . . . and, to my mind, in danger of losing its radical edge in relation to Western theories and theologies that privilege mind over body.

In moving to the farm, I wanted to act as farmer to St. Denis's seeds and midwife to Duncan's "new conception." I wanted to do so by relearning what Nietzsche described as the "small things" (1989, 256)—choices made each day about how to act. I wanted to help grow a dance-driven philosophical and cultural revolution—one that would impact how contemporary humans *conceive* of knowledge, ethics, religion, the earth, and dance itself; and so encourage humans to *act* in ways that honor the ongoing life of their own bodily selves and the vast network of human and "more than human" others (Abram 1996).[2]

WHAT I WANTED TO KNOW

The questions I carried sprang from frustrations I had felt in trying to make space for dance in the field of religious studies.[3] Instead of looking at dancing as one kind of ritual, practice, religious experience, or symbolic expression, I wanted to draw upon the experience of dancing to redefine these concepts altogether—to let dancing define them, rather than the other way around.

I wondered what difference it would make to my dancing and to my thinking about dancing and religion if, on a daily basis, I sought out the experience shift that I desire, and value so highly, of being moved in and by nature.

Could dancing in natural settings serve as a generator of theoretical insights into religion? Could some kind of dancing serve as a practice capable of guiding the evolution of human cultures in earth-friendly directions? Could the practice of dance encourage humans to take greater responsibility for what their ways of life create? And if so, how could dancing do that kind of work? Where, when, and under what conditions?

My most ardent belief was that it could.

ON THE FARM: A PHILOSOPHY OF BODILY BECOMING

Within three years of moving, our family had grown. We were three Jersey cows; a quarterhorse named Marvin; a magnificent cat queen; a rotating crop of chickens, ducks, and kittens; and two parents and four, soon to be five, children. Lessons, which came hard and fast, quickly jolted me out of any romantic reveries I had harbored about pastoral living. I was neck-deep in the gritty, earthen reality.

Nature was not all heart-opening mountain meadows, inspiring ancient oaks, and well-organized garden plots. Nature was rats eating fruit from the kitchen table at night; cows smeared in their own manure; wave after wave of insects hatching; and warm eggs speckled with chicken dung. Nature was thorns and thistles, burrs and nettles that clung, stung, itched, and burned. Nature was blistering cold mornings when the animals still needed food and water. Nature was the fox tearing the back off a laying hen and a favorite cow dying of a bloated intestine. My farmer neighbors were not living in primal oneness with the beautiful landscape; they were snarled in a daily struggle to eke out an income in a political economy that does not adequately value food or farming—a struggle that drives them to rely heavily on diesel engines, genetically engineered seeds, and immigrant laborers.

MOVEMENT ALL THE WAY DOWN

What impressed me the most about rural life, however, was less the dirt or death than the incessant *movement*. Life in the country is anything but calm. The relentless, irrepressible force of existence is constantly swelling, cracking, and breaking out in new bodies, new beings, filling any spaces I clean or clear, in a torrent of existence that rushes on indifferent to human life. Blink and the scene changes. Turn your head and wonders appear.

The first tenet of my philosophy of bodily becoming took root in this experience. *It's movement all the way down.*[4] Plants flex, spread, curl and climb; animals scurry, hoard, and hide; the ground heaves and splits. Movement everywhere at every dimension of shape and size, intrudes, invades, and colonizes. *What always is is always becoming, ever humming, itself overcoming, with no particular preference for human lives; oh we may come and go in time, but movement never dies.*

I was unprepared for the onslaught. I had to respond. I learned to make new patterns of movement. I learned to tend newborn calves, orphaned kittens, and baby chicks; milk a cow, churn butter, make hard and soft cheeses; fell a tree, chop wood, and start fires; plant, weed, harvest, and process all manner of vegetables and fruit; remove burrs and bugs; build strong doors and fences, and muck mounds of manure. I gave birth to my fourth and fifth children at home. I made all of our bread.

At a visceral level, I learned that what humans need in order to survive is nowhere simply given. It must be wrestled and wrested, dug up and cut, hunted and hauled, gathered and prepared. It is hard work. Nevertheless, every time—yes every time—I drag myself outside to feed, water, and tend— even in the wee hours of the morning—I am rewarded by a patch of sky, a rising moon, a big-eyed calf, or a hurrying hen that blasts my heart wide open and inspires me to move in response. On the farm, nature appears to me as this call, this demand, to move in response to its movement—to be moved by its movement—in ways that enable my life.

As anthropologists and evolutionary biologists note, humans have evolved into the creatures who are able to survive in the widest range of ecosystems and cultural systems around the globe. According to dominant models of evolution, individual organisms adapt to their environments by taking advantage of random acts of genetic mutation (Dunbar 1998). This interpretation, however, depends upon a worldview in which matter is real and movement is what matter does (LaMothe 2015, ch. 2). With a shift to consider that matter is what movement does—that movement is constitutive of all things, all nature, all life—the appearance of random activity disappears. *What if movement guides our destiny, not shapes of materiality; what if movement forms are to blame for ratcheting up the organismal game—not random acts of failed reproduction but movement tacks that secure greater traction?*

Humans, too, are movement all the way down. Humans are nothing more or less than an *impulse to connect* (LaMothe 2011). They evolved as creatures who maximized a capacity present across species: the ability to create and become patterns of sensing and responding that relate them to (the movement patterns that comprise) their environment in human-sustaining ways (LaMothe 2015, ch. 4). To a unique degree, humans have an ability to invite, receive, and follow through with impulses to move that arise in and for the moment. They can remember these movement patterns and teach them to other humans who are also able to create patterns of movement. Every movement a human makes animates potentials that then *become* who that human is—one who made that movement. One who can make that movement again. *Every movement made is a pattern laid. / Every reach, every curve a pathway paved, carefully saved / in muscle and nerve, equipping you with the nerve to swerve / in hot pursuit of whatever you choose to serve.* These movement patterns comprise a *rhythm of bodily becoming* that finds expression in technological advances and religious beliefs, as well as in the social and symbolic environments in which humans live.

My perspective on dancing shifted. I saw this boundless, complex interplay of human, culture, and nature as itself *dance*. This "dance of life" is *actual* and *ongoing*. It is a concrete process in which one movement gives rise to another across any nature/culture or mind/body divide according to a logic internal to movement itself.

From the perspective of bodily becoming, every known tradition or technique of dance appears as a collection of movement patterns that has succeeded in producing humans whose movements relate them to the movements of their environments in life-enabling ways. Dance traditions *create* situated, relational humans who survive to pass the tradition on. This dynamic is true whether those dancing are practicing jumps in a contemporary studio or stepping in a circle around a ceremonial fire. From this perspective, dancing is not a tool humans choose in order to accomplish a functional task; dancing is the dynamic that distinguishes the ways in which humans create and use tools, language, and culture, and become *human*.

KINETIC CREATIVITY

The rhythm of bodily becoming that dance articulates and humans are has a logic and an intrinsic morality. Its logic is given by the imperfect doubling that happens with every movement made; the morality is inherent in the trajectories of movement potential that result.

From the perspective of bodily becoming, every movement at every scale of shape or size unfolds along a trajectory that stretches back billions of years through trillions of other movements-made and forward into an infinite future. Every simple movement in time and space exists as multiple, inter-crossing, mutually impacting movements. A human, in turn, is a gathering of movement potentials that have been made by many human as well as many more-than-human others and passed on in the shape of an eye, spine, or egg (Shubin 2008); in a sequence of DNA; in the plan of a ritual or belief; or in the form of a shovel, knife, yurt, teepee, or barn.

More importantly, however, every "being" or "thing" is not only a history of movements made, "it" exists as a site where new movements emerge out of that history. "It" is an *ever-unfolding present*—a capacity for discovering and releasing new impulses to connect with whatever will allow the movement to continue. Humans, too. Humans *are* an ability to receive and follow through with impulses to move that arise in and for the moving moment—they are a locus of what I call *kinetic creativity*.

As both a set of inherited movement potentials (biological and cultural) *and* a potential for making novel movement, the rhythm of bodily becoming that a human is is never wholly conservative nor wholly new. Every movement that emerges is both an expression of movements made in the past, and a response to an utterly new moment.

Navigating this rhythm can be challenging. A bodily self can get stuck in habitual patterns or be swayed by the patterns made by others, and so create and become movements that do not respond specifically to the challenges of her own moment. In this case, a bodily self may respond by repeating what she knows, reactively or reflexively, in a knee-jerk fashion. Alternately, a bodily self can cultivate her *kinetic creativity*—her willingness and ability to sense and move with impulses born in the crucible of her own ever-unfolding present.

As my philosophy of bodily becoming took root and grew, dancing appeared to me as a primary means by which humans learn to exercise their kinetic creativity in ways that will support their ongoing bodily becoming (LaMothe 2015). Whether that dancing occurs within a hierarchical social order of a medieval European court or on the plains of West Africa, the logic is the same: to become a human is to learn to make the *right* steps—that is, the movement patterns that align one's kinetic creativity with the trajectory of life that people in that context have learned (by virtue of movements they and others have made) to value and to desire.

To be clear, I am not celebrating a "primacy of movement" in which an individual body is a material object whose movement is a source of cognition (Sheets-Johnstone 2011). From the perspective of bodily becoming, there is no such body. Any body is a rhythm of creating and becoming patterns of movement unique to its location amid webs of moving relations. Nor am I affirming, with new materialists, that entangled relationships constitute all things (Barad 2007). Often in these accounts, "relationships" appear as objects that are stacked up to make other objects.

While I hew close to Spinoza, Deleuze, and Guatarri in their identification of speed as differentiating things from one another (1987), it is not just speed that counts. Every thing is a movement potential unfolding along trajectories of movements made and remembered at every level of existence, imaginable or not. *Matter's no thing that moves. It's movement that chose to choose / a mark of stability, an arc of identity / a tight temporality, specific formality / and so it might seem to be real. . . . It's not. It's movement all the way down.*

Every human movement *is* a history, a relationship, a trajectory. Every movement *is* a discovery, a potential, a vulnerability. Every ever-unfolding

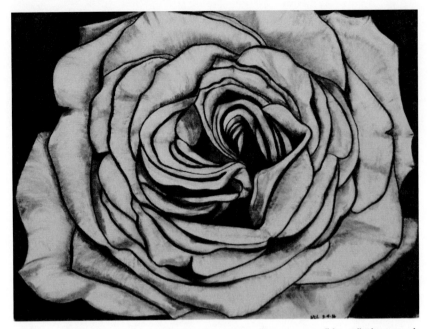

Figure 7.2. *White Rose* by Kimerer LaMothe, Charcoal on paper, 24" by 18." Photograph © 2017 by LaMothe.

present *is* a pattern of coordinated vectors that both expresses the multitude of movements that make it possible, and gives rise to another equally baffling multitude. And in this rhythm of bodily becoming lies the possibility of healing, wisdom, compassion, and love. *Life in me senses and responds to the strife in me, guiding me to move differently, along a trajectory of healing possibility that is always already at work in me.*

DANCING IN EARTH

As I watched my oldest children grow up and farm; as I read works of anthropology, evolutionary biology, developmental psychology, and eco-phenomenology; as I embraced the physical effort and the profound delights of living in a beautiful, spacious place; and as I initiated my own dance-in-nature practice, a new perspective on the importance of human dancing for the health of the planet appeared to me. Humans are not creatures who dance on earth; they dance *in* earth (Abram 2010). Even more to the point, earth dances in and through them.

Abram explains how our senses evolved to need the stimulation of the natural world for their proper development (1991). A philosophy of bodily becoming takes a step farther. What is a sense organ if not a capacity to move? What is sensing if not a movement pattern whose rhythm is impressed or interfered with by another movement, and so registers a change?

If the act of sensing and responding is first and foremost a process of creating and becoming movement patterns, then how humans dance—the patterns of movement they rehearse—educates their senses to particular possibilities and ranges of perception. Sensory awareness is not simply given; it is not something we can choose to turn on or not. Sensory awareness emerges in us as the fruit of making movements that guide us to attend to whatever those movements enable us to perceive as real—including the earth and even dance itself.

How humans dance, where they dance, and how they think about dance matter for their ability to conceive of the natural world as a reality of which they are one enabling part. Dancing provides humans with a lived experience of their own moving bodily selves, their own bodily becoming. For this reason, dancing has the potential to train humans to participate *consciously* in earth's ongoing existence. *Humans are animals who can submit / to the movement of others and so permit / their movement to move us to commit to helping them exist. We can let nature persist.*

From the Kalahari Bushman to Haitian voudoun to Native Americans to American modern dancers, humans dance to realize their power as earth creatures—the power to submit to the movement of others, to move with these others, and so serve as sites where new movements emerge that cultivate mutually life-enabling relationships with them.[5] Cultures who describe their dancing as religious or spiritual or sacred are often describing this efficacy. "Dancing" is not religious because it expresses a belief in a supernatural or transcendent Other. Rather, the sacred exists *in and as* a dance that quickens and mobilizes the power of human movement-making to heal and create along trajectories of movement that nurture the ongoing rhythm of bodily becoming. *Religion began in a dance that altered people's circumstance / pulling joy from misery by tapping a kinetic ability / to move with affinity, in proximity / to what they conceive as divinity.*

BREAKING FREE

In giving me a perspective on dancing as participation in earth, farm life also shed light on the notion it replaced. The understanding of dancing that I had carried with me to the farm was informed by movement patterns I had been making—patterns common to those living in a modern Westernized world. Most of us spend most of our days and nights thinking, feeling, and acting; reading, writing, speaking, and even dancing in cubes formed by four flat, still walls, a flat floor, and a flat ceiling. The room is still. The air is still. Temperature and light are controlled. People move within the space as the furniture allows. Sometimes there is a window. Sometimes the window opens.

In such spaces, humans learn to perceive nature as a "room" and themselves as objects that move within it. Nature appears as a relatively stable material context in relation to which humans adapt and for which they are responsible. "Dance" appears as one activity among others that humans can choose to do with their bodies in this room. Whether the human relationship to nature is conceived as one of control and use, or protection and care, both views represent the same reading-and-writing, room-enabled perspective.

Yet, in taking cover within walls that block exposure to the natural world, modern humans "protect" themselves not just from a varied wash of sensory inputs but also from the patterns of movement in relation to which their senses evolved *as* a capacity to move and respond in return. When culture acts as a wall, it serves to arrest this kinetic interplay that primes and stretches our sensory range. We learn to forget not only that dancing *is* a human's relationship to the natural world, but also that dance *is* the means by which nature creates itself as human.

While it is easy to understand why humans seek to insulate themselves from the wild vagaries of the natural world, too much protection puts them in danger of falling out of sync with the rhythms of the natural world that sustain their sense of themselves as individual minds. The practice of dance has been and still has the potential to be the missing link.

On the farm, dance broke free in me—what it was, how to do it, and why it matters for me and for the natural world. My mission shifted, and I vowed to serve this dance as its advocate in my writing, dancing, and living. I committed to generating a visionary definition of dancing that "remains faithful to the earth" (Nietzsche 1954, 125).

WHAT IS DANCE?

Any definition is provisional—the very streams of thought it makes possible will overcome it. Any definition is participatory—it exists as a moment in a person's rhythm of bodily becoming that both expresses and enables her complexly intercrossing experience. Any definition is thereby dynamic—proving its worth by the perspectives it opens, by the human action it defends, and by the thought it inspires.

Here is mine, for today.

Dance is an irrepressible rhythm of creating and becoming relational patterns of movement. It is a dynamic reality—a rhythm of bodily becoming—in which humans are always already participating. The question is how.

Any human event, action, practice, or performance that involves rhythmic bodily movement, whether secular or religious, spontaneous or rehearsed, choreographed or improvised, technical or free-form, marks a moment in which the rhythm of bodily becoming comes alive in a person or group to generate and coordinate thoughts, feelings, and actions. The movement patterns of any dance event are informed—but never wholly determined—by patterns of movement dictated by culture, directed by biology, or discovered by chance, patterns that participants have already made and become.

Further, a dance event participates in the rhythm of bodily becoming by educating the senses of those who do it or watch it in at least two ways. First, dance events educate the senses of those involved to specific patterns of movement known to guide effective, ethical action in relation to others, whether those others appear as humans, gods, creatures, or elemental forces (LaMothe 2015).

Second, as participants succeed in learning and re-creating movement patterns, the experience educates their senses to the power and potential of their own kinetic creativity—to their own ability to create and become patterns of sensation and response. They experience their ability to receive and follow through with the impulses to move that will align their bodily self in

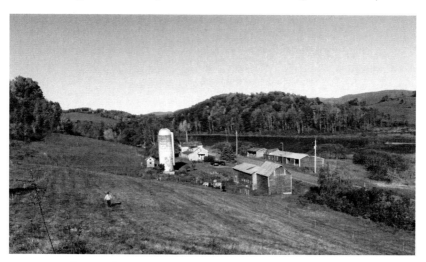

Figure 7.3. Hebron Hollow Farm. Photograph © 2016 by LaMothe.

the moment with the movements desired. A person does not just learn to do a plié; she learns that she can learn to do a plié. She learns that that plié will erupt in her as an answer for how to move in a given moment. From this realization sprouts a worldview—a philosophy of bodily becoming—in which dancing exercises the enabling condition of human life, learning, and culture.

Does the idea that every body dances threaten to obscure the distinctiveness of dance traditions and techniques? To the contrary. It serves to illuminate and mobilize the vast knowledge embedded in dance traditions across cultures and throughout history as theoretical, practical resources for how to create life-enabling relationships that remain faithful to the earth.

II

AN ECOKINETIC APPROACH

In order to identify and make use of the theoretical and practical resources enfolded in dance traditions from around the world, I offer an ecokinetic approach rooted in a philosophy of bodily becoming. This approach is earth-friendly (eco-) and movement-oriented (-kinetic). The primary goal of an ecokinetic approach is to discern and reveal the agency of dance action in relation to human persons, and their ethics, aesthetics, and religion. A corollary is to acknowledge the responsibility of a scholar for participating consciously in the ongoing life of the dancing he studies.

An ecokinetic approach meets both aims by guiding scholars to mobilize their *kinetic imagination* as a resource for *empathizing* with the *sensory education* that the practice of *specific movement patterns* affords, so as to assess the potentials for knowing and believing that such sensory education predicts. In the process, this approach illuminates how dancing, dance events, dance techniques, and dance traditions are relevant and even vital players in determining the fate of the earth and its humans.

PHENOMENOLOGY OF RELIGION

Ecokinetics draws inspiration from the phenomenology of religion—a branch of phenomenology that sprang from the tree of continental philosophy alongside Husserl. Phenomenologists of religion wanted a way to understand critically what appears in human history as "religious" or "sacred." For Gerardus van der Leeuw, often recognized as a founding voice in the phenomenology of religion, the task of the phenomenologist is to practice what humans do every day—their "true vital activity"—as they try to make sense of their own and others' experiences (1986, 676).

In van der Leeuw's hands, the phenomenology of religion took shape as a critical, self-correcting method for understanding other people's experiences of what they conceive as "power" that cannot be reduced to rational, verbal, symbolic, or material explanations. Because the phenomenology of religion attends so carefully to questions of power and agency that appear to exceed human ability, it provides rich resources for considering the ways in which dance techniques and traditions cultivate human relationships with the more-than-human world.

A PHENOMENON

A phenomenon, for van der Leeuw, refers to that which appears. That which appears *is* a relationship, not a subject or object but a "third thing" or "meaning" (1986, 673). In the vocabulary of bodily becoming, this "third thing" is itself a movement—a crossing of movement patterns—in which the movement of a scholar's senses bumps up against movements emanating from other directions to produce a new wave of thoughts and feelings that registers in the phenomenologist of religion as something that can be recognized and named as sacred or divine.

Given her understanding of a phenomenon as relationship, a phenomenologist of religion knows better than to try to discern the truth of whether or not the sacred exists. Rather, the phenomenologist essays to understand why and how and under what conditions something appears to someone as "sacred." For van der Leeuw, the mark of such a phenomenon is an experience of *being moved* by some force that disrupts and displaces, boosts or curtails, human intentions and actions. Such marks are often evident in dance traditions, for example, in the case of Haitian voudou where a dancer, after a period of sustained rhythmic movement, "is ridden" by a spiritual entity or *lwa* who then dictates the dancer's movements (Daniel 2005). Alternatively, in the case of the Kalahari Bushmen, after a period of sustained stepping and stamping around a fire-centered circle, an experienced healer will *kia* and enter into a state of heightened emotion where she is overcome with *n|om* or energized lifeforce, and impelled to touch and heal others in the circle (Keeney 2013). In such cases, then, dance *appears* to the phenomenologist as "religion."

Ecokinetics embraces this orientation to phenomena as a way to understand the agency of dance action. Its task in relation to what appears is threefold: 1) to invite and identify patterns of movement-making; 2) to assess the sensory education that such movement making affords; and 3) to map the potentials for thinking, feeling, and acting in relation to the natural world that this appearance represents (see also LaMothe 2014).

INVITING APPEARANCES: THE EPOCHÉ

To invite and identify appearances of meaning, a phenomenologist practices suspending or bracketing his preconceptions or judgments. The goal is to clear one's consciousness so as to be as open as possible to new perceptions. From the perspective of bodily becoming, insofar as any phenomenon is itself a crossing of bodily movements (of subject and object), it is not only mental space that needs clearing. An ecokinetic scholar aims to bracket the most basic patterns of bodily movement that subtend sensory perception.

Of course, complete suspension of such movements is not possible; humans are (inescapably) the bodily movements that they are. Nevertheless, as dance traditions throughout time testify, it is possible to awaken and to own a sensory awareness of one's bodily self as movement—as a rhythm of bodily becoming—and to practice staying as close as possible to that sensory space. With this quickened sensory awareness comes vulnerability—a kinetic responsivity. An ecokinetic scholar whose senses are so trained is more likely to notice patterns, more likely to identify with their impact, and more likely to respond by dedicating attention to their appearance. He is more likely to understand why given movement patterns appear to someone as sacred.

As the Bushmen of the Kalahari have insisted for years, their bodily movement matters: their dancing keeps the web of relationships that is the universe alive and healthy (Keeney and Keeney 2015). Rather than trying to determine whether this claim is true or false, an ecokinetic phenomenologist quickens her own sensory awareness to discern how the bodily movements of the Bushmen that appear to her are educating the senses of those who are making (or watching) them in ways that make this perception of a living universe possible.

For van der Leeuw, such sensory responsiveness is at the heart of the phenomenological method. To practice it is to love. As he writes:

> Understanding . . . presupposes intellectual restraint. But this is never the attitude of the cold-blooded spectator: it is, on the contrary, the loving gaze of the lover on the beloved object. For all understanding rests upon self-surrendering love . . . to him who does not love, nothing whatever is manifested. (1986, 684)

Insofar as a scholar approaches the study of dance techniques and traditions with this kind of movement-enabled sensory awareness, he enhances his ability to recognize that other people's bodily movements are similarly priming them to notice whatever meaning their movement patterns are training them to perceive.

EMPATHIZING IMAGINATIVELY

An ecokinetic scholar seeks to *understand* what appears by *empathizing kinetically* with the experiences of those who are making or watching or otherwise encountering those bodily movements. As van der Leeuw insists, empathy is and must be imaginative. As he avers, any appearance to me of someone else's experience disappears as soon as it happens. All I have is the memory of its appearing, and all I can do is reconstruct that appearance as faithfully as possible. As a result, the phenomenology of religion has one desire:

> to testify to what has been manifested to it. This it can do only . . . by a second experience of the event, by a thorough reconstruction . . . To see face to face is denied us. But much can be observed even in a mirror; and it is possible to speak about things seen. (677–678)

Van der Leeuw's use of the term "mirror" was prophetic. The discovery of mirror neurons in the mid-1990s not only reframed cultural conversations surrounding empathy in terms of neuronal activity, it also shed light on the role of bodily movement in a person's ability to empathize. As now known, mirror neurons fire when one person sees another making a movement. They fire in the pattern of coordination that would be required for the observer to re-create that pattern of movement (Ramachandran 2011). Yet the term *mirror* is misleading, for the mirror neurons' activity proceeds not by way of visual pathways alone, but by way of the observer's sensory ability to re-create movement patterns. When van der Leeuw affirms that an observer "interpolates" her own experience into the reconstruction of what has appeared to her and confirms "we can do no otherwise" (1986, 674), he implies that movement patterns and the sensory awareness they represent are the "stuff" with which persons engage in a thorough reconstruction—a second experience—of what appears to them.

From the perspective of bodily becoming, empathy does not proceed by way of feelings or thoughts, per se, but by way of kinetic experience. *To empathize is to move with.* Humans draw on their own experiences of creating and becoming patterns of movement in order to reconstruct the sensory education provided by trajectories of movement-making evident in others. *We move with to share a toy; move with to multiply joy. / Move with to see otherwise. Move with to apologize. / We move with to comfort hurt. Move with to convert despair into hope.*

In this task again, a scholar's practice of rhythmic bodily movement is an asset. As van der Leeuw confirms: "In writing about the dance, I discovered that, even more than in the other arts, participation is necessary if it is to be understood. With the spoken or written word, little can be explained when the point is to appreciate rhythm and imitate it" (1963, 12). Here, the value of participating in dance is not only to learn the steps of a given dance. The value lies in cultivating a sensory receptivity to patterns and variations in rhythm, including those within oneself (74). By dancing, a scholar learns viscerally that the movement patterns people create are integral not accidental to who they are.

With this visceral knowledge, an ecokinetic phenomenologist is primed to call upon her own kinetic experience as a resource for imagining how the movements that appear to her are educating the senses of those who are making them. By using her kinetic imagination in this way, a scholar is able to map the possibilities for believing and thinking that practicing those movement patterns makes possible, especially in relation to more-than-human powers. She is able to *understand* not only how and why a given phenomenon appears to her as *dance* but also how and why that dancing enacts a relationship to (whatever those movement patterns enable participants to conceive and know as) the *earth* in which they live. As noted above, from a perspective of bodily becoming, dancing *is* a human connection to the earth. The practice of kinetic, imaginative empathy enables a scholar to understand how and why and to what ends.

In ecokinetics, as van der Leeuw affirms, there is no goal, no arrival. There is only the ongoing process of inviting and then kinetically, imaginatively, empathically recreating what appears. As he writes: "Only the persistent and strenuous application of this intense sympathy, only the uninterrupted learning of his role, qualifies the phenomenologist to interpret appearances" (1986, 675). Such uninterrupted learning ensures that an ecokinetic scholar will keep assessing his success in bracketing his own kinetic, aesthetic preferences; that he will keep adjusting his imaginative reconstructions in relation to what appears to him; and that he will be better prepared by his growing knowledge of the options to re-create and understand the meaning of a single case (677). Finally, as noted, that uninterrupted learning involves some kind of *participation*.

Insofar as a scholar adopts this posture of self-critique and ongoing practice, she knows that each time a phenomenon appears to her as "dance," she is not just naming it. She is participating in *its* ongoing life in the world. She is drawing it into a new web of meanings and relationships and thereby altering its appearance for others. These new connections, in turn, affect the attention directed toward that phenomenon and influence its potential for development. Through her uninterrupted learning, then, an ecokinetic phenomenologist commits to paying attention to how her reconstructions of what appears to her are affecting the ongoing history and practice of dance.

Conclusion

The four walls of a study or studio educate human senses to an illusion that dance is one art among many; an occasion for self expression and perhaps political activism; a medium for asserting identity, nationality, ethnicity; and at times a catalyst for healing and entering altered states. It is and can be all of these.

On the farm, I have come to believe that dance is also the means by which humans become *human* bodily selves. *Humans are who they are, able to bond near and far, / by moving with others around and above, / wanting and needing to live in love, / equipped with the power to detect / the subtle moves of a dance dialect. / Nothing more or less, than an impulse to connect.*

A person is not a puppet. Dance involves steps, but can never be reduced to them. Steps are a means to exercise and expand sensory awareness along potential pathways of culturally specific, life-sustaining thought and action. Any steps a person makes quicken his or her inherent kinetic creativity, so that he or she has the opportunity to find not only feelings of joy, but unique, seemingly sui generis impulses of healing, intuition, understanding, and love. Insofar as dancing can educate people's sensory awareness to their own movement *as* the movement of nature within them, then the dancing may prime them to think and feel and act in ways that express this careful attention—that honor the earth as a *dance* in whose life their own ongoing movement participates.

In facing our current climate crisis, it is not enough for humans to *care* for the earth (Warren 1996), to dance for the earth, or even to *think* about the earth as a relational whole (Abram 2010). Humans are better equipped to participate responsibly in the ongoing life of earth when they cultivate the kind of sensory awareness that dancing can enable. By dancing, humans can build, within themselves and their societies, moral compasses that can guide them to act in ways that take care of the earthly conditions of their own ongoing existence.

On the farm, we are aware of how the movements we make on an ongoing basis perpetuate patterns of consumption, combustion, and waste that desecrate our earth. Yet, we *are* aware, and painfully so. Every day, this sensory awareness goads us to open to new impulses to move that will better express love for the earth in us and around us—whether that means hanging laundry outside on a clothesline, replacing another processed food with something homemade, reusing or recycling every possible item, relying on our wood stove for heat, helping each other thrive, or creating works of art that communicate participation in this sensory awareness of the ongoing dance in and around us.

The experiment continues.

Notes

1. I have described these dynamics in depth, most notably in the beginning sections of each chapter in *Why We Dance* (2015).

2. The ascetic ideal refers to the belief, equally scientific and religious, that truth exists over and against the particulars—the movement—of bodily selves (Nietzsche 1989).

3. Strenski (2006) and Vasquez (2011) offer two accounts of the field of religious studies and its contested bias toward belief-oriented, text-based theories and methods.

4. Sentences in italics are from "The Ever Unfolding Present," a concert of original music and dance that featured nine songs-poems, one for each chapter of my book, *Why We Dance* (2015). The piece premiered at the Southern Vermont Arts Center in Manchester, Vermont, on August 20, 2016.

5. In a forthcoming book project, I am working out this thesis in relation to particular cases, including Native American (Kurath), African Bushman (Keeney and Keeney), Haitian voudou (Daniel), the American Shakers, and others.

8

Filming Jitdance

Detroit Redux

JOANNA McNAMARA

Highway 94, which stretches between my hometown of Ann Arbor and Detroit, quickly narrows into three lanes as the first decaying structures of Detroit appear on the horizon. Semis hauling everything from steel or aggregates to hamburger and fireworks continue to press forward at harrowing speeds. The skyline looming ahead now enters my peripheral vision to become the present; the flicker of a crumbling hotel there, a row of burned-out homes here. Future meets present in a fusion of—*place*—Detroit. A city imbued by seemingly disparate phenomena: the old and the new, the abandoned and found, the natural and the urban, the adage and the allegro.

The concept of "place" has myriad scholarly interpretations. As eco-phenomenologist Edward S. Casey proposes, "place" is something "*at work*, something ongoing and dynamic, an *ingredient* in something else," such as history, nature, politics, gender, poetic imagination, sociology, architecture, or religion (1997, 286). As I enter Detroit's city limits these contexts converge, shaping my perception of this fascinating city; from my rear-view mirror, the highway behind me now melts into a distant past. *Place* is "the event of envelopment itself" (339).

Our Place

For the past six years, I and my troupe of dancers, musicians, and filmmakers, have enveloped ourselves in Detroit—rehearsing and filming dance in Detroit's museums, boathouses, locker rooms, city streets, beaches, and iconic, abandoned buildings. I first became curious about Detroit while listening to my husband's stories of growing up there. When he became ill, he often spoke of his childhood, and I wrote these memories down or recorded them on my digital voice recorder: "We would cross a bridge on Sunday afternoons [to Belle Isle Park] and everything was different on the other side. We could have been back in the fifth century for all we knew. We left the city far behind and entered an enchanted place. It was a quiet serenity and so much green. At night the fountain lit up in magical colors and we stood at its edges in absolute awe."

It didn't take me long to fall in love with this captivating city through my own experiences of dancing and making screendances there. Although we can never go back in time, except through memory, there are infinite and wondrous freedoms associated with moving into and out of, across, and through place. Place exists in the interval between body and landscape, says Casey:

> Unlike the double-bind of time, however, the double bound of place is open ended. Far from being constrictive in the manner of a deadline, the lifeline extending from body to landscape (and back again) is as porous as a sieve. Thanks to the mutual enlivening of body and landscape, a place constantly overflows its own boundaries. Uncontainable on its near edge, it flows back into the body that subtends it; uncontainable on its far side, it flows outward into the circumambient world. Place's inflow and outflow are such that to be fully *in* a place is never to be confined to a punctate position; it is to be already on the way out. (1993, 29)

From the small and functional locker room at the bathhouse on Belle Isle to the opulent and grand spaces of the Michigan Central Train Station or Detroit Institute of Arts, Diego Rivera Industry Hall, I've filled these places with the immediacy of dancing bodies and music and then captured these richly vital images and sounds on film. Spinning across the topography of the city, spiraling through its stories, my troupe of dancers form a moment-to-moment, unpunctuated partnership with Detroit, as if incorporeal beings in some future story.

In writing this chapter, I bring Detroit into an even wider circle of inquiry through a hermeneutic study of *Jitdance: Detroit Redux*, the screendance I am currently directing with Detroit Jit dancer, choreographer, and company director of Hardcore Detroit, Haleem "Stringz" Rasul, with music by composer Howard Cass and cinematography and editing by Andrzej Milosz and Ayhan Vostina, respectively. (I refer to my collaborators by their first names in the rest of the chapter in keeping with our working relationship.) I will say much more about Haleem, and his urban street dance of choice, Detroit Jit, which is surely the homegrown dancing body of Detroit.

My goal in this chapter is to let the making of this screendance, and the screendance itself, speak of Detroit and its transitions. I turn toward hermeneutic phenomenology—the perspective that experience structures the way we understand and make meaning of the world. Casey's ecological perspective furthers the centrality of place and body so integral to hermeneutics, and equally integral to my film and chapter. He explains that the lived body mediates both the "expressiveness" and "orientedness" of place (1997, 230, 231). As my dancers and I move through space, the space itself is remade, produced by our bodies in motion. It expands forward and contracts, coils inward and flickers up as we vitalize these empty spaces. Others produce this place-in-the-making as well. Locals, students on field trips, and tourists come and go, creating a social fabric wherever we film. Some linger awhile, others stay and ask questions: "What are you doing this for?" "Where are you from?" The dancers and I are energized by these exchanges as we rehearse and film.

From the locals we hear personal stories about the locations as we rehearse and film, and these stories sometimes inspire improvisations at the site. Fifty-eight-year-old Harrison Richardson, who lives near Michigan Central Train Station, hangs around on his vintage, French Peugeot bike as we rehearse, ready to share his stories with us and the steady stream of tourists who show up. Like others in Detroit, he has fallen on hard times, but has created a niche for himself, earning tips for his wide-based knowledge about the train station and Detroit. He is a steadfast presence there.

As is the case of many historical dwellings in Detroit, the train station, built in the Beaux Arts Classical style, is a spectacle of transformation. From what was at one time the tallest station in America, moving up to 4,000 people a day through its elegant, main lobby, to becoming an abandoned and vandalized building, the station is now on the rise to a complete renovation.

I ask Harrison if I may jot down some of his personal experiences inside the station, before the wealthy Moroun family bought it, rented it out for the *Batman v Superman: Dawn of Justice* movie, and then locked it up tight. He leans toward me and wipes his craggy face with his Detroit Tigers baseball cap. "Homeless people lived everywhere up in those office spaces and there was lots of gang stuff going on, too. One man had a weird altar up there and became this kind of spiritual leader."[1] Harrison points to an area of pavement obscured by weeds: "Guess what that manhole right there in the front of the building led to, years back," he whispers. "Part of an underground railroad system." Later as we improvise in the park, in front of the station, I ask the dancers to emerge individually from the tall, maidenhair grasses and imagine the gravel paths they're dancing on to be a maze of tunnels to traverse. They dart over the gritty surfaces, kicking up dirt, their outstretched limbs defining imaginary walls.

Phenomenological hermeneutics, in its ability to accommodate the personal experiences of the participants, as well as the historical, sociocultural, and aesthetic contexts of a work, is especially relevant for the interpretation of a screendance made in Detroit, a city misunderstood, and with Detroit Jit, an urban street dance not yet fully recognized, even though rapidly gaining in popularity. Hans-Georg Gadamer writes: "This is hermeneutics: to let what seems to be far and alienated speak again" (1980, 83).

Linking hermeneutics with the reflective approach in the description of lived experiences, I first explore the historical and sociocultural settings of *Jitdance: Detroit Redux*. This includes an inquiry into the Heidelberg Project, which is the name of the public art site where this screendance is recorded, and of Detroit Jit dance, the primary urban street dance style of this screendance. As the theme of this screendance emerges, I consider the voices of participants alongside the texts of writers and philosophers whose works oscillate with this hermeneutic. I anticipate that a blueprint for interpretation of their insights and experiences will emerge. Circling the multilayers of this project, I trust an expanding conversation and understanding of the relationships reflective of Detroit's ever-changing urban landscape to surface.

As dance and filmmakers working in Detroit, we are not alone in our efforts and contributions. All over the city artists are working and the arts flourishing: stately theaters, abandoned houses, and empty warehouses are fired-up with music, theater, and dance. The Kresge and John S. and James L. Knight Foundations have generously contributed to the developing art scene. The Knight Arts Challenge, Detroit, has awarded over twenty million dollars to arts organizations and individual artists in the past four years alone. Performing and visual artists continue to arrive from around the world to live and work here or just browse, dig, and spend time in this compelling environment. Rent is cheap and property inexpensive. At least for now.

In the past six years, Joori Jung, formerly a dancer in New York City, has founded ARTLAB J, a leading dance company and studio on Russell Street. She also directs Detroit Dance City Festival, an annual event for local, national, and international dance artists. Crossing over to Cass Street in midtown, local Detroiter, and my collaborator, Haleem "Stringz" Rasul, founder of a Detroit Jit dance company, Hardcore Detroit, rehearses dancers for an upcoming performance at the Light Box. Marcus White has developed a robust performance production company, Marcus White/White Werx, which seems to be everywhere both online and off since 2013. At the Carr Center in downtown, Jennifer Harge, director of Harge Dance Stories, choreographs dances promoting social change through storytelling and enhanced community engagement. Kristi Faulkner of Kristi Faulkner Dance has a similar aim, but with an emphasis on challenging gender roles, and Barbara Selinger, a founder and director of Detroit Dance Collective for thirty-eight years, has seen and experienced it all—the ups and downs, the coming and goings in Detroit—yet she has continued to see her company thrive. From a dance scene that is booming everywhere, to the Detroit Institute of Arts and the Museum of Contemporary Art Detroit, and for all the virtual spaces between the ebb of Motown and the rise of Detroit techno music, it is no wonder Detroit has been a hub for artists and the arts. Yes, even today, possibilities abound in Detroit.

Yet uncertainties about the place of Detroit continue to ripple out into urban myths across the regional, national, and international map. Listening to a panel of speakers at the *2016 Detroit Dance City Festival*, a studio owner claims that a parent of one of her students from the suburbs has said other parents in her neighborhood are afraid to bring their children into Detroit, no matter what the reputation of the studio in training young, preprofessional dancers. Instructors and studio owners in the audience nod their heads in understanding. What to do? The answers are not clear.

And so I continue to ask myself, "What can I do?" And what I do is this. I send my screendances out to a global, virtual village, satisfied that a wider sphere of intercultural dialogue takes place, lessening the remoteness of Detroit, making it more accessible, less unfamiliar. Because even though Detroit has been named a UNESCO City of Design and urban farms are prospering as the city has emerged from bankruptcy, Detroit is still a city misunderstood.

Location and Body: The Heidelberg Project and Jit Dance

It's a stinging-cold, late afternoon in January, when filmmaker and film editor Ayhan Vostina and I arrive at the Heidelberg Project to meet Haleem Rasul to talk about the screendance we're making here in August. Stepping into an enchanted streetscape of colorful, repurposed objects, we spot Heidelberg's founding artist, Tyree Guyton, on the other side of the street, smiling and animated as he chats with a visitor to the site. We all wave to each other.

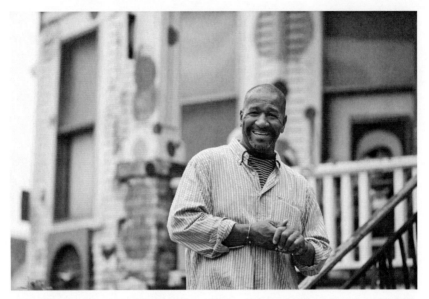

Figure 8.1. Tyree Guyton at the Heidelberg Project in Detroit. Photo courtesy of Heidelberg archives.

Described at various times as a painter, sculptor, outsider artist, urban environmentalist, or folk artist, Tyree, along with the support of his grandfather, artist Sam Mackey, founded Heidelberg Project in 1986 on Heidelberg Street, the street that three generations of his family has lived on. Watching the perils of a postindustrial calamity around him, the young Guyton, who eventually trained at the College for Creative Studies in Detroit and has been awarded a Doctorate of Fine Arts, decided to take matters in his own hands and, along with Mackey, began making something new out of the trash people dumped, the objects they left behind, and the burned-down or decaying dwellings surrounding him on Heidelberg. In an interview I had with Tyree, in October, 2016, several months following completion of the film, he remembers that moment: "It was like 4th of July fireworks that went off in my head at the age of nine and I knew it and I heard it. I heard my calling. It was a beautiful day. Some things you don't forget. And those are the kind of moments that can change your life forever."[2] Drugs and poverty surrounded Guyton but, with a hammer, saw, paintbrush, and some paints, he created a two-block, lush oasis of invention, here on the east side of Detroit.

This calling to recycle or construct an inventive exhibit out of residue left behind is not new to the American art scene. Artists of other times and places have reconsidered and refabricated the remnants of urban decay. New York City, for example, was hit in the early 1970s with the recession and residents fled to the suburbs. According to Philip Ursprung (2013, 239–240), as large parts of the city's infrastructure fell into a state of decay, artists began turning their attention to the idea of urban transformation. Architect and artist Gordon Matta-Clark began digging "layer by layer the material substance of buildings, rescuing the traces of everyday life as it had existed in the houses in and around the metropolis and simultaneously searched through the debris for the building blocks of the new" (240).

Land artist Robert Smithson also greatly influenced the processes and thinking of his contemporaries in the 1970s and beyond (Flam 1966; Ursprung 2013). Although mostly known for his later, large-scale land art projects such as *Spiral Jetty* (1970), *Spiral Hill* (1971), and *Amarillo Ramp* (1973), Smithson's early projects focused on discovering natural landscape materials such as rocks or sand at a *site* and exhibiting them elsewhere, such as inside fabricated containers in a gallery, or what he referred to as a *non-site*. These containers were accompanied by a drawing, map, or text about the *site* itself. What Smithson proposed, both explicitly in his writings and implicitly in his art projects, was that art, contrary to past traditions and beliefs, did not have to be exhibited in a formal setting, nor thought of as a commodity simply to be sold or acquired. Art did not have to be shiny, new, and finished to be art—a belief held by urban, environmental, and recycler artists of today.

How Smithson, Matta-Clark, and other contemporary environmental artists, both in America and abroad, have found, retrieved, recycled, and exhibited their discovered materials often speaks of artists with vast networks of contacts and resources. These artists have the ability to travel, often far away from home, with the financial support necessary to transport what are sometimes large-scale materials long distances. As Smithson says in a text he wrote to accompany his work, *Non-site (Palisades-Edgewater, N.J.)*, "Instead of putting a work of art on some land, some land is put into the work of art" (Schwendener 2014). Often, their work has been exhibited in galleries, museums, photograph catalogues, text, video, or films.

Far from the romantic concept of the distance between *site* and *non-site*, here at the Heidelberg Project, art and land are one in the same. In contrast, Tyree's recycled objects and abandoned, now repurposed, homes have been discovered in his immediate surroundings and have remained there. He recalls the wise words of his professor, Charles McGee, who many years ago told Tyree: "If you can do it at home, you can do it anywhere." Unlike other recycler artists, Tyree's home, place, and art are one and the same. "Persons who live in places—who inhabit or reinhabit them—come to share features with the local landscape; but equally so, they make a difference to, perhaps indelibly mark, the land in which they dwell" (Casey 1993, 305). Just as the human body is always immediate and present in dance, so, too, is the Heidelberg Project like a second skin to Tyree.

As Ayhan and I wander through the Heidelberg Project, we enter a strange land that is never quite new or actually finished and is at once both fun and thought provoking. Children must go! Tyree says: "I say to the parents it's okay for the kids to play with the things, the toys, it's okay. That's part of the magic of what art *can* be, to me." There are large, colorful polka dots painted everywhere, like big balloons waiting to be popped. They cover the People House (sometimes referred to as the "Dotty-Wotty" house where Tyree's mother now lives), bob down the street, and show up in the most unlikely places. Vinyl LP albums surface in odd locations, too. A nod to Motown and things past in Detroit? Across the street there's a mound of piled-up shoes. Who wore those bright yellow heels? Or the Nike athletic shoes? Where are those people now? And at the end of a row of houses, hundreds of shoes dangle from a chain-link fence. A fence: a location of human exchanges, of stories shared and boundaries scaled. The possibilities of narrative emerge, yet the images and narratives here are random, bouncing in from all different directions.

What Tyree Guyton may not have expected thirty years ago was that the Heidelberg Project would become the third most visited site in Detroit, with more than 200,000 people annually rambling around the grounds. What to make of these visitors? Will gentrification ooze into a neighborhood and with it a whole list of community ills? Will real estate property rise, along with the displacement of locals who can no longer afford their home or sustain their past lifestyle? Are *others*, such as screendance makers or visitors who enter and leave, seen as those who don't belong? What about the invasion of privacy wrought by an onslaught of tourists, eager to experience the art here? If gentrification is seen as the eventual funneling of money into a depraved area without understanding the social processes underpinning the fabric of that community, none of that is visible here. At least not for the past 30 years. And cafés? Boutiques? Nowhere to be seen, here at the Heidelberg, on the east side of Detroit.

Tyree is passionate about art as social change, building this art environment as a way of enhancing peoples' lives and his own neighborhood through the positivity of creative imagination. "It's like going to church and all of a sudden the spirit is so high that the people are starting to dance because you give them a reason to dance," he says. "You bring out the best in people. You do it at home. You do it in your own backyard. And you show the world what's possible out of nothing."

Unlike the tedious processes I've often faced in obtaining film permits and confirming schedules, Tyree and his staff, including artist Toni Nunn and his wife and executive director, Jenenne Whitfield, immediately and warmheartedly give me permission to rehearse and film at the Heidelberg Project:

"May we use the rusted wagon with the vinyl LPs albums in it as a prop, to be pulled around the grounds during the filming?" I ask. "We will return it exactly as we found it."

"Yes!" they answer.

"May we dance and record inside the *House of Soul*?" I add.

"Yes!" they answer enthusiastically.

As much as the Heidelberg lifeworld is about the art, it is also about the value placed on human interactions in the spaces between. Tyree explains: "It's my way of using art as a vehicle, a magnet to connect kindred spirits."

Ayhan and I continue walking around the site. Multicolored, abandoned cars are everywhere, along with the recurring images of stylized, two-dimensional clocks on plywood. When I ask him about the clocks later during our interview, he says, "I have placed them in a very methodical way all over the Project so that every place you look you see a clock. Because we are in a time zone, we are in a tunnel of time. And it's called life." There's one clock at the top of a tree and another on the ground over there. Then, surprise! Turning a corner everything changes; the atmosphere is now disturbing, poignant. Stuffed animals and dolls abound. Creepy, decapitated dolls; dolls with amputated limbs. The long leg of a black doll sticks out of a closed toilet lid. There's a mound of stuffed animals, but the four seasons of Michigan have zapped the luster from their fabric. Who were the children that gave up their warm fuzzy playthings? And bright-colored, polyester dresses are tacked onto walls. Remnants of those who fled? Or, perhaps worse? Birdcages; a small, plastic figurine of a black man inside a birdcage playing a trumpet. As Tyree says, "Life is about the changes that you're a part of and it's the changes that you're not a part of but you are a part of. It's the demolition, it's the fires, it's fighting with the government"—all of which Tyree has endured during the past thirty years at the Heidelberg Project.

Messages surround us. On a piece of plywood in the shape of a cross, *Soul Never Dies*:

> *Soul Never Dies*; I go back to the message again and again. Look at the red lettering. *Soul Never Dies*. I remember my husband's words about Belle Isle Park, "*We left the city far behind and entered an enchanted place.*"

Ayhan and I take different paths; I wander over to Ms. Bell's Yellowhouse Guestbook, where visitors to Heidelberg can sign the outside of her house. She's on her porch, as usual, eager to talk. Meet a couple from France who are here on an anniversary, chat with a family from Norway. Smokelike vapors stream from our mouths as we talk, form intricate patterns then quickly dissipate in the cold, harsh wind. We share some thoughts about the art and ask each other questions. As we wander over the space and take it in, we also produce the space, make it something different, a bigger, more expansive place than before. The tangible moments making the Heidelberg Project as *place* reflect not only the collected biographies of prior occupants "plowing into the present" (Ursprung 2013, 248) but also of the immediate, lived collection of those biographies side by side with the immediacy of the lived-community itself, including Guyton and the neighbors and visitors who come and go. "From being lost in space and time (or more likely, lost to them in the era of modernity), we find our way in place" (Casey 1993, 29).

Body

If the Heidelberg is the quintessential, homegrown arts environment of Detroit, Jit dance is surely its body. Haleem pulls up to the Heidelberg Project and parks his SUV, ready to talk about the screendance we're making here in August, *Jitdance: Detroit Redux.*

Tall and lanky, he's the artistic director of Hardcore Detroit, which he founded after graduating from Western Michigan University in 2001. The company is known for b-boying, and house dance, but mostly the Detroit cultural dance form known as "Detroit-Jit." Haleem, who grew up in Detroit, is deeply connected to the urban dance scene and has become a historian, spokesperson, and promoter of Jit dance. He is the recipient of both a Kresge Artist Fellowship and a John S. and James L. Knight Arts Foundation award and has become an international ambassador for Detroit Jit, teaching master classes and workshops in Europe, Africa, Indonesia, China, and throughout the United States.

Although the Jitters reflect distinctively individual styles, they all perform with the speed of a thrown dart. During rehearsals I attend, Gabrielle McLeod, Haleem's rehearsal assistant, rapidly calls out each step during rehearsals: "Kick, wiggle back, kick, kick, and kick. Wiggle, wiggle, shuffle back, jazzy, jazzy step."

They stomp into the ground, cross-laterally, front and back, kick at ankle level, step back with one foot and then the other. Knees lift into a sharp, side

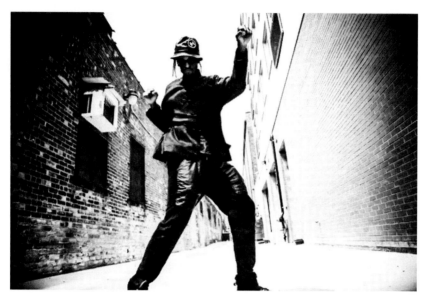

Figure 8.2. Haleem "Stringz" Rasul in Detroit. Photo © 2015 by Andie Mills.

attitude and wiggle back and forth. They fly into the air, pinlike, with ankles crossed, and then drop cross-legged to the ground, pop'n right back up to shuffle in a tight little circle, then pivot two times around in the opposite direction with bent knees. This mostly vertical, up and down movement is relieved with fast slides to the left and right, or sharp little under-curves through second position. In pleasing juxtaposition to these intricate foot patterns and strong lower bodywork, from the waist up, the torso and arms move fluidly, gliding through space. There's often a side tilt toward the working leg, with clenched fists meeting at the sternum and elbows pointing to the sides; then the hands drop quickly down and the arms circle from front to back. Sometimes sudden, percussive elbow flaps punctuate the movement flow. They flap up and down from the waist or, with the elbows bent at the side of the body, clenched fists frame the shoulders and vibrate sharply. The men do fast inversions and drop into a plank position, wiggle back into downward dog and push off the ground. And in a duet that Jai Hatcher and James Broxton are performing for the film, they toss in a couple of the acrobatic moves, commonly seen in Jit.

Ardent about the importance of understanding and preserving the history of Detroit Jit, Haleem tracked down the originators of Jit and interviewed them in a session that lasted more than three hours. Realizing how

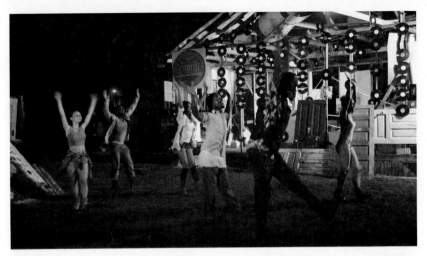

Figure 8.3. Dancers performing in *Jitdance: Detroit Redux* in front of the Soul Never Dies House at the Heidelberg Project. Left to right, Anna Shahinian, James Broxton, Gabrielle McLeod, Alonzo Walker, Haleem Rasul, and Jai Hatcher. Photo © 2016 by Andrew Milosz.

significant their story was to Detroit culture, he made a documentary about their lives and careers titled, *The Jitterbugs: Pioneers of Jit* (Rasul 2013). Hermeneutic philosopher Wilhelm Dilthey says that the ability to understand something becomes easier as historical consciousness is expanded. Lived experiences should not be considered isolated entities: "Knowledge of the mind-constructed world originates from the interaction between lived experience, understanding of other people, the historical comprehension of communities as the subject of historical activity, and insight into objective mind" (Mueller-Voomer 1985, 151, 152). As Haleem says during an interview with me in August, 2016, "Jit brings an understanding of where I come from and how we move."[3] Not only is Haleem's understanding of Jit broadened through his understanding of the historicity of Jit dance, so, too, is the world beyond Detroit.

Detroit Jit dance, not to be confused with the cool, swing dance of the '30s called the Jitterbug, was pioneered by three Detroit-based brothers who developed this style of urban cultural dance in the '70s and called themselves the Jitterbugs (again, unrelated to the Jitterbug dance). While the African American street dance form of breakdancing was developing in New York and locking in California, the Jitterbug brothers, Tracey, Johnny, and James McGhee—self-proclaimed thugs, thieves, and gangster criminals—started Jit dancing between cruising Detroit at night and stealing stuff. In *Acres of*

Diamonds, Johnny says the brothers would pull the car over at the end of the evening, get out, and separate the new loot under a street light (Cevallos and Scholl 2013). Once the loot was divided, they would hang out and start exchanging some box slaps and dance moves. Soon, they were refining their moves at home, and performing at basement parties. Two more dancers temporarily joined the group and opportunities followed: a wedding here, a nightclub gig there. And then soul singer Kim Weston saw the brothers performing and invited them to the Detroit *Festival of the Performing Arts*. It was there that they learned discipline and began crafting highly coordinated routines that were synchronized and entertaining. Tracey McGhee says of Weston: "She literally saved our life because she was able to pull us off the streets, put us in the program, *Festival of the Performing Arts*. That's where we had places to perform, people to perform in front of" (Chakrabarti 2014).

One of their instructors at the festival, Clifford Fears, a former dancer with Katherine Dunham who directed his own dance theater group in Detroit, impressed the brothers with a film clip of the renowned Nicolas Brothers, the dancing duet in Broadway musicals and Hollywood movies. The Nicolas Brothers combined tap with athletic acrobats, a little ballet, and highly innovative moves to create what was called *flash dance*. As the Jitterbugs continued to develop and refine their style, they drew from the athleticism and stunts of the Nicholas Brothers as well as Motown backup dancers but with an edgier, street feel that was at the same time seamless and elegant. What separated the Jitterbugs' new dance style from West Coast lock'n and East Coast break'n and hip-hop was an emphasis on fast, intricate footwork. Their music of choice? Funkadelic. The suits they wore? Chic and polished. The overall feel? Talented and hot. What better way to sell some of the drab, stale cars at the auto shows, such as the 1986 Chevrolet Spectrum and Nova?

The offer to dance at the auto shows came from the Gail and Rice Inc. production and entertainment company, and the Jitterbugs were elated. Suddenly, the brothers were making plenty of money doing what they loved to do: Jit'n in about eight performances a day and hanging out together, doing whatever they wanted at night. But, in time, these new opportunities also lavished a set of challenges not all the brothers could manage and the eldest of the trio, James, began missing performances and sleeping through important meetings. "We came from almost nothing," says Johnny McGhee, and "We grew to almost something" (Rasul 2013). The group was falling apart and it would be a couple of decades before Jit dance would be picked up by a new generation and gain the national and international acclaim that their counterparts of lock'n, break'n and then hip-hop had enjoyed since the '70s.

Their legacy, the brothers agree, is that Jit has been revived by the younger generation. When Detroit Jit came on the scene again, which side of Woodward Avenue you were dancing on distinguished it. The westside style was theatrical with dramatic facial expressions, the eastside style, known for its cool, more laid-back approach. No matter the location or approach, all Jit is based on competitions, usually consisting of two dancers battling it out on the dance floor, first one than the other. Whoever the judges deem most successful, that competitor then moves forward to another round, until an overall winner is declared. Haleem says, "Our community here is not so big and pretty much everyone is familiar with each other, if you have put some years into the dance, and with the help of social media. And there are so many places we all go as a community to dance." These places include clubs, dancers' basements, studios, and outdoor venues that are so prevalent in Detroit.

The Jit community is comprised mostly of male dancers but that's changing some. Gabrielle McLeod, mentioned earlier, is a strong, athletic Jitter who dances with such elegant ease that it's as if she never even walked, only Jitted. Gabrielle says that women Jitters bring uniqueness to Jit because

> obviously, we are women. But it's mostly personal and reflects who we are as individuals. When I'm dancing I feel like my body is moving powerfully, physically, as if frantic, but it's a smooth kind of frantic. Hard and smooth along with gritty and soulful and techno music brings those two together. It may look hard on the outside but it also has to be smooth and soulful on the inside. It puts you in another zone. It's not organic, not an easy technique to learn, and it has to become a part of you.[4]

One of the other dancers, Alonzo Walker, who directs Positive Surroundings, a dance and film production company in Detroit, is laserlike and precise in his attack, and thinks of Jit as both a mental and spiritual practice:

> Jit'n is mental, because you've got to be keeping your movement in mind, you know, what you're going to do next. But it's spiritual, too. When Jit'n, you're on a different plane and you're one with the music vibes.[5]

It's no surprise that Jit dance linked up with Detroit techno music, the electronic music spearheaded by the three musicians Juan Atkins, Derrick May, and Kevin Saunderson, who have experimented, worked, and played music together since their school days in Belleville, Michigan, a suburb of Detroit. At a panel discussion at the Museum of Contemporary Art Detroit in May 2016, Atkins, May, and Saunderson talk about the influence of Detroit-based

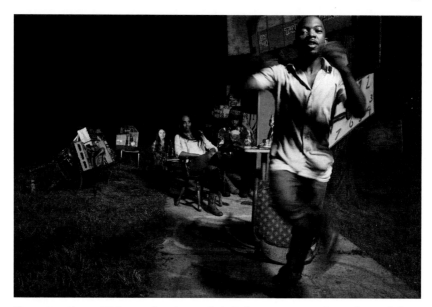

Figure 8.4. Alonzo Walker performing a solo in *Jitdance: Detroit Redux*, at the Heidelberg Project, Detroit. Photo © 2016 by Andrew Milosz.

experimental radio stations on their development as young musicians (Atkins 2016). As test markets for music, these loosely formatted radio stations such as WDRQ, WLBS, WGPR, and WJLB thrilled the three friends with a mixed-bag offering of genres and styles, including Kraftwerk, the B-52s, and Prince. DJ Charles Johnson, better known by his radio name of "The Electrifying Mojo," was a particular inspiration, giving Juan Atkins his first break when Atkins's pal, May, hung out at a diner Mojo frequented in the middle of the night, just to pass off Atkins's music to him. In its hypersonic tempo, techno music is the perfect fit with a dance form that is anaerobic and full throttle ahead, with lighteningspeed footwork. It also has its roots in Detroit culture so it *feels* right to Jit dancers.

Producing Place and Body

As Haleem, Ayhan, and I talk and walk around the Heidelberg we begin to interpret the environment and plan our screendance. By nature of the surroundings, our path is circuitous, our conversation rambling, irregular. We step up wood stairs to an open structure and peer down into the basements of burned-out dwellings; the shrill caw of crows pricks the steely gray sky overhead. Our exploration is yielding a screendance soon to be and mirroring the thoughts of Casey: "Between the extremes of exploration and inhabitation lies an entire middle realm, for the most part neglected in previous investigations of built space, that calls for our concerted attention" (1993, 120–121). No, we are not in the cultural hub of downtown Detroit or the cool Cass corridor. We are in East Detroit, surrounded by an area yielding the highest crime rate in the city. We are in an art environment produced by a local Detroiter, traversed by thousands and produced by all, including us. Here in this *place* we interact with each other in certain ways as we stroll across this well-planned wilderness.

Then, out of nowhere, Haleem laughs, starts to say something, and then stops.

"What, Haleem?" I prod.

He starts laughing again and gets me laughing, too, although I have no idea what I'm laughing about. Then he tells me. He envisions one of the dancers wearing a teddy-bear backpack.

"Um . . . whhhaaaaat . . . ?" I ask. "A teddy-bear backpack?!"

We both laugh.

"Really!" he confirms. "I mean it! I brought a friend from out of town here a couple of weeks ago and ever since I've been having this image of the dancers wearing teddy-bear backpacks."

Now I know he's serious.

"Um," I smile, "Do you think Alonzo and James will agree to wearing a teddy-bear backpack?"

We both start laughing again, but from Haleem's initial image the screendance takes off. Anna Shahinian, our petite dancer with the large, expressive eyes, will wear the backpack, and move from place to place in Heidelberg, watching as the other dancers are Jit'n. "I envision abstract forms of dancers merging with the art-sculpts, as if in some sort of surreal cemetery," I offer.

"Sounds like a night film to me!" Ayhan proclaims.

We look at each other, all in agreement that a night shoot at Heidelberg is crazy thinking. But . . . we must! My mind speeds forward, dodging around one red flag after another. Arriving, filming, and departing the Heidelberg Project at night could be challenging. Haleem, Ayhan, and the dancers all agree it would be safe, but I recall that there have been some arsons at Heidelberg in the dark hours. Would the dancers be in jeopardy? The film crew? What about the equipment? Would we even be allowed to film at night? The Heidelberg staff says "Yes" and they tell me that there are security cameras now in operation at night. Still, I figure security guards are a must. Obtaining the correct lighting equipment for night shoots will be an additional expense. My husband's words come back to me. *At night the fountain on Belle Isle lit up in magical colors, and we stood at its edges in absolute awe.* I think to myself, Yes, we must do this.

Months later, when I drop off Ayhan at 5:00 a.m., following our first night of filming *Jitdance*, I remind him that the night film was his idea.

"Yeah," he laughs, "But you didn't say 'No,' Joanna!"

It's Almost All about Time

During frequent visits to the Heidelberg Project, I keep returning to the small, open-air structure called the *Soul House*, comprised only of wood beams, and covered with vinyl LP albums. I keep looking at the sign there in the shape of a cross: *Soul Never Dies*. On the inside, in the middle of a fascinating mise en scène, there's a rusted wagon holding a huge pile of dusty, warped albums in it. I imagine Anna pulling the handle behind her as she proceeds from vignette to vignette of the Jit dancers performing solos, duets, and trios.

At rehearsal I put an old stereo on top of the warped albums in Anna's rusted wagon and she uses it at each stop along the way to "play" the music. This idea beautifully integrates the vignettes of the Jit dancers. Also, Anna is a contemporary and hip-hop dancer and, although she adroitly picks up Haleem's Jit phrases, she doesn't possess the subtle stylistic nuances conveyed

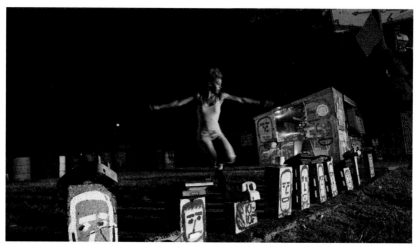

Figure 8.5. Jai Hatcher performing a solo in *Jitdance: Detroit Redux* at the Heidelberg Project, Detroit. Photo © 2016 by Andrew Milosz.

by the professional Jit dancers, even though it's quickly becoming her favorite dance style. As a talking point, a directing point, Anna becomes an Alice in Wonderland figure who observes the fantastical Jitland around her. The dancers dazzle with their moves when she plays one of the warped albums. Sometimes she struggles to learn this puzzling, quick-footed movement; sometimes she simply watches and observes. In the last scene she discovers the *Soul House* where soul never dies, a place where all the Jit dancers, now gathered together, hover in a state of temporary repose. Anna tosses her backpack aside, unties her hair, and enters. When she shakes the arm of one of the dancers the entire group begins to Jit. They point to Anna, no longer the observer, the naive amateur, who at last joins them in their dance for this magical moment sometime before the sun rises and she must leave her new friends behind.[6]

Haleem, Ayhan, the dancers, and I talk about our shared project and its meaning during rehearsal breaks. Essential themes emerge in conversation, go into hiding for a while, and then reappear in mutated forms as rehearsals progress. Will the screendance serve as a metaphor about the silence of Jit dance and its current resurrection? Of the rich history and current transformation of Detroit arts and culture in general? Of the evolution from soul to techno music in Detroit? But I'm curious to hear what others have to say about this: Anna is Caucasian, and the other five dancers are African American. What to make of the white girl, moving among the Jitters, motivating them to dance when she plays the music? Once the film is edited and complete, could the tone be unintentionally menacing? Jit dancer Alonzo Walker says the meaning is about the influence of whites over black music. He also thinks it suggests the historical ebb and flow, the rise and fall and rise again of dance and music in Detroit. For Haleem, the mystery behind the night shoot in this surreal location, along with the distinct dance moves, will invite many interpretations. There'll be a lot of different ways to think about it. Mostly, he feels that "the piece speaks on the state of our dance Jit—that it's somewhat dead or nostalgic—to now having this outside character stumbling across and uncovering a dance form that is full of life, movement, and open to being embraced." He likes the narrative that has emerged and thinks it complements the look and feel of the individual dancers and the different scenes we're using. So, much like the random, serendipitous conversations and qualities discovered at the Heidelberg Project, *Jitdance: Detroit Redux* takes on a spontaneous direction of its own, and then powers full speed ahead to fulfill its cohesive destiny.

The time has come, but the first night of filming unfolds like a comedy of errors. As we are stepping out of the car onto Heidelberg Street, the large, heavy limb of a rotted tree crashes onto the hood. Our cinematographer arrives two hours late because a special project he's shooting for a local TV station runs overtime, and an artist living on Heidelberg Street becomes angry that we won't be including footage of his art work in the dance film. The police arrive and are friendly, but they would like to know what we're doing. I pull my IPhone out of my pocket and quickly scroll to a series of email exchanges between me and the Heidelberg staff that clearly confirms their support of this night film. The police approve. Turning back to the film crew and dancers, I mumble to myself: "I will love you, my little Apple, until the day you drop into my bathtub, I will." It's now 11:30 p.m.

At last, as we film one night after another, we settle into the rhythm of the shoot, totally embracing the weirdness and exhilaration of working late into the night at the Heidelberg Project. The police, now interested in our project return from time to time, serving as a pop-up audience. Also joining the audience are the dancers' friends, some of the neighbors, our security guards, and onlookers who come and go. But just as we're finishing our last night of filming at about 4:00 a.m., a car cruises by and then abruptly circles around to park, even as the security guards walk in their direction. The police have already left, the street is strangely still, and the once hauntingly beautiful artscapes now appear as ghostly aberrations under a couple of yellow-tinged street lights. Five people hop out of their car faster than my 4 a.m. brain can register and my heart starts kicking in my chest. "Hey," yells out Brandon Thomas, one of our security guards who stands six feet and six inches tall. "What's going on over there?" And just as quickly, my heart slows down. It's a group of high school students here to enjoy the Heidelberg in the dark.

Only a week has passed since filming when big news breaks in Detroit. Tyree Guyton announces that he has decided to dismantle Heidelberg over a period of two years. All outside activities at Heidelberg will be stopped immediately. Haleem, Ayhan, and I are ecstatic that we made it just under the wire before this unexpected turn of events, but we're dismayed, too, that the Heidelberg will close. Tyree says that after thirty years it's time to do something new, something different. A couple of months later, in October 2016, Tyree grants me an interview, parts of which have already been cited in this chapter.

"Thirty years!" he says. "I've been traveling in the same direction, and I woke up one morning and it hit me—that it was okay to travel in a different direction. We don't know what tomorrow will bring, but we take it for granted. Today you're here. Today you're dead. Just like that."

I nod, fully comprehending.

He continues, "I welcome change, I need it. You're going to lose your hair. You're going to lose your teeth. Your body's going to start changing. Your diet is going to change. Things you used to eat a long time ago, you can't eat anymore. Change. So I've got to change the Heidelberg."

Tyree wants to shake things up at the Heidelberg, make it different, and he will become the alchemist, the magician once again, ready to move out of life's way and let it take him where he needs to be.

"Don't stop dancing," he says to me.

"Never!" I smile. "*Soul never dies.*"

Meanwhile, in writing this chapter, I have rediscovered the place of Detroit, beginning with a reflective description of my biases and interest in the screendance project and the employment of hermeneutic phenomenology as an approach to better understand the process. Eventually, I addressed the historical, sociocultural, and aesthetic basis of both the Heidelberg Project and Detroit Jit dance, followed by an exploration of the making of the film in collaboration with other artists. Our collective efforts have followed a circuitous road of dead-ends, detours, and side streets, offering a heightened understanding of filming *Jitdance* and the fluid, ever-changing urban landscape of *Detroit Redux*.

Notes

1. Richardson, Harrison. Personal interview. August 5, 2015. In front of the Detroit Central Train Station.

2. Guyton, Tyree. Personal interview. October 28, 2016. The Heidelberg Project office, Watson Street, Detroit.

3. Rasul, Haleem Stringz. Personal interview. August 6, 2016. The Heidelberg Project, Detroit.

4. McLeod, Gabrielle. Personal interview. August 4, 2016. The Heidelberg Project, Detroit.

5. Walker, Alonzo. Personal interview. August 3, 2016. The Heidelberg Project, Detroit.

6. To see the screendance, *Jitdance: Detroit Redux*, go to https://vimeo.com/211224648 (accessed July 16, 2016).

9

Being *Ma*

Moonlight Peeping through the Doorway

CHRISTINE BELLEROSE

In my body when I dance
when I am still
in the way I move—*Ma*, moonlit memory
was *ma* with me all along?

> "Do not think flowing is like wind and rain moving from east to
> west.
> The entire world is not unchangeable, is not immovable. It flows."
> —Excerpt from *Uji* by Dōgen, *Zen Sourcebook* 159.

Uji (*The Time Being*) by Zen Master Dōgen (1200–1253) is "a rare Zen study of
the complex question of time, in which Dōgen asks his followers to actualize
all time as being, which can only be accomplished by vigorously abiding in
each moment" (Kasulis 2004, 141).

In this chapter, "Being *Ma*," through dance and performance moves alongside continental phenomenology and Shintō Zen philosophies. In doing so,
it reveals but the tip of the relationship between being human and being a
human spirited-body as part of the world's body.

Serendipity played a role in tracing the path of my research on *ma*, as
it continues to do so today. I remind myself throughout to keep an open
mind, as phenomenologists do, and allow myself to be surprised by multiple
encounters with performers and scholars in dance and Japanese / Chinese
philosophies. I began my movement practice in Montréal, where I was born.
Movement observation brought me to Hanoi in 1999, eventually working with
Dr. Vu Thi Thanh Huong at the Centre for Linguistics and Vietnamese Studies

in Hanoi. From there, I moved to China where I lived until the 2008 Beijing Olympics. By another twist of faith, I met, in December 2014, with scholar, dancer, butoh-ka (butoh dancer), and somatic teacher Sondra Fraleigh during her workshop and conference in Utah. I further had the opportunity to dialogue with favorite topics of hers: *ma* presence, the lived body, conscious movement, and the somatic approach as they bear world-memories and embodied narratives. During the week, I explored solo eco-performances in mountains, rivers, and barren lands. At the time of my meeting with Fraleigh, I was beginning my *ma* journey and had very little understanding of *ma*. Fraleigh became a touchstone for *ma* inquiry as she imprinted on me her *savoir*. The significance of her guidance on my existence, and on my understanding of Japanese aesthetics through phenomenology and somatic arts, resonates within.

Ma, concept of space-time, has a long history in Japan and also translates into some Western performance philosophies. As a space-time concept of embodiment, *ma* exists at the threshold of corporeal experiences. *Ma* permeates the cosmological flow of Shintō Zen divinities' order, and it enters the contemporary dance philosophy of butoh as embodied flow. Butoh, the dance form originating in post–WWII Japan, migrates as a spatio-temporal and ecological perspective adopted by a number of movement art practitioners outside of Japan. This chapter on being *ma* aims to describe a conceptual space-time as experienced in its relationship with artistic intent in performance, with examples from butoh and durational performance practice. My *ma* journey also draws upon my own performance experience and philosophies of existential phenomenology. *Being Ma* resides at the nexus of *ma* and the *lived body*.

Approaching *Ma*

Being ma is a condition I strive to attain in my own somatic performance practice. It is no coincidence that my embodied research grew from an imprint of phenomenological space-time and space-time conceived in Shintō (神道) and Zen (禅) / Chan (禪 or 禅). My own path is a mix of original and displaced roots. French-Québecois is my mother tongue. I live to the East and to the West. Once, a longtime resident of Beijing, now at the time of writing these lines, I live in Gatineau (Québec). Author Sarah Bakewell's recent depiction of philosophy as "a discipline for flourishing and living a fully human, responsible life" resonates with my worldview on artistic practice and research (2016, 16). Bakewell tells the story of how Friedrich Nietzsche and Søren Kierkegaard pioneered what would become existential phenomenology, with French philosopher Jean-Paul Sartre as the bridge (16–25).

My way of living *ma* accords with the Sartrean position that "I exist" (1963a). I invent myself through freedom, a theme of Sartre's. Freedom of movement exists in my dance. In recognizing that such freedom comes with responsibility, I live in "good faith," a term that Sartre made famous. My somatic practice of *ma* is an expression of my being—"existence precedes essence" (Sartre 1963b). Sartre's insight that existence comes first means that nothing is "in essence" pre-given. The existential position in accounting for reflexive and embodied research methods opens the possibility of "connecting to what might crossover my own experience" (Fraleigh, personal correspondence, 2015). In living a dimension of in-between places, my encounter with *ma* shapes how I approach research and how I dance. "*Ma* is an experiential definition" (Kasulis 2004, 11). And like the experiential somatics of *ma*, phenomenology makes sense when experienced in the flesh.

My approach to *ma* emerges from experiential journeys in life and performance. My positioning of self between East and West, by definition an ontological study of being, opens the possibility for what Edmund Husserl at the root of phenomenology terms "empathy," or "experiencing someone else" (1960, 146). In a state of empathic awareness, I connect to myself and to my surroundings, to humans, nonhumans, and elements of nature. Connectedness allows me to "create a sense of place," how architect and Japanese garden aficionado Günter Nitschke explains this Shintō philosophy, an expression implicit to architectural design ("ma-dori" 間取り) (1993, 56).

I gained my first meaningful insight on *ma* in 2015 in Québec city when friend and dancer Amélie Gagnon shared with me the story of a choreographer asking her for "more *ma*." The anecdote stuck with me. I wondered: What is this *ma* that cannot be explained, yet which is key to enliven dance? I let the process inform me: "I am peeling away at something deeper that I am missing" (Fraleigh, personal correspondence, 2015).

MA IN SPACE-TIME

Ma is challenging to explain in English for all the reasons involved in translating a historical and cultural concept. It does not help that very few writings exist about *ma*, let alone in a Western language. For practical reasons, the knowledge of *ma* is transmitted via practice. *Ma* is first a Shintō concept originating in Japan, which evolved through layers of Zen Buddhism influences. Philosopher of religion Thomas P. Kasulis writes of Shintō that "it is particularly difficult to explain, even for most Japanese" (2004, 1); yet, in his teaching, he shows that there is nothing so alien in the ordinary spiritual experience of Shintō that most people cannot understand it (38). I have a sense that it is not so much *ma* that is difficult to translate but the space-time dimension in which it lives.

In this chapter, I aim to accompany the readers on a journey of *ma*, not directly through its historical or cultural identity, but rather through the way it moves and its affect. *Ma* cuts across time-space experience, and also holds perspectives of temporality and spatiality. *Ma* ferries aliveness between bodies and through bodies. In turn, bodies move with *ma*. However, *ma* does not remain locked in one body. Waves cycle *ma*, entering and exiting *ma* in a never-ending echo of its undulation. Space-time is moved through *ma*; in turn, beings absorb and liberate its movement affects. *Ma* dynamic is that of flow connecting spaces (of place and bodies). The phenomenologist Maurice Merleau-Ponty says that "our body is not primarily in space: it is of space" (1962, 171).

Spatial-temporal awareness is key to engaging with the etherealness of *ma*, while action is key to activate it. The ebb and flow of *ma* is embodied in human movement and action, encouraging connective awareness. Such awareness of *ma* acknowledges an empathic sense of *one-self* and *other-as-self*, a perspective I develop later through Merleau-Ponty's phenomenology of *entrelacs* (entwining).

The Body Portal

An original collage of *ma*, in the *Kanji* of Figure 9.1, reveals the meaning of *ma* as "moonlight peeping through the doorway" (Nitschke 1966, 116). Nitschke draws back to the original Chinese pictorial, the sign for the element "moon." In its early form, the pictogram for "sun" had, in its center, a dot rather than a dash. The dash, explains sinologue Wang Hongyuan, signifies "light" (1994, 31). The cover art for the exhibition catalogue, *MA: Space-Time in Japan*, depicts a calligraphy of *ma*. At the center of one lattice is a sign for light not yet transformed as sun. *C'est à dire*, the moon is in its transformation toward becoming the sun. It is a turning of the day into night and the night into day. It means "not moon" or "day sun" (Nitschke 1966, 116).

The elements of the sun and the moon; the interval and in-betweenness; light and dark in their glow, all point to layers of change and traces of ancestry. The change of meaning for the same idea, and the ideogram change for one idea are parts of the ebb and flow of *ma*, as meaning-in-the-making. In a poetic sense, *ma* is a verb because *ma* functions as a journey.

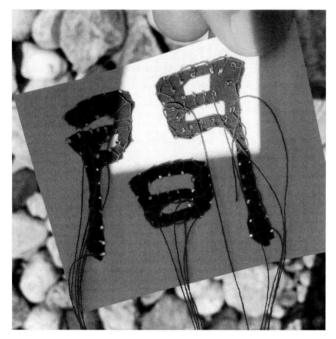

Figure 9.1. Collage of *Kanji ma.*

Through embodied practices of dance and performance, Merleau-Ponty's philosophy of flesh and folding moves and entwines (1968a). Chiasm is a crisscrossing of intention or material. For the example, we can think of fabric in light of *entrelacs* to illustrate the dynamics of chiasmic connections and intervals, considering the possible twinings of warp and woof. Intertwining—Chiasm—is Merleau-Ponty's philosophy of somatic (experienced) connectedness. It is significant to this essay that Chiasm and the philosophy of Shintō Zen are similar. Through *entrelacs*, the relation between the material and spiritual may be external, internal, and/or both. "But, the material never exists without *some* relation to the spiritual" (Nitschke 1993, 16).

The complexity of intertwined elements, inner/outer and material/spiritual, is key to understanding the complexity of Japanese/Chinese pictograms, just as one difficulty of defining *ma* resides in the structure of Japanese language where words overlay ideas. *Ma,* for instance, describes "a channel of communality of creation" and, at the same time, "the demon's possession," explains poet Shuzo Takiguchi (qtd. by Isozaki 2001, 11). Japanese words and stories are inscribed in written ideograms that evoke imagery. Accordingly, *ma* evolved from a two-lattice door within which, at times a moonlight, and at other times, a sun appears, as I have mentioned. The story of *ma*'s meaning resides in an evolving cosmology and adapting ideogram. The cosmology of *ma* is best addressed in contextualizing key actors in the story of *ma*. These would be *kami*, divinities in eternal flow drive; *himorogi*, which alters serving as temporary bodies for the *kami*; and the idea of *hashi* as "in-betweenness," as architect and installation artist Isozaki Arata likes to frame *ma*. I consider each of these more fully in the next sections.

There is a wealth of stories related to the cosmology of *ma* in "Man TRANS-forms" exhibition at the Cooper-Hewitt, National Design Museum (1976–1977) designed by Japanese architect Isozaki Arata and curated by Hans Hollein. The exhibition is documented in "MA: Space-Time in Japan," produced by The Smithsonian Institution (1979). In complement to the documentation of the art aesthetic of "ManTRANSforms," Isozaki's theoretical writing on Western and Eastern architecture offers a popular, yet rich, historical and cultural explanation of the experienced space and time of Japan. In the early 1960s, Western architects, like Günter Nitschke, turned to Eastern cultures with the aim to broaden not only architectural research but also to "define a new anthropological field of human inquiry" (1993, 7). These readings show how the Western concept of place relates to the concept of space as it exists in the Japanese imagination.

The writing of these scholars and artists re-center *ma* in its space-time environment. For the purpose of this chapter, I condense the cosmology of *ma* described by architect Isozaki, photographer Futagawa Yukio, artist Kuramata Shiro, editor Matsuoka Seigow, dress designer Miyaki Issey, and sculptor Miyawaki Aiko, and Nitschke, identifying a few of the essential concepts of *ma*: *kami*, *himoroji*, *hashi*, *utsuroi*, and *michiyuki*. These orient us in environmental nature, while linking to the unseen as well, as we see later.

KAMI (SPIRIT)

Understanding *ma* first requires us to consider *kami* divinities in Japanese cosmology. *Kami* are divinities that permeate the cosmos. These entities have no bodies, nor do they take the shape of a body. *Kami* have no shape, nor does *ma*. They exist and appear in shape-specific objects. In nature, objects that *kami* favor are identified as emblematic of the presence of *kami*: pine trees, bamboo shoots, plum flower trees, round boulders, conical sand piles, waterfalls, the full moon, and so forth. *Kami* descend or ascend through these objects.

Kami are responsible for ruling the ebb and flow of all creation. They eternally flow through and out. A *kami* is contained only in passing. To invite *kami* in, there needs to be a material object serving as its temporary body.

Through this imagery, one can sense *kami* in the creative juice of dancers. Poetically, *kami* are present in a dancer's flow. This brings to mind *chi* or *q'i*, the essence of life, as believed in Chinese traditional medicine, and *en*, a concept of transactional space that Nitschke writes about. However, similar to *chi*, the ebb and flow of *kami* through *ma* has an essence of its own.

HIMOROGI (BODY)

Himorogi is an altar that is built to offer such a temporary body to *kami*. The *himorogi* is a coded structure. At its rudimentary shape, it has four pillars. A rope is tied to its central pole. The *himorogi* altar recalls the anatomy of the human body: the four limbs, the heart, and the nervous system. Butoh Company *Dairakurakan* founder, Maro Akaji, explains that gods and humans meet within the human body; "there are those who believe that the body is moved by unseen forces that inhabit the flesh" (Blackwood 1990). Altar of wood, altar of flesh: *ma* regulates a flow between bodies thereby connecting bodies.

Himorogi range from temporary makeshifts to fixed elaborately decorated structures. Its architecture continues to influence urban planning and design of entire cities in Japan. Sidney Pink, an American artist who lived in Japan in the 2000s, shared with me anecdotes of having to walk around *himorogi* because in some places *himorogi* would obstruct a way of passage. Pink showed me a photograph he took of his residence where such *himorogi* lodged in the way of the car park, according to its Shintō Zen specific placement. Pink reflected that *himorogi* affect the walking flow of urban dwellers, in turn imprinting the passersby with a Shintō Zen *ma* walk (Sidney Pink, personal correspondence, 2016).

HASHI (INTERVAL)

As interval, *ma* flows between and connects bodies. *Ma* as perspective serves to expand an understanding of its in-betweenness quality. Isozaki, creator of the exhibition entitled "ManTRANSforms," describes in his essay, "*Ma* (Interstice) and Rubble," his frustration of expressing in English ideas that "could adequately be constructed only in Japanese" (2001, 91). Out of this frustration was born the design of the exhibition. Isokazi's own piece, *Angel Cage*, is an installation of winged statues inside a larger-than-life birdcage. The largeness of the structure allows the spectator multiple perspectives of in-betweenness, by walking through and seeing from above. In Isozaki's words, "the ambiguity of this 'membrane' or interface that divides interior and exterior," permeates the many meanings of the homophone *hashi* (93). *Ma* in-between sits between *hashi*.

In a passage from "Ma (Interstice) and Rubble," Isozaki explains his belief of the *ma* interstice as it relates to ancestral time and space: "I believe it necessary to return to an undifferentiated time and space. In Japanese, when the concept of time (時間) and space (空間) were first written down, the Chinese ideogram *ma* (間)—an interstice—was used as the second character for both. I determined the search for clues in this space in between" (90).

The idea *hashi* describes is a space between two edges. *Hashi* translates to the real world into things like chopsticks ("hashi" 箸), ladder and stairs ("hashi go" 梯子), and ideas of bridge, border, steps, the end, margin, and so forth. In an image sense, *hashi* borders the *ma* unseen, revealing it. It delimits *ma*, as it also delimits the void/cosmos where *kami* live. It is *hashi* that gives *ma* its in-between quality. "So it is possible to understand *hashi* as

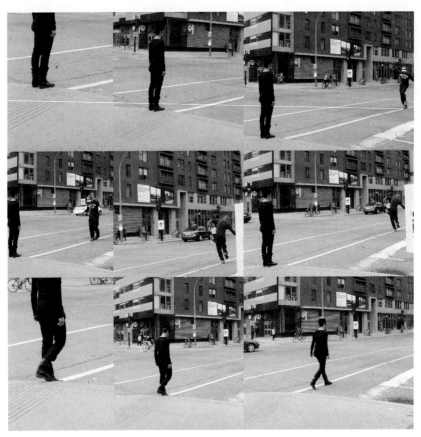

Figure 9.2. Martine Viale. Durational Art Performance: *Chronology of an Action, Ma Intervalle.* Photograph © 2014 by Martin Dufrasne. Courtesy, Martine Viale.

a concept that relates couples of contradictory terms; the term disjoins and also connects two worlds," Isozaki explains (93).

Artist Martine Viale, shown in Figure 9.2, trained in her early adulthood in Japan under master Tanaka Min and his son at the Body Weather Farm, which was originally for butoh experiential performance but now has branched into other forms. She has carried the strict discipline quality over to her practice of durational art performance. Since 2013, Viale has been exploring the interval, through performances she calls *Ma Intervalle (actions infiltrantes)* and *Ma Intervalle.* Based in Montréal, Canada, since the early stage of her artistic career, she currently lives in Perpignan, France.

In an interview (February 20, 2015), I asked Viale about her work with *ma* and her play on its various themes. For each performance, she deconstructs *ma*, negotiating one aspect of it while composing with it. Through this process, Viale performs her recollections of the connections and disjoins of an interval. In one of her performances, the artist composed with *ma* as possession, playing on the French language ("adjectif féminin possessif de la première personne du singulier"), the feminine possessive adjective of the singular for the first person. The artist understands *ma* cannot be held; it really is a play on words and perceptions. She also works on the interval between female and male, seeking hybrid qualities over uniqueness. By choosing to work in public spaces, Viale looks for spaces that are benign, like fringe spaces without much of a sense of meaning or purpose. She then activates their meaning in the process of working with the interval between purpose and possibilities.

The artist speaks of the difficulty of pinning down the interval: "There is so much that eludes me in the interval. It is a perspective of every 'possibles.'" Viale makes use of empty space, hidden space, and the silence of the interval, remarking on there being possibilities within the act itself. During one of our meetings, she demonstrates this by pouring out the liquid from her drinking glass into another glass. In this demonstration, Viale explained that *ma* is the act of not filling up the glass to the brim. The void, the empty space at the top, is the interval, the space of possibilities.

An existentialist philosophy guides her from the start of the project in 2013, when she asked herself if it was possible to simply *be and remain* in the interval. By her own account in our interview, Viale connects her *ma* interval journey with her visit to Japan a long time ago where she first encountered *ma*. The *ma* that was introduced to her in Japan had stayed with her all these years. And eventually, in its own time, Viale came back to it. *Ma* existed within, exerting a will of its own. The interval between life and art is a thin one.

Her work is comparable to butoh and contemporary dance practices, yet unique. Viale moves with spatial awareness of self and body, and her movements have very little embellishment. The aesthetic function of a movement, for Viale, is in its function of composing space through her intervention in space. Penetrating, cunning, and extremely receptive, the performer seeks the interval; yet, through her space-sensitive work, she transcends the interval of an interval and embodies the *hashi*, the edge.

With site-specific performances, Viale looks for a relationship of contrast between herself and the space. For the *Ma Intervalle (actions infiltrantes)* project, the artist performed in the wooden staircase at Place des Arts, the Café Van Houtte, the red bench facing Complexe Desjardins, Le Chemin de la Reine, and all recognizable landmarks in the city of Montréal. By doing so, Viale was seeking a contrast to the proposed convention. The artist confesses that at times her work is performed in a spirit of intentionality. At other times, it is in a state of awareness (fr. *présence*). At still other times, her work is performed as an intuitive act of removal (of art, artist, and place). *Ma Intervalle (actions infiltrantes)* took place in the same seven spaces over the course of four seasons, thus putting emphasis on time, and the passage of time.

During a workshop I took with Viale in Montréal ("Laboratory of the Body / Butoh," 2015), she confessed to the group that if she were to perform one more day of this piece, she would stay out of the picture. After four seasons, the performance had reached a point in time where it had accomplished its wholeness. After four seasons, the interval itself had become an artifact imprinted by the artist's performative legacy. The distinct purpose of the piece, filling intervals, had reached its satiety. Of course, there are many more gaps to fill, cracks and holes and dents in the sector Viale operated on. Not being present on site would have been a performance consecrating the echo of *ma*. Not being on site plays on the visible-invisible interval paradox generative of an art-intent.

Such a play on appearance and disappearance is at play in a performance of *Ma Intervalle (actions infiltrantes)*, which she did at a public bus stop. Viale, half hiding herself inside the bus shelter, let passersby see her double—the hidden revealed by her reflection in the glass window, and the visible revealed plainly in sight. In this work, Viale explores multiplicity of presence: "I am, and I am in the reflection of the glass panel," Viale says. Her work of rhythm, pace, and reflection explores the interstice of the interval.

It is of note that appearance and disappearance is a signature butoh process taught by Nakajima Natsu, who was a female founder of butoh (Fraleigh, email conversation, 2016). For Viale and in butoh, it is the mover who holds the power of appearing and disappearing.

How *Ma* Moves

UTSUROI (CHANGE)

To illustrate what Isozaki describes as "*ma* coordinating a moment from one place to another," I turn to rhythms and pace as I found how Isozaki illustrates the role of *ustsuroi* and *michiyuki* (2001, 17). *Ma* is a sort of bellboy for *kami*. When the divinities enter *hashi*, *ma* sets off the bell. "*Ma* is the way of sensing the moment of movement" (14). Two phenomena signal the moment and the interval between moments: the moment is *utsuroi*; its measure between manifestation is *michiyuki*. *Utsuroi* corroborates transformation and movement. It develops as *utsuru* meaning "change" (ibid.). *Utsuroi* is a compound-sign meaning "activated cosmos" (ibid.). By breaking down the idea, we can understand the role of *ma* as both spatial and temporal activator, and as an actor of change.

The moment of change in movement is echoed in the butoh of Takenouchi Atsushi through his practice of the art of transforming or shape-shifting. His performance of *Skin* at the 2012 Seattle Butoh Festival (October 27) stands out in this regard. Takenouchi is a master of shape-shifting, of "alchemy in motion" (Fraleigh 2010, 41). He dances his humanity, as also other beings and nonbeings. Takenouchi's worldwide influence extends to majestic landscapes of ice glaciers in Alaska and pained grounds of the Killing Fields in Cambodia. His performance *ma* yokes dance and healing. A disciple of butoh founders Ohno and Hijikata, Takenouchi eventually evolved his own branch, the Jinen form of butoh. "Jinen Butoh" celebrates the healing of the self in relation to the landscape (Takenouchi, website).

Invoking *ma*, Takenouchi shapes space as land and nature. His embodied impulses extend in movements of great power and urgency. Dancing with a feeling for liminal space-time *ma* and projecting a sense of magic, the dancer transforms from human-dancer to the storied bodies he dances—whether these be plant, mountain, or animal. Fraleigh writes of Takenouchi's dance, "its butoh alchemy moves through ineffable spaces 'in between'" (2010, 76). The ability of a dancer to process coming and going between worlds, of space and place, creates the possibility to shift time and space.

The shape-shifting his performances afford inheres in his ability to play with moments in time. Speed and near stillness create images of shifting time. Takenouchi activates temporal possibilities contained in the cosmos of an amphitheater, or in the execution of his site-specific performances. His Jinen butoh connects human consciousness to nature as *Skin*, and to the skin of the cosmos.

MICHIYUKI (CREATIVE RHYTHM)

Dance critic Goda Nario explains *ma*, "when the dancer is with rhythm, it is thin. When the dance is off the rhythm, you can selectively perceive the whole in the gaps" (Fraleigh, 1999b, 176).

Earlier in my research, I had the great luck of connecting with Iwase Kanako, a Japanese Classical Dancer of *Nihon Buyo*. She was born and raised in Japan, where she began studying dance at an early age. During her graduate studies in New York City, she continued her training of *Nihon Buyo* with Master Sachiyo Ito. During our interview of March 7, 2015, Iwase spoke of her experience from an embodied point of view, drawing from her own dance practice through childhood in Japan and the dance company she belonged to in New York City. "How did you experience or encounter *ma*?" I asked Iwase.

Ma, as I have said, is integral to butoh sensibility, and Iwase explained that *ma* also integrally exists in *Nihon Buyo*. By her account, the definition of *ma* as interval-space and the body as a vessel inviting spirits is in much more researched contemporary somatic practices than in traditional indigenous Japanese dances. Iwase spoke about her understanding of *ma* and how it regulates a time interval of being with-rhythm and off-rhythm.

Iwase's experience as a practicing student of the *Nihon Buyo* began as a child. She danced eighteen years with the same teacher in Japan. All this time she followed and copied her dance teacher's every movement. The pedagogy of her childhood teacher offered no space for creative rhythm, tempo, or self-expression. This type of teaching is called, "shadowing" the master. In contrast, the experience Iwase had while studying a very short time with Sachiyo in New York City allowed her personal signature into the dance.

In her experience of shadowing the teacher's dance, *ma* meant following the tempo of a song. This *ma* rhythm was on time with the tempo. When the teacher asked a pupil to find *ma*, the dancer was expected to find the tempo. In this way, Iwase danced with the tempo. She describes the experience as a meditative exercise, as the body dances in time with the regular and cyclical rhythm of *ma*. Precision and codes reflect the structure of the movements of *kami* passing through *himorogi*. Such codes are reflected in Western classical ballet, and *Nihon Buyo*. *Ma* regulated represents an alignment of "together with."

Paradoxically, breaking the rhythm is also another element of Japanese Classical Dance. *Ma* represents perceptual attunement to the irregularities of time. When performances are opened to the public, they enlarge the space of perceptual resonance to include a much wider place for *ma* to echo through. As the ongoing dynamic exchange between dance and audience begins, dancers take agency of the pacing of the tempo and flow, executing the specific movements. A stage performance must involve the audience's sense of projection and recuperation of flow for them to pay attention to the dance.

In our interview (March 7, 2015), Iwase explains *ma* off-rhythm. *Ma* off-rhythm offsets the audience's expectation of tempo and flow. Dancers and musicians together activate space through dissonance and off-rhythm, playing with possibilities of *michiyuki*. Thus, the audience is kept in a state of participatory alertness. In such cases, space is transformed by the timely action of the mover. Isozaki explains that "space is divided invisibly by one's movement and breathing" (Isozaki 2001, 17).

In attunement to irregularities of time (as explained above), *ma* is to time in space what rhythm is to movement. It is the mover who holds the agency of regulating tempo: running, skipping, gliding, stepping one foot at a time (or both), and so on. The dancer punctuates the melodic phrase through movements: brisk, largo, speeding up and slowing down, syncopating and holding off until the chosen moment. While *utsuroi* signs the moment of change, *michiyuki* signs the interval between times. In the realm of dance, *usturoi* and *michiyuki* may be understood as rhythm and pace. In the living paradox of being on and off rhythm, *ma* resonates in motion.

BEING DANCED

The crescent moon
becomes full and wanes
until nothing is left—But there it is again
the moon at dawn.

> Excerpt from *The Secret Skill of Great Peace*, by Zen Master Ikkyū Sōjun (1394–1481) *Zen Sourcebook*, 2008, 204.

The *kanji* of *ma* in Figure 9.2 paints perspectives of *bodily becoming through movement*. The body in this image is expressed as *ma* portal. For the dancer to experience being a portal is to experience *being danced*.

Merleau-Ponty describes a phenomenology of body as portal, with the qualities of "obverse" and "reverse, or "flesh and folding," as I stated earlier. Rather than concentrating on a two-dimensional duality, he develops two parts of a whole, or the wholistic body-portal, as I understand it. Dancing as portal, I evolve and change, understanding that all creations are in a state of becoming.

As a somatic image, Merleau-Ponty's idea of being inside and outside draws on a perception of *irréalizer*, the nontranslatable French word Merleau-Ponty invented, possibly with a close meaning of "more-than-realizing." He used *irréalizer* to explain the lived-connection experienced by touching another as if touching oneself. Where connection draws on existentialism, the image of myself as the inside and the outside is also inspired from a celebrated existential thought put forth by Sartre, "by choosing the self, one being choses [*sic*] herself as all beings" (fr. *en se choississant, on choisit tous les hommes*) (qtd. in Guigot 2013, 5).

Dancing the body as portal involves becoming the dance as channeling experience through *ma* connectivity. Poet Shuzo speaks to this wide possibility, "*ma* is a channel opened to all, everywhere and always" (qtd. by Isozaki, in 2001, 11). Channeling is the action of connecting with essences of beings, human and other, earthly and otherworldly. For the earthbound dancing body, channeling translates as somatic awareness activation, enlivening, perhaps, a spirited-dance. One process of channeling involves breathing-in the world and breathing-out in the world. It is a process that involves bodily transformation, which we have said exists in the cosmology of *ma*.

When a choreographer asks a dancer for "more *ma*," the dancer is asked to perform vitality. A dancer who yields *ma* brings qualities of aliveness to an otherwise neutral, or unborn, space-time. Fraleigh exposes space and time as neutral, "until we move them" (1987, 185). Beyond a perfectly executed movement, the dancer channels magical spirited qualities. To witness Takenouchi's dancing with awareness is to witness a whole space vibrating with energy. His being appears a portal through which flows trans-species connection. The channel by which he travels turns outward to move back inside, as he himself transforms on stage. Takenouchi, like the lung of the world, appears to receive *ma*, and to send out *ma*, reflecting the moon and the sun.

MA SENSE

Nitschke expresses beautifully the richness of *ma* meanings, as the objective sense of place, the subjective felt sense, and the metaphysical sense. The architect proposes *ma* as possibly an additional human sense. *Ma* carries a felt sense that can make movement beautiful.

Nitschke's description of a metaphysical sense is comparable to theorist Rudolph Laban's weight buoyancy praxis, which is neither heavy nor light. In terms of impulse, buoyancy is neither fixed nor is it reactive. A sense of freedom and a sense of tension exist together with the idea of buoyancy. *Ma* exists in both freedom and in tension. *Ma* lodges in the liminal moment between facing a decision and being transformed by action on the decision. Dance theorist Irmgard Bartenieff writes, "without tension, there is no change, no life, no experimentation, no communication, no dance" (1980, 192). Buoyancy acknowledges tension while freely allowing it to go on.

A Personal Encounter with *Ma*

Accordingly, in 2014, I explored rivers and canyons of Southwest Utah, for the first time in the towering cliffs of the Ancestral Puebloans at Mukuntuweap National Monument, also known as Zion National Park. Later over the course of two years, I had the opportunity to experience embodied affects of freedom and tension in a buoyant *ma* emanating from this environment.

In late December of 2014, I performed *Healing my Mother*, alone with my surroundings and a video camera (see Plate 7). The following year, I continued my exploratory dance of dynamic exchange between landscapes and the human. In the series *Healing my Mother* I put myself in a perspective of acutely sensing incoming and outgoing influences. I gave myself freedom to intentionally imprint and be imprinted. The heat of my body impacted the ice, and the ice melted. My body became colder upon touching the ice. My dance resonated out of my body into my surroundings, and they echoed back, regenerating my narrative. In a Sartrean perspective, I invented both self and otherness through my actions. My freedom built on artistic intention, and not on thinking an act that I had to do.

I entered in a conversation with the ice. In the interval between the landscape and me, I experienced what I will call "a somatic radiance-echo." I experienced *ma* in action as a frequency and organic modulation. I remained there for what felt like a long time, almost still—but for a spirited and agitated body *vibrating* at the speed of ice! In his workshops, butoh teacher Mario Veillette speaks of movement echoes, which is how I sensed *ma*. As I performed slow buoyant flow, I received and gave out energy, connecting to my surroundings.

I understood my wholistic relationship to the land without the conviction of having thought an answer; I pained to wait for the next impulse, yet I never grew bored because waiting itself is a moment already full of *ma*. A sensation of regeneration permeated my body and soul. I felt what Fraleigh explains as, "a dance existing through the body" (1987, 50). Through my own experience, and listening to artists sharing their own experience, I observe that artists in their creative processes create from something (fr. *à partir de quelque chose*) while at the same time create from nothing (fr. *à partir de rien*).

On the premise that creation is a personal and a collective interweave, there is also the promise that the personal serves the collective, and the collective serves the personal. The collective is already an *entrelacs*, as is creativity. Because *ma* exists in-between, *ma* is in continuous and eternal creation. In Sartrean existential philosophy, this condition refers to the "exigency of creation" (fr. *l'exigence de la création*) (in Guigot 2013, 9). *Ma* exists in a slippery in-between; paradoxically, as it passes, it is born. This "necessary moment" (fr. *ce moment nécessaire)* (6) is the moment where creation is actualized and the essence of *ma* becomes. This elusive moment of time being (moonlight peeping through the doorway) is also discussed in the *Uji* masterpiece of Zen of Master Dōgen, as I cited at the start of the chapter. *Ma* creates itself by being in the process of creation. *Ma* constantly creates and re-creates itself in the metaphysics of being and becoming.

Shintō Zen philosophy, the existentialism of Sartre and the phenomenology of Merleau-Ponty, allow me several frames of reference in studying dance and performance through *ma*. As I look back on the exploration of dancing on ice at Weeping Rock, I might desire a different dance, not one of freezing hands, with knees and feet wet and shivering, as I glide prudently across the ice-over ledge. The dance I experienced was of body as elemental: of flesh, cave, and ice coexisting. Through *ma*, I did not stop at the failure to love the freezing and slippery surface I crawled on, and I made no attempt to ornament my dance with gestures that would look aesthetically stunning.

Dancing this way, I recognize I am a human, and the wall I dance my life on is ice water over rock overlooking a precipice. I do not become ice (unless I stay out too long and freeze to death!), and I also don't expect the ice to be something other than it is.

Merleau-Ponty's proposition of *entwining* explains my feeling of belonging to the ice. The fold of my flesh into the flesh of the world is, in his words, "realized by the doubling up of my body into inside and outside—and the doubling up of the things (their inside and their outside)" (1968, 264). Furthermore, Merleau-Ponty develops the flesh (more-than-a-body) as two leaves. His very last notes for the work on *The Intertwining—The Chiasm* describe the insertion of world and body as: "the insertion of the world between the two leaves of my body the insertion of my body between the 2 leaves of each thing and of the world. By studying the 2 leaves we ought to find the structure of being—" (ibid.).

Ma eternally flows between and through me, as I invite *chiasm*: "by reason of this mediation through reversal, this chiasm, there is not simply a for-Oneself, for-the-Other antithesis, there is Being as containing all that, first as sensible Being and then as Being without restriction—which means there is not only a me-other rivalry, but a cofunctioning. We function as one unique body" (ibid., 214–215).

Among its other meanings, *ma* is a point of departure in performance. The artist can go anywhere outside of the original *ma*. For the artist Viale (as we saw earlier), personal encounter with *ma* and working in public spaces changes how she approaches her work. As a result, Viale transforms. In completion, she passes over her role of *agent activator*. The modified intervals will go on as modified essence, and those unfilled intervals will continue as unfilled invisible essence. The artistic intervention resides in the acknowledgment of a possibility. Once the meaning-in-the-making is achieved, the artist turns to other journeys, other spatial compositions and performances.

MA AND LIFE

My interest in pointing to Viale and butoh resides in their ability to cross over cultures in their appeal. Butoh, unique in its aesthetic, expanded to be practiced by dancers and performers of many different backgrounds via their own aesthetic. Butoh has reached beyond Japan because of its affinities with basic movements and experiences—like squatting and reaching, walking, holding, and falling—and in paying attention to feelings and experiences—to plants and animals, atmospheres and landscapes, and particularly environments in peril, an original ecological concern of Ohno Kazuo and now his student Takenouchi Atsushi. Butoh takes its cues from life in varied tempos of fast and slow, while often favoring very slow movement. The formulation of butoh involves nature and shape-shifting as part of its aesthetic power. In performance, the power of the dancer lives in her aliveness, invoking the dance as fundamental phenomenon in time-space and movement:

> As dance exhibits phenomenal presence through the creative, it invokes free agency, intention, and initiative. A dance exists through the human body; it derives through the body's aesthetic form and psychic life. As dance exists within the condition of human movement, it involves lived human time and human space. (Fraleigh 1987, 50).

In light of *ma*, a morphic power of aliveness can be unlocked by practicing slow-flow in butoh, as the *kami* flow eternally in and out of objects, changing them. Butoh's *slow-ma* flow eternally between objects as it enters and leaves. This flow, if observed in an optic of slow pace in butoh, explains in one aesthetic example how *ma* moves in dance.

Butoh, in its original aesthetic, is a dance that stands out as disarticulated. In the *Routledge Performance Practitioners* book series, Fraleigh and Tamah Nakamura trace back to the *Daruma* doll that butoh founder Hijikata Tatsumi pointed to as a source of his butoh dance. "The *Daruma* doll is a limbless figure weighted so that it bounces back when knocked down" (Fraleigh and Naka-mura 2006, 6). The Daruma doll has no choices in performing her movement. Her way of being is determined by the doll maker who has built the doll with the ability to bounce back when knocked down, a symbol of resilience and persistence, like slow movement in butoh. As in most performance, move-ments in butoh are intentional. The intention to be direct or indirect has not to do with spastic uncontrollable jerking but with moving consciously through choices of flowing or breaking flow. I have experienced butoh as a dance of deliberately breaking codes.

Dance scholar and butoh-ka Joan Laage writes about the genesis of butoh and the historical context during which butoh's cofounder Ohno Kazuo and Hijikata Tatsumi lived. In the mid–twentieth century, German influences were felt internationally, especially through Mary Wigman as can be observed in Ohno's re-creation of Wigman's Witch Dance (1993, 6). Hijikata Tatsumi also imported foreign influences by studying modern dance and flamenco. Over time, Hijikata questioned "the nature of dance itself, and the meaning [of it] for him" (9). Eventually, Ohno and Hijikata broke with dance tradi-tions that reproduce codes of movement, including those of Japan, thereby putting an emphasis on creativity in dance (8).

My study of butoh has been liberating, and it also commits me to an evalu-ation of codes and gestures. As I allow movement to come "naturally" and without thought, no movement is predetermined by forms I expect. Hijikata called butoh "dance experience" (Fraleigh and Nakamura 2006, 33–34). Bu-toh teacher Mario Veillette posits butoh to be a state of dance, rather than a dance of codes (2005, 11). The reality of butoh lives as an experience, that of the dancer and the audience in relation. At once individuation and unifi-cation, butoh is more accurately considered *Being Butoh*, an evolving form of dance morphology. Each butoh (dance step) born is an expression of an ecology of elements interconnecting.

IN THE END

The experience of documenting *ma* is unquestionably an individual and unique story in itself, one that resonates with *ma*'s open-ended definition. As per Iwase's account, there are at least two kinds of *ma*. Iwase suggests the possibility that *ma* has a meaning, and at the same time, it also means noth-ing. *Ma* is an experience realized through intentional creativity, wherein complex layers of space-time can be created and realized (made real). Pos-sibilities—of being and becoming—flow in *ma*. *Ma* flows in actual movement and perceptual echoes, reverberations of embodied moments that open possibilities of feeling the world empathically.

Ma also holds tension; as without tension, movement becomes absent. Thus, inherent dualities exist consistent with the meanings of *ma*. Such dualities are created by the manifestation of intention in the choices and purposes that performers express. The sun is the sun because it is daytime, and so is the moon nighttime. They exist in relation. *Ma* exists in elements of time and space where the dancer moves in cadence with the music along a sinuous path or changes paths at a seemingly off-tempo beat, moving at odds with her own joints. In every moment of the dance, there is a moment of *being* and a moment of *becoming*. *Being danced* is a realization of *ma*, the sun and moon abiding in each moment.

Now I'm left with a question: Can *ma* be meaningful outside of its Japanese context? For me it is. I find it a fascinating way of understanding what goes on when I dance—in imagery, connectivity to nature and to others, and in space-time variables. Nevertheless, *ma* remains a unique culture's embodied experience. I relate to *ma* as a cultural phenomenon that occurs naturally in transformative experiences of the dancer and audience. Space-time serves as a container for this study of *ma*, reflecting and describing a specific culture and my relationship to it. Observing *ma* in movement allows me to cross over and make sense of another culture through an experiential phenomenon.

And yet another question: How does *ma* enlarge the discourse of dance studies? I write in the belief that *ma* expands understandings of the dance itself. When I move, I am more than a moving body; I am a part of all that moves and exists. When I summon *ma*, I am: and I affirm that I am.

IV

Questions of Self-Knowing

10

"What If . . ."

A Question of Transcendence

HILLEL D. BRAUDE AND AMI SHULMAN

The central pivot for this chapter's analysis of the phenomenology of dance and performance is the relation between the invited sense of possibility in *Free Fantasy Variations* (FFV) and Husserl's concept of "*I can.*" We explore the tension between a dancer's corporeal "immanence," or indwelling, and the dancer's desire for "transcendence"—in moving beyond perceived self-limits. Stated in full, our chapter invites "Possibilities of Self through Free Fantasy Movement Variations."

Introduction

Of all art forms, dance is the most paradoxical in its material immateriality. A dance performance emerges from the body of the dancer. The materiality of the dance is the actual corporeal form. The body is the dance, yet the dance is not the body. Dance as a performative art arises from the elemental human desire to express through the realm of the physical and beyond the limitations of language. Much dance performance plays with a dancer's exploration of the inherent freedom within bodily movement through touching the limits of physical possibility. The tension that exists between these two states of being, between a dancer's corporeal form and the desire to move beyond it, is often most evident in the analysis of transitional moments in a dance performance. There are many kinds of transitional moments, for example, when movement emerges, when nonintentional movement becomes intentional, and similarly when a dancer shifts from a nonperformative sensibility to a performative one.

Another kind of shift occurs in terms of how a dance is observed or experienced by another, in other words, when a private dance becomes a public performance. These transformations, occurring through a change in kinesthetic perception, require a certain reflective distance, either internally in the self of the dancer, or via the presence of an external observer of the dance. Moreover, the transitions between these different threshold states may not always be fluid, especially when the mover becomes cognitively preoccupied with the components of a particular kinetic action. Hence, transitional moments may also represent tensions or points of stress between different threshold levels of lived experience. The shift between transitional moments, as mentioned, for example, between the private self and the performative self, and between the technical action and performance, are clearest in the moment of discovering or appropriating a new movement phrase. (A movement phrase does not necessarily refer to a clearly choreographed repeatable form but represents a quintessential movement score, a "structure of tasks.") In performing a movement phrase, the dancer moves in a fluid spatiotemporal reality, suspended between conscious reflection on the components of the dance, and the qualitative dynamics of the dance that reflect the dancer's individuality. The more the dance is internalized as part of the dancer, the more the dance assumes its own life. The Irish poet W. B. Yeats alludes to this phenomenon, asking at the end of his often quoted poem, *Among School Children*, "How can we know the dancer from the dance?"[1]

This chapter, a collaboration between a philosopher—Hillel Braude—and dance and movement educator—Ami Shulman—who are also both certified Feldenkrais practitioners, examines Yeats's question from the phenomenological perspective of *Free Fantasy Variations*. As explicated by Edmund Husserl, FFV refers to an "as-if experience" in consciousness, the ability to provide an "always-possible" modification of any actual experience (Husserl 1969, 206; Zaner 1981, 39). FFV represents a relatively neglected component of Husserl's phenomenological methodology. Yet, arguably, FFV is the fundamental method of *eidetic* description, even more than the famous phenomenological *reduction* and *epoché*. Richard Zaner claims that FFV is "far and away the most significant and important phenomenological method, the most powerful and the most fruitful" (*1981*, 244). Husserl claimed in his *Cartesian Meditations* that FFV is "*the fundamental form of all particular transcendental methods* . . . [and gives] the legitimate sense of a transcendental phenomenology" (1960, 72).

Reflecting its two authors' experience and expertise, this chapter traverses the relation between the invited sense of possibility in FFV and Husserl's concept of "*I can.*" Our analysis emphasizes how correlating movement with FFV grounds phenomenological exploration in the lifeworld, the realm that people inhabit through the body rather than simply becoming a free-floating act of consciousness unmoored from its human and earthly origins. In terms of structure, throughout this chapter Ami Shulman provides first-person reflections on her teaching approach interwoven alongside Hillel Braude's phenomenological reflection. This methodology aims to capture something of the performative nature of both movement performance and phenomeno-logical reflection. The authors focus on the sense of kinesthetic "possibility" as revealed in the distinct moments of creating, teaching, and performing a movement phrase. In particular, we reflect on the first-person description by Ami of her own performative experience as dancer, rehearsal director, and movement teacher, informing her creative processes eliciting "performance presence" from a dancer. Ami's class is a contemporary technique class with a somatic perspective. It is highly dynamic and integrates the floor as an es-sential component for full body connectivity and proprioceptive awareness. It is a structured class that explores the HOW of movement rather than the WHAT, looking at how movement efficiency and clarity liberates the form, enhancing the movement potential of the individual.

Our analysis pivots around the transitional moment when a movement or series of movements finds a performative quality, especially the transition through which the performer's movement becomes realized, facilitated by the imaginary visualization cue "what if." Besides drawing on Ami's teaching process, we will also refer to insights from the Feldenkrais Method. Keeping with the theme of this book, *Phenomenologies of the Body in Performance*, our conceptual approach is phenomenological. Transcendental phenomenology allows a fascinating entry into examining the relation between dance and performance. The aim of phenomenology, as developed by Edmund Husserl, was to provide a methodology of revealing the correlations between objects, and the way they are presented in consciousness, i.e., between experiencing and what is experienced. Phenomenology provides an exemplary method-ology for our analysis of performance, moving back and forth between the kinesthetic event and its reflective analysis.

The phenomenological method is itself performative, characterized by being a cognitive act that points toward the investigator. Elizabeth Behnke observes that the "radical freedom from suppositions" achieved by phenomenological reduction requires "inquiring back into our streaming life of action and af-fection" (2010, 50).[2] Phenomenological inquiry requires, therefore, a process of self-reflection analogous to the introspective process of inquiring into the kinaesthetic constitution of a dance performance. There is, therefore, a deep structural link between phenomenological inquiry and dance performance. Taking into account this link, we consider that Husserl's concept of FFV provides the most fitting phenomenological conceptual tool for our analysis of dance movement performance. As mentioned, FFV refers to an "as-if experience" in consciousness, the ability to provide an "always-possible" modification of any actual experience. For example, toward the beginning of *Ideas I*, Husserl writes:

> The Eidos, the *pure essence*, can be exemplified for intuition in experiential data—in data of perception, memory, and so forth; but it can equally well be exemplified in *data of mere phantasy*. Accordingly, to seize upon an essence itself, and to seize upon it *originarily*, we can start from corresponding experiencing intuitions, *but equally well from intuitions which are non-experiencing, which do not seize upon factual existence but which are instead "merely imaginative"* (§4, 1).

Our project uses *FFV* to explore dance phenomena in context of lived situations, not merely the imaginative. While "as-if . . ." *fantasy variation* is associated with the production of pure possibilities, Husserl's "*I can*" is associated with the "practical possibilities" of concrete individuals. We invite both possibilities into play.

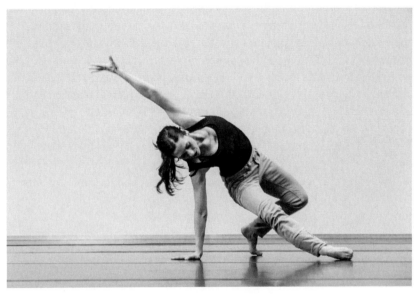

Figure 10.1. Ami Shulman. Photograph in Berlin © 2016 by Jubal Battisti.

Knowing the Dancer from the Dance:
A Phenomenological Inquiry

Ami: As a rehearsal director, I have witnessed incredible performers who have embodied movement in such a way that I was no longer aware of the dance, but instead, I had a visceral experience of it. The performer enters a magical unfolding of time and possibility, where my presence as an observer is interwoven in the fabric of the performance. This experience is as much mine as theirs, and I am as changed by observing it as they are by doing it. Witnessing these kinds of performances is rare.

Hillel: As noted by literary theorist Paul de Man, Yeats's seemingly innocent question about dance can be legitimately interpreted in two opposing ways. First, understood *figuratively*, Yeats affirms the "potential unity between form and experience, between creator and creation. It denies the discrepancy between the sign and [its] referent . . ." (1973, 30). According to this straightforward figurative reading, the dancer and the dance form an indissociable unity. De Man notes, however, that read *literally*, the "two essentially different elements, sign and meaning, are so intricately intertwined in the imagined 'presence' that the poem addresses" (ibid.) that it is not possible to make the necessary distinction to avoid the error of identifying what is essentially nonidentifiable. De Man notes further that Yeats's poem is "about the possibility of convergence between experiences of consciousness . . . and entities accessible to the senses such as bodies, persons or icons" (ibid.). These kinds of questions, exploring the possible relation between the experience of consciousness and embodied senses are phenomenological rather than rhetorical. Thus, the last line of Yeats's poem asks the kinds of phenomenological questions about self, body, and consciousness addressed by modern phenomenologists following the explorative methodology developed by Edmund Husserl.

The body is central for Husserl's phenomenological project. He describes the body as the "zero point," the "ultimate central here" around which every experienced object is oriented (1950, 158–166). The appearance of every object for consciousness, every "thing-appearance," is correlative to certain "perceptual circumstances," including kinaesthetic "circumstances," such as directing and moving my eyes in seeing, moving my arms, hands, and fingers in touching, bringing my ear closer in order to hear better, etc." (*Husserliana* 1950, 20–22, 56–61) For Husserl, the body is characterized as being "freely moving" (*Husserliana* 1950, 68–73), in other words, as being able to move immediately and spontaneously (*Husserliana* 1950, 152–159). This body potentiality is summarized by Husserl in terms of the phrase "*I can*."[3] This sense of the "*I can*" finds its apotheosis in the moving body, surpassing conceptions of the self in the freedom of the dance.

Ami: A sense of *possibility* frames my view as an educator/teacher. To access possibility, you need to have physical and mental availability in cultivating the sense of "I can." Our perceptions can change such availability, however unconsciously. As Husserl and Feldenkrais both held, perception is at the root of movement potentials. The potentiality of the body, afforded by the sense of "*I can*," is primarily a state of availability, a felt sense of one's capacity that affords diverse options in the dancer's ability to adapt, respond, and articulate. To be "freely moving," one must ensure that the mind or the thinking does not interfere with that process. We can have some very fixed ideas about ourselves, life, and movement, some of which are not true; nor do they serve us well. While we strive for integration of the whole self in dance, attuned integration involves the capacity to differentiate the parts in relation to the whole. For example, dancers can be *identified with the concept of the "midline."* In their thinking, it can be a zero point of such fixity that when they start to move they hold this line still even when the movement is asking something different of them. I challenge dancers' thinking by bringing new perspectives to the movement that they are doing, both sensorially as well through structural connectivity. The fundamental issue underlying this thinking is that there is not just one way to do something, nor is there one way to think of something. So, if your movement could encompass any *possibility*, what then would you be able to do?

Hillel: It is sensible that philosophers of dance have applied the tools of phenomenology to analyze dance and performance. As an object of consciousness in its own right, dance provides a specialized realm for phenomenological investigation. Dance performance can be explored phenomenologically for the relation between the subjective givenness of the dance, and its ever-extending circle of choreographer, dancer, audience, and world. Sondra Fraleigh in her essay "A Vulnerable Glance: Seeing Dance through Phenomenology" has noted that the phenomenon of a dance can include not only the "changing sense impressions of the dance as it flows through time but also insight in the essence of the dance. . . . It arises in consciousness as the motion reveals the intent of the whole and its parts" (1991, 12). Similarly, in her analysis of the relation between movement and dance grounded in Husserl's exposition of phenomenological methodology, Maxine Sheets-Johnstone observes, "The dancer is not moving through a form; the form is moving through her. How, indeed, 'can we know the dancer from the dance?'" (2012, 52).

Rather than being a "mere" rhetorical device, Yeats's question, "How can we know the dancer from the dance?" is entirely valid phenomenologically speaking. Yet at the same time, the rhetorical paradox inherent in Yeats's line also affirms the inherent tension between the phenomenological possibility and impossibility of intuiting the givenness of the dance performance. Investigating the relation of the dancer to the dance can be performed only via an act of reflective distance. The "brightening glance" of critical reflection already presupposes a tear in the living fabric of the dance. Yeats's question, interpreted figuratively as an ontological impossibility, might also speak to the cognitive phenomenon whereby explicit, conscious attention on the components of a skilled motor performance, such as playing the piano or dancing, interferes with its optimal outcome (Dreyfus 2012).

Phenomenology from its outset has provided a method of paying attention to lived experience, reflecting on the body simultaneously from "inside" and "outside" perspectives, even possibly without jeopardizing kinetic action. To perceive one's body from the inside and outside simultaneously is to experience the "physicality" and "subjectivity" of one's bodily self. Analyzing the phenomenological constitution of this dual experience, Dorothée Legrand and Susanne Ravn argue that, "one's body's physicality may express one's body's subjectivity, and . . . that the body's subjectivity can be experienced by the subject itself, through the nonreifying perception of its physical states" (2009, 390).

Ami: I recall a moment I experienced during a dance improvisation: I paused, turned my head, and perceived not only a new spatial dimension that was now available to me, but the entire configuration of my body represented to me with an array of possibilities that were previously hidden. I was in a workshop guided by Deborah Hay, with her seminal work, "Turn Your F^*cking Head"; my entire perception of my body, its organization, and what became possible to me was completely influenced by my selective visual field. I had been in a particular configuration and by the simple, yet epic, act of turning my head, my perception of my own physical body was completely renewed. My brain seemed rebooted and I was in a different place. What became available to me in my movement completely changed simply by the difference of the angle of my head and viewpoint. The Feldenkrais perspective calls this a shift of habitual organization, which also shifts one's self-image, giving rise to previously unexplored possibilities.

Hillel: Legrand and Ravn are interested in the intrinsic experience of consciousness and embodiment expressed through the dance. They "underline a structure of experience that is there before the dance, allowing the dance to happen" (2009, 15). Legrand and Ravns's analysis of the perception of subjectivity in bodily movement is noteworthy for highlighting the fluid relation between the dancer's body and the environment. The analysis of perceptual subjectivity in bodily movements requires paying attention to the capabilities of the body as "*I can,*" as well as the conditions inviting movement availability by both internal physical and external environmental factors. The actual possibilities for embodied "*I can*" arise in the face of these internal and external conditions. The "*I can*" is always inner-directed toward the organizing force of the body, and outer-directed toward the external world, shaping the contours of its affordances.

Ami: I have seen good dancers become exceptional performers literally overnight, and I noticed that it was primarily a shift in the thinking that facilitated this—a certain permissiveness that aligns receptivity, responsiveness, experience, and action all at once to make something that is greater than the sum of those things. It is the mind that gets in the way of this process more than physical capacity. We don't need to be aware of our unconscious limiting beliefs to have a sense that we feel somehow limited. "You can't outperform your self-image." Our unconscious self-perceptions affect the options that become available to us. If you work thinking that you are limited, you will be. In the genius work of the Feldenkrais Method, the concept of limitation is used as a tool, subverting its restrictive nature into one of affordance, by allowing a person to discover what else they can do within that given situation. This ingenious concept of creating a constraint affords a greater capacity for movement articulation in the parts that are available to move, affording new possibilities and perspectives to a movement.

Hillel: One of the most important points of contact between phenomenology and dance performance is the relation between possibility and impossibility. Similarly, the theme of possibility was a central preoccupation for Husserl in developing his philosophy of transcendental subjectivity. In this regard, Husserl distinguished between "pure possibility" and "real possibility" (quoted by Mohanty 1984). "Pure possibility," following Leibniz, refers to objects that are independent of spatiotemporal being. They pertain to only *eidetic* species or essences and are not capable of real existence—for example, the abstract idea of a triangle. "Real possibility," on the other hand, refers to the possibility for individual existence of an ideal actuality. FFV, through "as if . . ." consciousness transforms every actual object into a possible as-if object. As J. N. Mohanty explains, the possibility of perception may provide the basis for bringing to intuitive givenness the pure eidos of "perception" (1984, 24). In contrast with the pure possibility achieved by FFV exists the "practical possibility" achieved by the expression "*I can.*" "What I can, am able to, that of which I know myself as capable, . . . that is a practical possibility" (Husserl 1950, 258). Husserl's method of FFV is crucial in providing the phenomenological methodology enabling moving between "pure" and "practical" possibilities.

FFV is crucial for Husserl's project because it provides a means of navigating between perceptual empirical data and imaginative variations. A *"fact* of perception may be 'transformed' in phantasy, into a *possible* perception" (Mohanty 1984, 24). However, this is not a one-way street in the direction of abstraction. While *"as-if . . ." fantasy variation* is associated with the production of pure possibilities, Husserl's "I can" refers to "practical possibilities" of concrete individuals. There is, thus, a living tension between the abstraction into pure possibility afforded through FFV and practical possibilities achieved through the consciousness of "*I can.*"

We will return to elaborating "pure possibility" and "practical possibility" in relation to movement and kinesthesia later in this chapter. In summary, meanwhile, we argue that movement and dance provide the practical embodied realm where the phenomenological method of FFV finds its

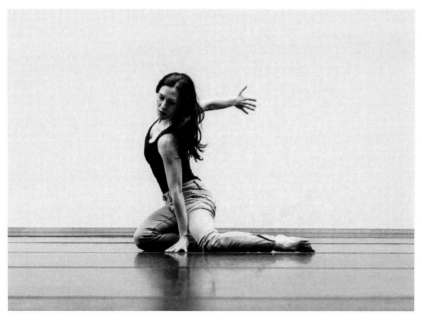

Figure 10.2. Ami Shulman, *In the Moment.* Photograph in Berlin © 2016 by Jubal Battisti.

ideal expression. Hence, Maxine Sheets-Johnstone writes in her seminal study, *Primacy of Movement*: "What phenomenological analyses bring to our understanding of perception are decisively deeper understandings of the process of constitution, including deeper understandings of both the relationship between movement and perception as indicated by if-then relations, by an "I move," and so on, and the possibility of self-evidence" (1999, 190). In what follows, we investigate the living tension between pure possibility and practical possibility, between FFV and "I can," through describing aspects of perceptual experience from the performer's point of view and later analyzing the phenomenology of creating and appropriating a new movement phrase.

Possibilities in Performance and Pedagogy

Ami: Memories of my most liberating experiences as a performer have a dreamlike sensibility, a sense of boundlessness, where I am physically in relation to the environment and myself. I experience a state of optimal choice-making while discovering new and vital possibilities in the moment. There is no separation between my thinking-self, my sensing-self, and my doing-self. I am in a complete state of presence, able to command my movement choices, though the movement itself is in a state of becoming, and its destiny remains yet undefined. I experience the unfolding of a process of articulations and possibilities available through my body, a conduit shaped by my unique life experiences.

My recollection of this has a paradoxical twist. On stage, I had no sense of the distinction between what was happening to me, what I was actively participating in, and what was transpiring in the moment (the dance itself)—I experienced it as a completely integrated gestalt. However, in self-reflection, I identify these three distinct elements mentioned earlier as existing separately from the whole; my first-person experience of the seamless unity of the dance becomes ever more elusive—being part of me, moving through me, and having its own sense of existence.

This place of ecstasy when I dance, when I'm in my element, is not something I own or have. It is something that passes through me, filtered through the intelligence of my kinesthetic system, which is both completely accessible and also completely informed by my personal life journey. There is something about this aspect of dance, where it is not "me," and yet it is the most "me" I will ever be. I know myself there, and also, I don't. There is a remove that is almost voyeuristic. In the moment itself, I don't feel myself a physical body but a dynamism of energy. How can I access this sense, and my memory of it, if it is so ephemeral?

There is more to say on this as I find it a phenomenon in its own right, but for now, I leave just a glimpse of this description in order to speak of the magic of movement, the intelligence of the kinesthetic system, and how it must bypass language-based rationality and perceived certainty of knowing. I don't think dance is something that can be "captured." Movement, like air, will be there and serve—and the brilliant human brain, as depicted by science, will never be able to hold it.

*   *   *

I came into teaching with a choreographic eye. I was interested in choreography at that time and was compelled by the state of presence that a performer could evoke on stage. I wanted to cultivate a state in the performer that could move the dance beyond the perceived realms of the physical. What became apparent to me was that the aspect that made a difference to the embodied presence of a dancer was paradoxically the way we thought about the movement—how we would think about what it was that we were doing. It wasn't driven by the content of the choreography, but the way we engaged ourselves with it that made all the difference. My methodology involves how diverse aspects of "possibility" function as a means of accessing performance presence through embodied intention.

The way I begin teaching a class is intuitive. The initial directives I give to bring the dancers' attention toward a felt sense of their body appear almost like ritual. They are immediately drawn into a state of greater conscious sensory awareness, exemplifying Husserl's notion of "*I can*." Then, I guide them into movement explorations, challenging and expanding their perception of the movement, and cultivating a curiosity, which keeps them engaged in the unfolding moment.

When I begin teaching a class, I challenge preconceived ideas immediately. Starting on the knees I suggest to the dancers: "What if this was the dance." "What if you had to be here for 30 minutes and this was the dance." It is remarkable how this question shifts attention in a particular way. Clarity of thought often redefines the entire class.

My suggestive manner has a remove from an instructive manner and invites the dancers to take more responsibility for their choices. This empowers the dancers, simultaneously bringing them deeper into their thinking body.

In teaching technique, I am not as interested in the movement itself as I am in how it interacts in different situations. When preparing my classes, I spend hours improvising in the studio. At some point in the improvisation, I do a movement that intrigues me, and I instinctively know that I want to make an exercise leading out from this point of entry. Sometimes it's the quality and flow of the movement that draws my interest, and sometimes it's a clear articulation or a pathway of a movement that draws my attention, but in its essence, it is what that movement affords me—what "I can" do with it. I begin to notice how that initial movement is implicated in other movements. It is as if I don't fully understand the movement until I have experienced it in different situations. I am exploring that movement in action. This process has fundamentally informed my perspective on teaching technique, emphasizing the process of a movement within the structure of the body.

My work introduces somato-sensory and kinaesthetic principles within structured and highly dynamic movement phrases. The movement phrase itself, serving only as a vessel, falls into the background, allowing me to engage with the individuals, guiding them more intuitively toward accessing a deeper level of embodiment. I have developed a series of classes called "Playing with Possibility." The most poignant aspect of this series reframes the dancers' perception of movement giving rise to imaginative thinking through suggestive directives. This affordance of new possibilities in movement speaks to Husserl's discussion of FFV.

In the spring of 2015, I taught a series of contemporary dance technique classes to a group of pre-professionals in a workshop in Montreal. I took a movement phrase that I created for the floor and used it as a conduit through which I introduced new movement concepts. Each day I would teach this same phrase from a new perspective, so much so that it seemed like different movement material one day from the next, providing new perceptions about the invariant. On one particular day, I decided to redirect the movement from a sensory perspective.

We "sloughed" down the surface of the skin, an organ that has no beginning, middle, or end. As we did so, I spoke about the continuity of the skin. We slid the skin surface of our arm along our own bodies "as if" we were putting on a long glove, allowing that same gentle rotation to include the dimensionality of the arm as well as the sensitization of the skin's surface. We then slid the surface of the skin along the surface of the floor; this gave an embodied presence to the arm as well as to the action. Then we did the same movement phrase as we had done each day of the series.

After having worked with the sensibility of the skin surface, I said, "what if . . . there were no seam between the movements? How smoothly can you pass from one moment to the next?" I demonstrated this sense of continuity through the surface of the skin sliding my arm along the floor. "What if . . . the end of this movement was actually the beginning of the next one"? Demonstrating a seamless transition, I linked the movements like a long thread. "Who is to say where one movement ends and the next one begins, what if this phrase is one long movement? What if . . . the movement never arrives in any one destination but is continuously in transition, in a continuous state of becoming." When the dancers did the phrase, they became engaged in a particular way that brought a new dimension to the movement. The quality of the movement became smooth, pouring like a liquid through the space, seemingly expanding the territory of the body itself through its kinaesthetic sensibilities of touch and listening. I could no longer see the choreography of the phrase. It was an integration of the moving sensorial body in space.

The invitation to "what if . . ." brings the dancers into a state of active exploration. It requires a heightened state of responsiveness favoring movement as a process rather than a form. It sets up the conditions in which dancers can cultivate awareness, sense, discern, and select for themselves. This kind of experiential learning is rooted within the anatomical structure, yet it suggests a corporeal imaginary realm within which to play rather than an outcome on which to focus. This is an invitation to possibility in movement through embodied thought.

Integrating Conceptual Analysis and Embodied Experience: *Free Fantasy Variation* and Somatic Movement Exploration

Hillel: In the previous section, Ami provides an introspective auto-ethnographic description of her methodology for devising and teaching a movement phrase. The main stages involved in this procedure include: self-movement explorations in order to find a kinetic idea that she developed into a movement phrase, and transmission of kinesthetic sensibilities that animated the kinetic properties of the phrase, using it as a "way-in" for the dancer to explore the kinesthetic richness of the movement. Each component requires close observation and attention to the lived quality of a particular movement or series of movements. The transformative aspect to this process of self-discovery is ignited through the invitation to imagine "what if."

Ami's approach is analytical, constantly informed by processes of self-reflection and analysis, yet is not cognitivist in trying to impose a defined choreography. Instead, the pedagogic methodology is intended to help dancers move with more integration than they might and even "discover" themselves through the movement. This is facilitated by exploring material affordances in relation to conceptual fantasy variation metaphors, "what if."

Ami's process is phenomenological in eliciting the essential structure of a movement phrase, though she does not consciously apply formal phenomenological methodology. In particular, her method highlights the centrality of FFV in her work, in the way that she plays with movement variations, while exploring connectivity through functional and spatial relationships and then integrating a kinetic availability and responsiveness to the movement through her poignant use of the phrase "what if."

Ami's teaching approach is also strikingly similar to the somatic methodology developed by Moshe Feldenkrais. (*Somatics* refers to first-person experience of the lived body.) In a group-based Awareness through Movement Lesson (ATM), the Feldenkrais teacher will direct an intricate series of visualized movements. These lessons are constructed to enable the student to explore many different variations around a movement theme. Typically, these lessons will increase in their gradations of complexity and may elicit fundamental neuropsychological experiences associated with core functional movement patterns. During an ATM lesson, attention may be directed to at least three broad categories of the experience of the self in action: (1) the kinesthetic qualities of movement (2), the body in relation to the environment, and (3) attitudes to one's action that may arise (Smyth 2016).

Feldenkrais first described this technique of exploring different variations of a single movement in his early book on self-defense, *Practical Unarmed Combat.*[4] In his later work, *The Potent Self*, drawing on his experience in developing his therapeutic and educational somatic approach, Feldenkrais develops this insight further:

> The earliest learning consists in the exploration of our own body possibilities to move and act. In the multitude of undifferentiated muscular contractions, we soon learn to recognize configurations that have a bearing, a meaning, or relatedness to the exterior world of which our body is a part. Slowly these recognitions become definite acts. In this way we learn to walk, to speak, and to use a spoon. To acquire better posture, it is necessary to restart and further this process of learning and bring it to a higher level of excellence. (1985, 110–111)

Feldenkrais is describing a kinaesthetic methodology to determine perceptual invariants. The object of perception, the perceptual invariant, remains the same in itself, but becomes clearer to the perceiver through shifts in the observer perspective. As Carl Ginsburg notes, "The percept is an invariant because in moving the relationships between object, and perspective in relation to the position of yourself as an observer, follows an invariant set of relationships. Thus, the percept is a higher-level extraction of construction" (1970, 56). Ginsburg associates Feldenkrais's exploration of movement with the psychological work of J. J. Gibson, who in his research on perception also realized that the invariant becomes revealed through movement, similar to Ami's description of the improvisation class, where she had turned her head and discovered an array of possibility previously unavailable to her. There is a deep psychological basis to Feldenkrais's work (Braude 2016). However, additionally, the methodology behind Feldenkrais's exploratory movement variation patterns is scientific in nature. Indeed, as a young man, Moshe Feldenkrais (1904–1984) worked as a quantity surveyor, mapping out the geographical outlines of then British Mandate Palestine and subsequently studied engineering and physics in Paris, working in the laboratory of Joliot-Curie (Reese 2015). This scientific background characterizes all of Felden-krais's subsequent research and writing, providing shifting perspectives on what is invariant in functional movement.

There is something akin to the scientific method in Feldenkrais's (and Ami's) approach. Maxine Sheets-Johnstone has productively compared the scientific method of the brilliant nineteenth-century physician, physicist, and philosopher von Helmholtz (1821–1894) with Husserl's phenomeno-logical methodology. Von Helmholtz also independently discovered the importance of the correlation between perception and movement for his scientific investigations. What von Helmholtz called *presentabilia*—percep-tual invariants—and what Husserl called *presentiations*—possible percep-tions, according to Sheets-Johnstone are essentially synonymous. She notes they are both the "equivalent of 'free variations' arrived at through modified kinesthesis" (1999, 196). Feldenkrais's exploration of movement variations practiced and performed on his personal self, and then formalized in his many ATM lessons, provide a triadic link between Helmholz's science of perception and Husserl's phenomenology of perception.[5] (One ATM lesson, for example, builds on the theme of spontaneous movements of one's eyes in relation to moving one's head in various directions—up and down, down and up, left to right, right to left—while lying on the floor, so as to negate the effects of gravity on the work the nervous system has to perform.) As an exemplary somatic practice, the Feldenkrais Method has been described as "phenomenology in action" (Fraleigh 2015). Hillel Braude (2015) argues that somatics practices provide the corporeal bridge between the phenom-enological study of subjectivity and the naturalistic sciences. In integrating a methodology of investigation derived from the naturalistic sciences, i.e., physics, with the object of investigation being conscious awareness and the phenomenology of perception, Feldenkrais's ATM lessons encapsulate the embodied connection between *presentabilia* and *presentations* that Sheets-Johnstone refers to in her comparison of Husserl's and von Helmholtz's' respective research methodologies.

As we reach the concluding section of this chapter, it is apt to reflect on the following questions: How best to integrate the theoretical analysis of *FFV* and "*I can*" with Ami's first-person description of her teaching approach in which she elicits the embodied presence of the dancer at the suggestion of new kinaesthetic thinkings using "what if." What is the significance of this teaching experience of movement for phenomenology of dance and performance more generally? Finally, how does this phenomenological investigation shed explanatory light on the experience of transitions, from movement appropriation to performance, and on the experiential correlation between the dancer and the dance? In responding to these questions, it is helpful to review fundamental aspects of FFV.

First, FFV is the basic phenomenological method in eliciting the presupposed structure of an act of consciousness. Through playing with as many different possibilities in which an object may be represented to consciousness, in order to elicit what is invariant, the *eidetic* form of the object in question will become highlighted. This phenomenological method is analogous to that of the geometer, who abstracts from spatial reality ideal mathematical forms (Husserl 1970b, 21–59). Yet, as explicated by Richard Zaner, this phenomenological methodology is not limited to that of geometry, but is applicable to any *eidetic* science, including mathematics, geometry, and *eidetic* phenomenology itself (2012, 47).

Second, FFV signifies a liberating relationship with empirical reality. As Husserl writes, the "*method of eidetic description* [FFV] . . . signifies a transfer of all empirical descriptions into a new and fundamental dimension" (1960, 69). This *eidetic* transformation from the region of facts, from empirical reality, to the freedom of focusing on *any* actual or possible individual—within the kind of example under investigation—in terms of *fantasy* variation, is encapsulated in terms of the "as-if experience" (Husserl 1969, 206).

Third, while perception and kinesthesia are not the only realms where FFV may occur, Husserl emphasizes them as explanatory examples. In his *Cartesian Meditations*, Husserl writes:

> Abstaining from acceptance of its being, we change the fact of this perception into a pure possibility, one among quite "optional" pure possibilities—but the possibilities that are possible perceptions. We, so to speak, shift the actual

perception into the realm of non-actualities, the realm of the as-if, which supplies us with "pure" possibilities, pure of everything that restricts to this fact or to any fact whatever. As regards the latter point, we keep the aforesaid possibilities, not as restricted even to the co-posited de facto ego, but just as completely free "imaginableness" of fantasy. Accordingly from the very start we might have taken as our initial example a fantasizing [*sic*] ourselves into a perceiving, with no relation to the rest of our de facto life. Perception, the universal type thus acquired, floats in the air, so to speak—in the atmosphere of pure fantasiableness [*sic*]. Thus removed from all factualness, it has become the pure "*eidos*" perception, whose "*ideal*" extension is made up of all ideally possible perceptions as purely fantasiable [*sic*] processes. (1960, 70)

The example of perception links FFV with kinesthesia and the sense of embodied-beingness epitomized by Husserl's phrase "*I can*" (1970b, 161–162). As Maxine Sheets-Johnstone writes in *Primacy of Movement*, "What phenomenological analyses bring to our understanding of perception are decisively deeper understandings of the process of constitution, including deeper understandings of both the relationship between movement and perception as indicated by if-then relations, by an 'I move,' and so on, and the possibility of self-evidence" (1999, 190). This process of "constitution," therefore, does not only reveal the invariants of objects of consciousness, but is inherently self-reflexive. The exploration of possibilities of functional movement also allows the constitution of the core-self, what Husserl calls the ego (*Ich*), to emerge.

In *At Play in the Field of the Possibles*, Zaner provides an in-depth analysis of this process of constitution of self through FFV via what he calls "*exemplification*." Key to this process of *exemplification* is the shift of personal attention away from the individual affair for its own sake, to its consideration as an example of a phenomenon comparable with other *noetic* phenomena. However, shifting of the exemplar in this manner brings to the fore the awareness of the thing in relation to *my* awareness. Exemplification thereby reveals the "mode of givenness to my experiential subjectivity" (Zaner 2012, 53). Thus, through processes of exemplification, the contours of the *I* are constituted and not just the phenomenological object of consciousness.

The full relevance of these insights for phenomenology of dance and performance cannot be fully addressed here. Yet, the phenomenon that Ami Shulman describes wherein the dancer suddenly disappears in the movement of the dance, and a new self emerges, refers precisely to this process of self-discovery and even creation through the process of FFV in movement. It epitomizes the simultaneous conflation of physical immanence and experiential transcendence, of dance and phenomenological performance. The living tension between the factual conditions of being-in-the world, and its endless affordances rendered possible through infinite possibilities of exploration of movement variations as the key for self-transcendence, is exemplified in the somatic teaching process of Shulman, as well as the Feldenkrais method more generally. No doubt there are similar somatic, variational methods in dance processes. Such examples demonstrate how FFV plays with the relation between inner self, external bodily self, and the environment—what Husserl calls the "perceptual world."

FFV encapsulates the tension between its conceptualization by Husserl as the *eidetic* methodology par excellence to become free from the constraints of *empeira*, and its practical exemplification in terms of perception and kinesthesia. This tension has not escaped the perceptive gaze of Sheets-Johnstone, who was perhaps the first to detail the relevance of Husserl's concept of *FFV* for the phenomenology of dance and performance. Thus, she observes that Husserl privileges the possible over the actual in the service of the eidetic. Sheets-Johnstone's analysis is worth quoting at length and tentatively unpacking:

> To attain to what is essential demands a methodology proper to the task. But an imaginative free variation of self-movement can only be a *spectated* imaginative free variation of movement. In other words, the *kinesthesis*, the very stuff of an "I move," of an "I do," of an *organ* body, and so on, can be freely varied *imaginatively* only as a *visual* phenomenon. What appears in such an imaginative free variation is the visual phenomenon of oneself—or, as it turns out on close scrutiny, some body or other—moving. The resultant phenomenology of movement is a phenomenology of movement seen (Sheets-Johnstone 1999, 199–200).

She touches upon the apparent paradox of *free-fantasy* of self-movement, whereby FFV is for Husserl, arguably, the essential *eidetic* methodology for transcendental phenomenology; yet, as such it is inherently visual or speculative and is thereby not a fully embodied kinesthetic experience. Thus, Sheets-Johnstone considers that the "pure possibility" of FFV misses a vital kinaesthetic element associated with the "practical possibility" of the body in terms of its sense of "*I-can*." Therefore, Sheets-Johnstone further grounds her perspective of *fantasy variations* in movement seen, felt, and done:

> A concerted attempt to run through *imaginative kinesthetic* variations consistently involves the *actual tactile-kinesthetic* body. To imagine oneself slamming a door, for example, or swaying, or running, or doing whatever involves

incipient kinesthetic feelings of slamming, swaying, running, and so on. Accordingly, when Husserl writes that "There are reasons by virtue of which in phenomenology, as in all other eidetic sciences, presentations and, more precisely, *free fantasies acquire a position of primacy over other perceptions and do so even in the phenomenology of perception itself, excluding, to be sure, the phenomenology of the Data of sensation.*" (Sheets-Johnstone 1999, 199; italics in original)

Her work points out that *hyletic* data from sensation forming the embodied basis of actual kinesthetic experiences are necessary for the possibility of imaginative kinesthetic variations. Thus, imaginative kinesthetic variations cannot supersede actual lived experience. Recall the dance teaching technique described by Ami where she invited her dance students to "slough" down the surface of their skins. A key unstated aim of this technique, often included other senses such as hearing, touch, and proprioception to clarify the image or the perception of the possibility of movement, enables the movers to experience a novel kinesthetic action that elicits other *kinesthetic* and *perceptual* data. Moreover, Ami's accompanying invitation, to slide the skin surface of one's arm along one's body "as if" putting on a glove, only attains its significance as a free-variation of movement via the actual kinesthetic experience of sliding the arm on the skin. Actual possibility and real possibility are played out in this metaphor of embodied sloughing and seamlessness.

Sheets-Johnstone considers that Husserl affirms an alternative *kinesthetic* methodology in relation to *imaginative* free variation, even though he does not specify its details:

Clearly, though Husserl himself does not so specify, the phenomenology of kinesthesia presents itself as just such an exception to imaginative free fantasy. In effect, active self-experimentation is essential to understanding *the kinestheses.* In this respect, it is in fact doubtful that Husserl could possibly have arrived at his rich (if less than full explicated notion) of the kinestheses by way of imaginative free variation; he undoubtedly would have arrived at it through first-hand active self-experimentations, . . . In effect, active self-experimentations were the point of departure for phenomenological analysis; they were what Husserl elsewhere calls "the transcendental clue" grounding an investigation outside the natural attitude. (Sheets-Johnstone 1999, 199–200)

Sheets-Johnstone intimates that exploration of actual kinesthetic variations, analogous to those described in relation to von Helmholtz and Feldenkrais, led Husserl to his discovery of FFV in relation to movement. In other words, the freedom from conceptual constraints inherent in FFV is dependent on

Husserl's prior lived experience of the relation between "pure possibility" associated with "as if" imaginative fantasizing, and the myriad variations and constraints associated with the "*I-can.*" An apt analogy might be the attainment of flight by a young bird, who achieves the freedom of flight only through sensing its material weight through the at-first asynchronous flapping of its still immature wings.

Reviewing her underscore of Husserl's phenomenology of kinesthesia and the limitations of fantasized movement succinctly, Sheets-Johnstone continues:

> Given this clarification of free variation with respect to freely varied movement, we can appreciate the peculiar challenge that movement presents: fantasized movement can enlighten us only so far. To get at the essentials of movement, and, in turn, to arrive at fully fleshed out understandings of an "I move," of an "I do," of an *organ* body—structures into which Husserl gained initial insight but which he did not fully explore—it is essential to move. (1999, 199–200)

In summary, exploration of movement presents a realm necessary for phenomenological exploration that is independent of *eidetic* visualization but requires the kinesthetic experience of movement itself. Sheets-Johnstone helps explain why sensitive explorers of movement such as Feldenkrais and Shulman can stumble upon the richness of somatic explorations in order to free the self, using the affordances of embodiment, without being formally trained in the methodology of phenomenology. It also provides explanation why firsthand experience of movement is essential for phenomenology, without kinesthetic experience becoming fully reduced to phenomenological analyses of conscious experience. This "independence" of the kinaesthetic realm also explains why somatic practices provide important data for phenomenological analysis and yet are differentiated from phenomenology in representing a set of practices that enables the practitioner to be present with the pre-reflective self, without the imperative of phenomenological reflection (Braude 2015).

Finally, in moving between the groundedness of kinesthesia and perception and the freedom from the constraints of *empeira*, FFV presents one important means of mediating between logical possibility and practical possibility, symbolized by the expression "*I can.*" According to Mohanty, the kinesthetic "I can" consciousness, such as "I can move my hand," may be considered the "most primitive awareness of possibility on which the distinction between the actual and the possible is founded" (1984, 27–28). The "as if . . ." consciousness, associated with kinaesthetic variations provides the possibility for the theoretical pure possibility to become via *fantasy* free of all embodied limitations.

Yet, this practical possibility in kinaesthetic awareness is still a form of phenomenological consciousness that always reflects back to and upon the self. It is not simply free exploration caught up in the pleasurable *jouissance* of movement, as vital as pleasurable sensation is for movement exploration, but is equally dependent on the theoretical possibility encapsulated in the conceptual possibility "as if. ." In her dance class, Ami's suggestion, "what if . . ." emphasizes the importance of thought in structuring the infinite possibility within movement—hence, the importance of the FFV guidance by Ami in bringing the dancer's awareness back and forth between practical and theoretical possibilities of the self in relation to movement.

Finally, we wish to mention a third possibility of "*I can*" that opens up the possibility for further explorations of the relation between phenomenology of performance, or *phenomenology as performance*, in relation to the unfolding of the self in relation to thought and movement. Thus, Mohanty posits a third possibility, another kind of "*I can*" consciousness not "tied to

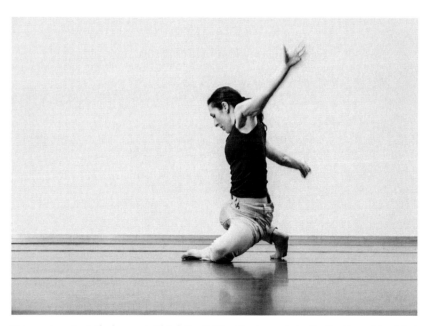

Figure 10.3. Ami Shulman, *A Third Possibility*. Photograph in Berlin © 2016 by Jubal Battisti.

corporeality in the manner kinaesthesis is" (1984, 27–28). We have seen in this analysis how active choice making in movement variations inevitably lead to the unfolding of the kinaesthetic self and assist the mover to become fully present in realization of intention, freeing the movement from its form. Mohanty suggests that for Husserl there is an even more "originary" form of "open possibility" in which the "structure of world-experience dissolves itself" (Mohanty 1984, 13–29). Moreover, this open possibility, in which the self strives to free itself from "world experience," is constituted theoretically in terms of conceptualization and not practically. Of course, there is no real possibility of nonbeing within conscious experience. However, this most primal of possibilities indicates the desire for the self to free even the self from itself, from the "*I*" in "*I can.*" This third possible "*I can*" stumbles upon the core existential issue associated with FFV's process of freeing thought in order "to take anything actual or possible as examples" (Zaner 2012, 169), i.e., that the "self is at stake" in the abstraction of exemplification (Zaner *At Play in the Field of the Possibles* 157). Exploring movement variations may free self-potential, but it may also help to dissolve the boundaries between inner and outer, between self and world, between immanent and transcendent. It is possible that the creative force propelling the shifts between transitional states in movement and the possibility of self-transcendence arise from this unconscious striving for the self to become free of itself, to dissolve itself in the pure freedom of thought in its own movement. "As if" movement was thought, and thought was movement with no self in between . . .

Notes

1. Sondra Fraleigh refers to this phenomenon as the realization of intention in movement. For her study of intention in dance, see "Witnessing the Frog Pond" (1999).

2. In support of her statement about the self-affectivity of phenomenological reflection, Behnke references *Husserliana Materialen* (1950).

3. For a more in-depth analysis of Husserl's "*I can,*" see Behnke, "Edmund Husserl's Contribution" (1996).

4. See, Feldenkrais, (1942, 9), as well as the autobiography of Feldenkrais by Mark Reese (2015, 182, 282).

5. See, especially, Merleau-Ponty, *Primacy of Perception* (1962, 194–196).

11

"Me, a Tree"

Young Children as Natural Phenomenologists

KAREN BOND

Sue Stinson and I began our first collaborative publication focused on young people's lived experiences of dance with the following commentary:

> Work by children in every art form has been both romanticized and criticized by adults. . . . it often seems that educators view children as incomplete adults, in need of education and training to make them mature as well as civilized. . . . This may be why the ideas and opinions of children are rarely found in research literature, even in education. (2000/01, 52)

While qualitative research on children's learning has grown since the 1990s, phenomenological inquiry into children's meaning-making as a source of theoretical and practical knowledge remains limited. Research continues to highlight the extent to which children meet values, theories, and developmental standards established by adults. Extending the adage that children should be seen and not heard, when it comes to dance scholarship as a whole, young people are seldom seen *or* heard, in spite of their peerless sensitivity to the ineffable (Bond 2014). Child psychologist Alice Miller predicts, "Someday we will regard our children not as creatures to manipulate or to change but rather as messengers from a world we once deeply knew, but which we have long since forgotten" (Miller 1990, xiii).

Other notable thinkers have acknowledged children's unique intelligences and contributions to knowledge. Critical theorist Terry Eagleton observes that in their "wondering estrangement" from accepted practices, "children make the *best* theorists" (1990, 34, emphasis mine). Antoine de Saint-Exupéry also admired children's agency and intellect (1943). Speaking as his semiautobio-

graphical aviator character in *The Little Prince* (voted the best book of the twentieth century in France), he states: "Grown-ups never understand anything for
themselves, and it is tiresome for children to always and forever be explaining
things to them" (4–5). Alluding to children's "naturalistic intelligence" (Gardner
1999), near the end of *The Little Prince*, Saint-Exupéry exclaims:

> Look up at the sky. Ask yourselves: is it yes or no? Has the sheep eaten the
> flower? And you will see how everything changes. . . . And no grown-up will
> ever understand that this is a matter of so much importance! (1943, 62)

Like Saint-Exupéry's prince, I suspect that most if not all children enjoy
explaining things to adults (especially when encouraged). Visionary social
scientist and cyberneticist Gregory Bateson featured philosophical interactions
with his daughter in a number of publications. In *Steps to an Ecology of Mind*,
he presents them as a collection titled "Metalogues," defined as conversations
"about some problematic subject" (1972, 12). Held with Mary Catherine Bateson when she was nine-to-fourteen years old (1948–1953), problematic subjects
included muddles, Frenchmen, games, being serious, knowing, outlines, Why
a Swan? (a conversation about ballet), and instinct (12–69). Maurice Merleau-
Ponty also enjoyed an intellectual connection with his daughter, for whom he
would inscribe his books, "Marianne, his favourite philosopher" (Bakewell
2016, 237). More recently, theoretical physicist Karen Barad acknowledged her
daughter, Mikaela, as her closest collaborator, writing:

> The way she meets the world each day with an open and loving heart-mind
> has taught me a great deal. Her insatiable sense of curiosity, unabated ability
> to experience pure joy in learning, wide-open sense of caring for other beings,
> and loving attentiveness to life (taking in the tiniest details and textures of the
> world (which she re-creates through poetry, drawings, paintings, sculpture,
> stories, dance, and song) are key ingredients to making possible futures worth
> remembering. (2007, xiii)

This chapter follows Edmund Husserl's (1982) call to go "back to the things
themselves" by returning to the young child's pre-theoretical universe of
dance. It endeavors to "explain" dance and dancing to adults through children's captioned drawings (collected over many years in a variety of settings)
in dialogue with scholarly autobiographical reflection and selected phenomenologies. Drawings were all created in response to a phenomenological
prompt immediately after sessions of improvisational, or creative, movement/
dance, for example, "What did you do in dance today?" As noted by Janet
O'Shea, "Dance can ground philosophical assertions . . . in the specifics of
practice" (2010, 11).

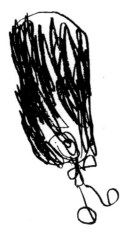

Figure 11.1. Pure Joy.

According to Talia Welsh, Merleau-Ponty sees the child as a "natural phe-nomenologist" who stays connected to experience and does not require "a resolution in theory" (2013, 110). Acknowledging that there is no way to grasp or interpret the full complexity of thinking of the three philosophers foregrounded in this chapter—Leonard C. Feldstein (1922–1984), Max van Manen, and Maurice Merleau-Ponty (1908–1964)—I also am not looking

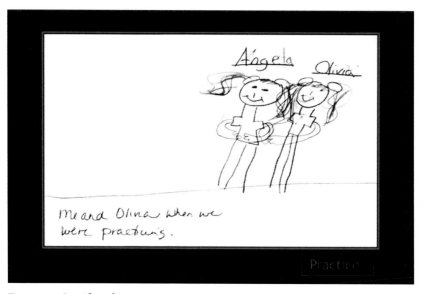

Figure 11.2. Specifics of Practice.

for resolutions in theory. Instead, I consider how children's lived experience drawings and utterances about dancing might strengthen a collection of empirical and philosophical ideas from literature.

Ultimately, this chapter is a heuristic project: I held a profusion of possible starting points and at this moment of writing am unclear how it will close. I am grateful to those who have led the way to restoration of transparent, first-person writing as a method of inquiry, in particular, anthropologists Ruth Behar (1996) and Deidre Sklar (2001) and sociologist Laurel Richardson (1994).

The next section presents a narrative of my own "becoming phenomenologies," beginning with early professional practice, moving through remembered serendipities, and, finally, concluding with theoretical commitment to phenomenology as an ethical-aesthetic practice in dance and life. Moreover, I endeavor to restore a measure of utility and grace to some of twentieth-century academia's contested constructs such as *essence*, *universal*, and *ideal* for a new millennial reader whose plurality of racial, ethnic, gender, class, and other social affinities motivates interest in the integration of personal agency with intersubjective resonance in a world that seems obsessed with difference and status.

Becoming Phenomenologies

During the 1990s, I was part of the Arts Forms of Enquiry study group at La Trobe University in Melbourne, Australia. Composed of artists, academics, psychologists, social workers, teachers, and combinations of these, the group shared an interest in questions of meaning in the arts. Many of us turned to phenomenology. I've reflected that if the group had been convened prior to my completion of dance doctoral research with six nonverbal children born with deaf-blindness (1991), my naively phenomenological approach to working with them might have been articulated as such at least a decade earlier.

Signs of an "inner phenomenologist" started to appear in the mid-1970s. As a newly hired dance tutor at Melbourne's State College of Victoria, Institute of Early Childhood Development, I began to formulate a philosophical framework for teaching dance with young children—not teaching *for* or *to*, but *with*. In retrospect, I realized that I had embraced this horizontal perspective through "apprenticeships of observation" (Fortin and Siedentop 1995, 9) with progressive educators, notably Anna Halprin and Betty Backus, whose teaching methods emphasized "starting where the student is" (Bond 2013). Influenced also by early developments in contact improvisation, I wanted my teaching to emphasize what I later came to know as *intersubjectivity*, created through somatic engagement with and between other(s) in shared environ-

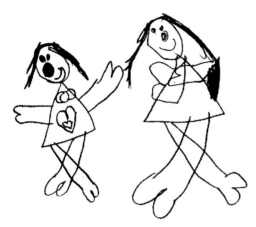

Figure 11.3. "It's her heart."

ments. Neurophenomenologist Shaun Gallagher explains intersubjectivity as a direct perceptual field:

> In seeing the actions and expressive movements of the other person in the context of the surrounding world, one already sees their meaning; no inference to a hidden set of mental states . . . is necessary. When I see the other's action or gesture, I see (I immediately perceive) the meaning in the action or gesture. I see the joy or I see the anger, or I see the intention in the face or in the posture or in the gesture or action of the other. (2005, 542)

In 1978, motivated by the challenge of a debut conference presentation, I wrote "Receiving the Dance of the Child: An Application of Developmental and Humanistic Learning Theories to Teaching Dance" (Bond 1978). Four years later I began doctoral research with psychologist and aesthetician Warren Lett at La Trobe University. I framed the study theoretically as humanistic, developmental, aesthetic, and therapeutic, but the center of its energy was experiential—twelve weeks of intensive dancing with the six children (three at a time, each with an adult partner) four times a week, systematically documented through video and field notes. During close analysis of video-recorded sessions, I began to conceptualize "receiving the dance of the child" as *kinesthetic empathy* (after McCoubrey 1987), a phenomenon first applied to dance theory by John Martin (1933).

Since the 1990s, kinesthetic empathy has been deconstructed by historians and cultural theorists, and Martin has been critiqued for idealist, universalist, and essentialist views on how dance is perceived by the viewer (Foster 1998, 2011; Franko 2002; Reason and Reynolds 2010). As a practical phenomenologist, attributions of idealist to Martin's theory of "kinesthetic sympathy" and "metakinesis" seem potentially overdetermined. Martin takes accountability for his values on the "ideal education" (1933, 15) (education being one context where a twenty-first-century form of embodied idealism experienced as radical pluralism might hold ethical possibilities), but I have not yet found him using the term in relation to viewing dance.

I question also how epistemologies of historical determinism or cultural relativism are any less universalizing or essentializing than Martin's psychobiological lens. Merleau-Ponty scholar Talia Welsh asserts, "Cultural relativism, like scientific psychology, depends upon a God's-eye view of existence. I stand disconnected from my own experience and note cultural differences between various groups" (2013, 148). She suggests further that for Merleau-Ponty, children's visual art has more to say about "essential engagement with our embodied selves and the world than a theory where our isolation from any common experience is asserted as a universal truth" (149).

Thinking further about *essence*, for me the construct has a certain "je ne sais quoi" and I wonder if this might be the case for others. Here, I spin a loose analogy with Robert Pirsig's (1974) front quote in *Zen and the Art of Motorcycle Maintenance*: "What is good, Phaedrus, and what is not good— need we ask anyone to tell us these things?"

While Karen Barad, like feminist philosophers Simone de Beauvoir (2010) and Judith Butler (2011) before her, deflates naturalistic assumptions that "reality" is composed of *fixed* essences, she uses the word liberally in her writing to reference "essences" of theories, for example, the "very essence of quantum physics" is "quantum entanglement" (Barad 2007, 386).

Returning to *kinesthetic empathy*, in the mid-1980s the notion had bodily, pragmatic, and explanatory value in my dance work with nonverbal children. Through mirroring, shadowing, echoing, and other modes of resonance, we danced with each child's unique gestures, postures, rhythms, spatial patterns, energy qualities, and vocalizations, and they "talked back." I was full of pedagogical hope that, supported by nonauthoritarian, "dialogic" relating (Freire 1994), these observably asocial or "acultural" children (Goode 1994), would create a group experience while living together in their residential educational setting.

In essence, I was committed to "allowing children to follow their own impulses and designs . . . uncluttered by external standards (even tacit standards) of performance" (Bond 1991, 99). I later came to understand this as the practice of epoché, or phenomenological bracketing (Van Manen 1990), but at the time saw it only as recognizing each child's right to express their dance. I knew this way of working departed from prevalent behaviorist methods intended to extinguish or normalize "atypical" behavior, but I explained that in dance, behavioral idiosyncrasy is an element of invention. One participating adult, however, confided that accommodating children's manneristic (i.e., "abnormal") behaviors in dance felt like heresy in the context of their training in behaviorist practices.

During the 1990s, Max van Manen's methodology workshops in Australia strengthened my sense of who I desired to be as a dancer, educator, and researcher, as captured in the following: "Research is a caring act: we want to know what is most essential to being" (Van Manen 1990, 5). He elaborates, "Phenomenology is a philosophy or theory of the unique . . . the nonreplaceable" practiced with awareness of "the evasive character of . . . *other*, the *whole*, the *communal*, or the *social*" [emphases mine]. Further, this process of pathic engagement enables possibilities of transformation, or what van Manen calls "true education" (7).

Peter Willis notes van Manen's emphasis on "reflective open attention," a kind of "aesthetic 'dwelling'" that seeks to uncover meaning "before the knower moves to analyse and name the phenomenon" (2014, 64). Young children's spontaneous dance drawings offer such openings to meaning, as can their spoken and written captions. Such lived experience descriptions of dancing might shed light on a problem that continues to perplex philosophers, psychologists, cognitive scientists, and dancers alike: the relation between experience and representation (figure 11.4).

One of van Manen's analytic prisms that gifts the dance scholar is what he calls the lifeworld existentials: lived body, space, time, and human relation or communality (1990, 101–106), which, without the qualifier *lived*, can be understood as elemental categories of dance (along with energy or force). Figures 11.5–11.8 exemplify how young children can show affinities for a particular "existential" in their graphic reflections on dancing.

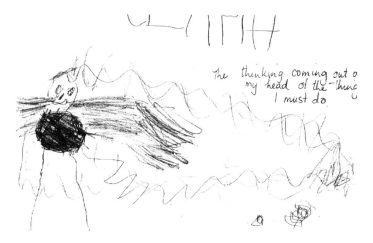

The thinking coming out o
my head of the thing
I must do.

Figure 11.4. "Thinking."

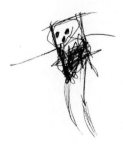

Figure 11.5. Lived Body.

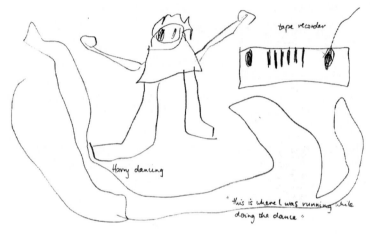

Figure 11.6. Lived Space.

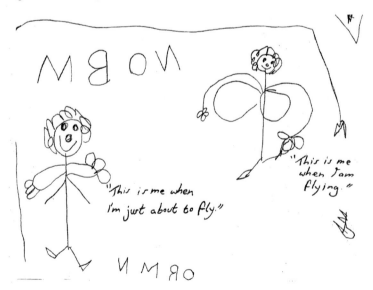

Figure 11.7. Lived Time.

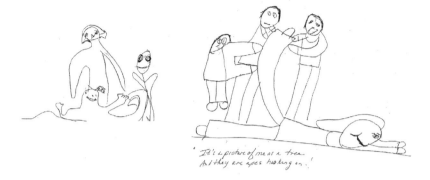

Figure 11.8. Lived Relation/Communality.

As a guide to illuminating lived experience and human possibility, life-world existentials can strengthen phenomenological viewing, writing, and dancing, evoking "a wondrous landscape . . . a feeling of disorientation . . . confusion . . . strangeness, of being struck with wonder" (Van Manen 2014, 359). This perspective complements Maxine Sheets-Johnstone's notion of phenomenological method as "making the familiar strange" (2015, xxiv).

Prior to encountering van Manen in person and in theory, I had been practicing "reflective open attention" (Willis 2014, 64) with six nonverbal children with deaf-blindness. Seeking to understand their observed trans-formations in dance, I discovered philosopher of science and psychoanalyst Leonard Feldstein's (1979) *The Dance of Being*, a biological-to-spiritual ontology of the person in which *rhythm* is an integrative theme. Feldstein identifies the "universal rhythmic theme of personhood" as *searching* (45), a premise that connects rhythm to existential creativity. In spite of impairments of both distance senses, children showed numerous instances of self-initiated exploration in dance, lending credence to Feldstein's "universal person" as a dancer.

Despite his clear metaphorical affiliations with dance and music, I have not yet found references to Feldstein in dance scholarly literature, including dance philosophy. Is this because he was a philosopher of science, a classical dualist (although not a binarist), a cosmologist spinning "designs of a daring imagination . . . yet somewhat cloudy and hard to make out" as Corinna Delkeskamp (1978) viewed his suggestion that the unconscious "glows" through the integrated person's actions, making them "luminous" (191)? Feldstein's transcendental empiricism with its base in biological rhythms, immanence, "flows," and poetics reminds me of Gilles Deleuze and Felix Guattari, whose

A Thousand Plateaus: Capitalism and Schizophrenia (2002) also includes dance metaphors but, unlike *The Dance of Being*, is a focus of growing interest across numerous disciplines, including dance studies (LaMothe 2015; Markula 2006; Rothfield 2011). Perhaps the "abiding religious conviction" that Feldstein identifies as influential to his thinking—a synthesis of Christianity and Judaism "as they are wedded to the astounding intellectual achievement of the Greeks" (xi) has alienated serious attention (see also LaMothe's [2006] commentary on the reverse—philosophy and religion's neglect of dance meanings in Nietzsche's writings).

My greatest challenge reading Feldstein (and many twentieth-century philosophers) is stylistic, for example, his persistent use of "man" to represent humankind, as flagged in *The Dance of Being's* subtitle: *Man's Labyrinthine Rhythms*. While I would prefer to interact with a more gender-neutral presentation (as Massumi makes available for *A Thousand Plateaus*) (Deleuze and Guattari 2002), the author's detailed, subtle, and "daringly designed" (Delkeskamp 1978) depictions of the "infrapersonal spectrum of biologic activities" (Feldstein 1979, 2), coiling and meeting in human action and being as "dance," helps me suspend gendered unease. *The Dance of Being* is full of movement, body, rhythm, space, and poetics, also illustrating being's "affinity, a sustained and inexorable attunement, to the inanimate" (56), prefiguring contemporary discourses in new materialism, eco-phenomenology, and object-oriented ontology (Bennett 2010; Morton 2015). Congruent with Feldstein, Ian Bogost (2012) writes, "Objects try to make sense of each other through the qualities and logics they possess" (66).

In relation to my study of nonverbal children with deaf-blindness, though, I did not feel equipped to align theoretical analysis of their observable transformations with Feldstein's full cosmological design, despite one boy discovering a state of "ecstatic being" in dance (Bond 1991, 311–322), which I likened to spiritual awakening. It was a single sentence in *The Dance of Being*, however, that allowed an empirically grounded finding of the study to take flight: "Through the unfolding of profoundly intimate rhythms, a personal style is engendered for each individual" (Feldstein 1979, 45). The empirical finding that personal style mediated children's engagement in dance had developed beyond rhythms to include body (gesture, posture, shape), space, voice quality, dynamics, affect, sensory preferences, and more (Bond 1994, 2008), but Feldstein's ontology of the essential-person-as-rhythm has continued to intrigue.

Specifically, Feldstein understands the person as a *ferment* of "incarnating rhythms" unfolding through phases of highly determined processes that, after Alfred North Whitehead, are nevertheless "pervaded by spontaneous self-enjoyment" (6–7). From each center—each singularity of rhythmic fer-

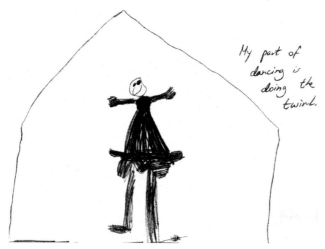

My part of dancing is doing the twirl.

Figure 11.9. Personal Style.

ment, person constructs identity amid forces of nature, events, and sociality, seeking novelty and variation (39). Moreover, center is "supremely reflexive . . . counterposing the germ of already formed identity to resistances ceaselessly encountered" (273). Feldstein's person is "a well-executed dance; every part, in its very mobility, congruent with . . . entire being," while subtle, complex rhythms emanate from and pass through other animate and inanimate entities—with fluctuant motility, "like so many concentric circles." Into this "orchestration of rhythm" breaks silence, stillness, and pause, over and over, brief or extended (41). I wonder whether to deny essence, to deny the universal, is to deny silence.

Through systematic philosophical inquiry, Feldstein identifies three interdependent categories that frame the dance of being—agency, power, and rhythm, which seem applicable to the *actual* (nonmetaphoric) "universal dancer," along with the qualia he attributes to each category. The following diagram provides a selection of language that I find pertinent to phenomenologies of dance and performance.

I invite you to engage intersubjectively with Feldstein's concepts, applying van Manen's reflective open attention. This, as dance philosophers who understand aesthetic indwelling and the possibility of silent, ahistorical knowing even amid words like *power*, with its load of social-cultural appropriations. Feldstein's *power* is a biological given and potential: the ability to do, act, move, resist, and search—Husserl's "I can," capacities that exist in particle and cell (1982). Considering the word's applications in discourses of human politics and war since at least 900 ACE, however (*Oxford English Dictionary*),

Table 11.1

Being as Agency	Being as Power	Being as Rhythm	
unity	ferment	*Orchestration*	*Invariance & mutuality*
essence	resonance	flux	space, time, matter
plurality	action	emotionality	vibration, pulsation
existence	identity	part-whole consistency	rotation, spiraling
center	potentiality	silence, stillness, pause	flowings
boundary	potency	personal style	crystallizations
sociality			transformations

I agree with Sondra Fraleigh that "we can find better words than 'power' and 'empowerment' to value dance" (forthcoming). Feldstein's theme of *agency* supports current studies in developmental psychology that emphasize its reflexive, interpersonal construction, as observed in infants' behaviors of spontaneity, creativity, and delight (Deans et al. 2015), qualities I associate with aesthetic autonomy (Bond 2001, 2008).

The concept of *ferment* interests me in relation to essences of dance as known by a young child living her/his unique rhythmic motility within endowed and shaped morphological boundaries and in association with events, organisms, and persons—Feldstein's modalities of rhythmic being (1979, 43). He invites us to consider Virginia Woolf's dancing moth for an account of how the powers of ferment shape life, reflecting, "Watching its flittings and its meanderings and its minutely humble motions, not however without a certain dignity, one might so easily forget it" (14). Yet, as Woolf portrays:

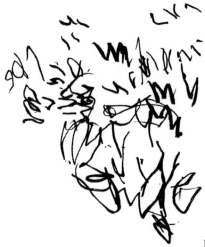

Figure 11.10. "I am dancing."

"ME, A TREE" · 217

What he could do he did. Watching him, it was as if a fibre, very thin but pure, of the enormous energy of the world had been thrust into his frail and diminutive body. . . . He was little or nothing but life. . . . It was as if someone had taken a tiny bead of pure life and decking it as lightly as possible with down and feather had set it dancing and zig zagging to show us the true nature of life. Thus displayed, one could not get over the strangeness of it. (1974, 4)

Consider, then, the person: 7.5 billion of us inhabiting Earth in 2017 (1.9 billion children) (www.unicef.org/statistics/; accessed June 1, 2017), all a ferment of searching. Consider some four million years of bi-pedal evolution, advancing the "roaming propensities of leg and foot" through which, according to Feldstein, "dance burst forth" (1979, 272). Does not each person contain the "enormous energy of the world"? Do not each of us contain the essence and existence of dance?

Feldstein exclaims:

The dance of being! The person is ferment; the interplay of persons is ferment; the community . . . is ferment. Yet the pattern of ferment is elusive . . . the invariant structures that endure across transmutations; the person is a manifold in flux. (38)

In my sense making, Feldstein's "enduring invariant structures" enable a unique person who can never be replicated completely, even at the intra-personal level; an existential sociality that encompasses events, organisms, and persons; and a transcendental cosmological epistemology. Rhythmic essence-as-unity remains reflexively centered on each being's potency toward

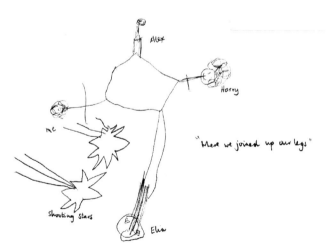

Figure 11.11. Roaming Propensities of Leg and Foot.

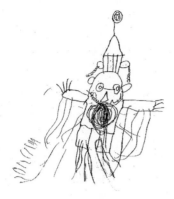

Figure 11.12. Ferment.

action, while existence is a plurality—affording paradoxical persistence with ceaseless possibilities of transformation. Feldstein acknowledges the problem of essence: how as a unity do I become a plurality? (21). But returning essence to its lived etymological roots, as essence, I am both *being* and *to be*.

Thinking further about the power of *ferment as rhythm*, Feldstein was not isolated during the 1970s and early '80s in his interest in rhythm as an ontological category, including in science. Physicist Fritjof Capra (1982) (still teaching at age 78) described life as a rhythmic dance, observing that human rhythmic facility allows expression of the distinctive person. Similar to Feldstein, he suggests that this "inner impulse . . . is the essence of personal identity" (327). Around the same time, poet and essayist Henri Meschonnic (1982) published his massive treatise on rhythm, *Critique du Rythme*, continuing to theorize rhythm ontologically for the remainder of his life:

> For rhythm is a subject form(er). The subject form(er). That it renews the meaning of things, that it is through rhythm that we reach the sense that we have of our being undone [défaire], that everything around us happens as it undoes itself [défaire], and that, approaching this sensation of the movement of everything, we ourselves are part of this movement. (2011, 165)

Dance and arts scholars have also theorized rhythm in existential terms. Sheets-Johnstone (2009b) locates dance's origins in the early rhythmic play of pre-hominids, identifying possible "kinetic markers" such as rough and tumble action, running, falling, jumping, and ballistic movement (322).

For dance analyst Laurence Louppe (2010), dance's "profound autonomy and originality," grounded in bodily rhythmic states of breath, time, and space, make dance the "art of extreme freedom" (135), a possibility overlooked by most existential philosophers (Nietzsche is a notable exception), including Merleau-Ponty, although he once portrayed painter Henri Matisse

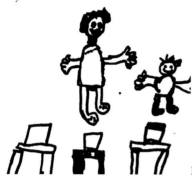

Figure 11.13. Ballistic Toast.

as dancing before the canvas (Wiskus 2008, 142) and has been credited as the best dancer among the Parisian Left Bank thinkers of his time (Bakewell 2016, 237). Approaching Feldstein's infrapersonal, Ellen Dissanayake (1995) states that "existence equals pulsation" (83)—respiration, brain waves, and circulatory rhythms provide the background to our being (240).

Merleau-Ponty (1968) and Sondra Fraleigh (2004) propose a rhythmic basis for the human ability to attune to others and to the world, the former stating that body is our "living bond with nature" (27).

Fraleigh suggests that the human capacity for "relational embodiment" (25) is particularly strong in children:

> Our dances are made of nature, the rhythms of our bodies . . . even as the
> dance itself is made possible through that same body rhythm, whether we

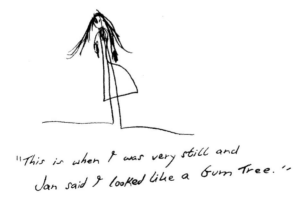

"This is when I was very still and
Jan said I looked like a Gum Tree."

Figure 11.14. "Me, a Tree."

decide to listen to it or not. The nonhuman forms and rhythms around us
also help to root our sensibilities and movements. Children know this as they
swing their linked-together arms like elephant trunks and unfold their dancer
arms like the wings of a lark. (118)

Being "natural phenomenologists," children experience these bonds intimately, enacting their multisensory, somato-cognitive intelligence—their
"synesthetic" perception (Welsh 2013, 114), their agency of power and flux
(Feldstein). Regarding Merleau-Ponty's thoughts on rhythm, Irene Klaver
(2005) suggests that though it was not thematized in *Phenomenology of
Perception* (a volume that refers to dance only three times), rhythm "sub-
tends the entire analysis" (41), like Feldstein's ontology of the person three
decades later. Merleau-Ponty (2002) states, "Biological existence is synchronized with human existence and is never indifferent to its distinctive
rhythm" (185).

Merleau-Ponty said little about dance per se, and his minimal treatment of
it as a "motor habit" has been critiqued, notably by Sheets-Johnstone (2015,
xiv). Nevertheless, the recent translation of his *Sorbonne Lectures (1949–1952)*
on child psychology (Merleau-Ponty 2010) became pay dirt for this chapter,
along with Talia Welsh's (2013) in-depth commentary, which elucidates his
views on the philosophical relevance of early childhood to the person's construction of self. Diverging from prominent developmental theories of the
time, notably Jean Piaget's, which tend to write the young child as "internally
occupied, passive receivers of culture," he describes the child's experience as
"unique, organized, and socially interactive" (xiv).

Staying with his interest in visual embodiment established in *Phenomenology of Perception*, Merleau-Ponty (2010) engaged with children's drawings
empirically:

> *The study of . . . drawing leads us back to . . . its ground: perception.* We have
> seen that drawings express affectivity rather than understanding. . . . we must
> pay close attention to what the child's perception . . . consists of when encoun-
> tering things . . . as affective stimulants. (171, emphasis original)

For example, he observed that children distort the comparative sizes of objects and persons depending on their affective relations, a phenomenon sub-
stantiated in the following drawing in which teacher "Elly" holds gigantic
proportion; further, in "measurable" reality, the artist "Me" is a fair bit smaller
than her friend "Grace."

Merleau-Ponty suggests that drawings of the very young offer unique insights into the nature of human perception, showing greater integration of

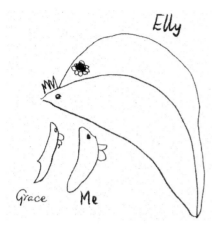

Figure 11.15. Teacher.

sensation, emotion, and intellect than do adult drawings. Moreover, sensory categorization is unusual; instead, children's drawing reveals perception of "totality," including nonvisual aspects of lived experience (Welsh 2013, 118). This is evidenced, for example, in the motion indicators appearing in drawings presented so far, some of which remind me of Feldstein's "glow" (Delkeskamp 1978). Philosopher of aesthetics Paul Crowther draws on Merleau-Ponty to state that vision is "a function of all our sensory, motor, and affective capacities operating as a unified field" (1993, 103). Moreover, children are not as conditioned into cultural styles of representation (Welsh 2013, 115) or the "conventional attitudes" held by adults (Merleau-Ponty 2010, 171). Their capacity for holistic perception opens them to essences of experience, one might suggest. Van Manen reminds that essence is not a mystical notion but pertains directly to quality of life:

> A good description that constitutes the essence of something is constructed so that the structure of a lived experience is revealed to us in such a fashion that we are now able to grasp the nature and significance of this experience in a hitherto unseen way. (1990, 39)

Children are exemplars of this kind of essential construction, where a good description can be a dance, a drawing, a story, a song, and so forth. In their structure, children's dance drawings reveal a fluidity of sensation. Children depict pre-reflective awareness of both center and mutuality with events, organisms, and persons (Feldstein 1979, 43). According to Welsh, Merleau-Ponty argued that without this kind of primary evidence, "we would be hard-pressed to explain the genesis of intersubjectivity" (2013, xviii). Both Merleau-Ponty (2010) and van Manen (1995) have asserted that any consideration of existential meanings returns us to the qualia of early childhood.

As alluded to earlier, Merleau-Ponty stressed the importance of not over-valuing the intellectual and representational abilities of children but instead suspending overdetermined cultural and scientific assumptions, or "natural attitude" (Husserl 2001). In doing so, we may discover "forms and styles of engagement that are not always found in a more developed sense in the adult," for example, intersubjectivities that are not based on mental processes (Welsh 2013, 106). Children's drawings reveal both persisting and evolving quali-ties of personal style, throwing light on the human capacity for perceptual continuity and self-organization. Feldstein's ontology of person-as-rhythm suggests that the child reflexively retrieves and re-physicalizes vivid moments of experience while seeking variation. These ideas will be pulled together in the next and concluding section of the chapter.

Crystallizations

On the whole, the materials and philosophers (child and adult) included in this project have educated me further on "the essential dancer," whom I understand as a child. The remainder of the chapter gathers materials and themes into a composite of language and images, starting with a visual rep-resentation. Figure 11.16 highlights what I consider the central contributions of van Manen, Feldstein, and Merleau-Ponty to the study. I then foreground thematically the tag cloud's layer of medium-font text, extending this with other phenomenological meanings accumulated in the chapter.

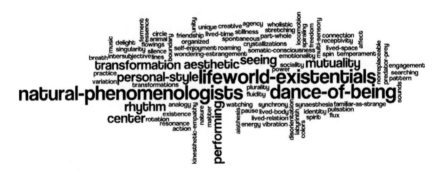

Figure 11.16. Essence, Existence, Perception.

CENTER

One of the topics I considered for this paper was "phenomenologies of center," an area of inquiry known experientially to most, if not all, dancers from a young age. Of the 72 drawings short-listed for this chapter, phenomena of center—rotation, spiral, circle, center, swing, spin, balance, imbalance, and fall—feature in almost half. Closer observation reveals that children's drawings emphasize consciousness of center through intensity of drawing gestures or inclusion of a "belly button," their own and others'. Feldstein describes center as "a singularity toward which all parts . . . [of body] are in some sense oriented . . . a locus of spiritual dynamism" (1979, 174) through which rhythms of animate and inanimate environment and of sociality radiate and flow (41).

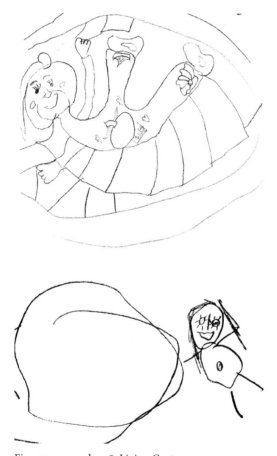

Figures 11.17 and 11.18. Living Centers.

Stephen

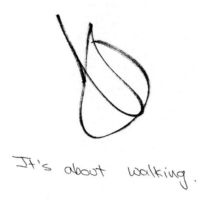

It's about walking.

Figure 11.19. "It's about Walking."

In addition to children's pre-reflective knowledge of center as both essence (singularity) and existence (plurality), some carry personal stylistic preferences for bi-pedal locomotion of walking and running (Figure 11.19), often integrated with awareness of orientation, rotation, and action. Sarah Ahmed observes that "body gets directed in some ways more than others" suggesting a connection between personal style and lived space, where "direction is organized rather than casual" (2006, 15).

The following sequence of drawings illustrates a young girl and her friends' persistent practice of running in the dance space, along with the artist's consciousness of center. Figure 11.20 illustrates somatic awareness of body center, a motif that recurs throughout her drawings. Figure 11.22 illustrates her unique logic of experiential representation: two "Annie's" and two "Me's" appear to progress in lived time as they run or perhaps observe "where the people run."

Returning to the study of nonverbal children with deaf-blindness, without consciously thinking "phenomenologically," I depicted an empirically grounded theory of personal style as a mediator of engagement in dance as a spiral, as reproduced in Figure 11.23 (Bond 1991, 353). Now, partnering Merleau-Ponty's observations of the young child's organized perceptual field—their unique phenomenal core of multisensory unity, or *aesthetic perception*, with Feldstein's notion of rhythmic being ceaselessly searching outward to community and receiving back from world, enables me to understand young children as natural phenomenologists and dancers of stylistically unique essence.

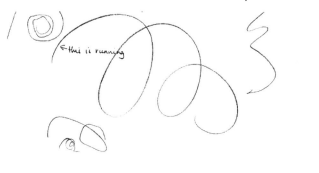

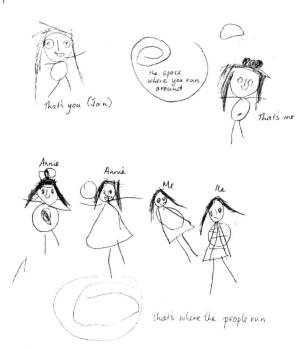

Figures 11.20–11.22. Perceptual Continuity.

SEEING

Working with persons living with visual and other sensory and emotional challenges also fostered an enduring interest in dance and dancing's visual aspects—what it means to see and be seen. Noticing the deaf-blind dancers' persistent attraction to light—their quiet passionate search for the visual—only 5 percent of those with deaf-blindness are totally blind—I imagined that

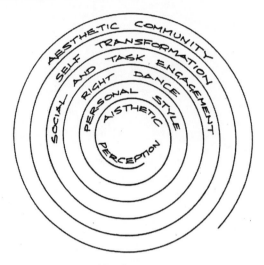

Figure 11.23. Spiraling Self and Community.

each saw the world through a distinctive kaleidoscopic lens. I learned new ways of dancing with light as I tried to see and feel the way the children did.

Times in dance when a child would seem to forget about light-seeking were usually associated with sharing rhythms or weight with other participants. When children were able to integrate the visual and kinesthetic, a quality of performativity emerged that had not been observed prior to dance. Without being taught formally (i.e., there seemed to be something about the "movement itself"), children learned to take turns being lifted, spun, and swung, and to "watch" each other moving, focusing their asymmetrical gazes to converge on a peer performer, sometimes clapping between turns.

As for the "normally sighted," I've long held a sense that *seeing* is a more concrete theme in children's dance drawings and captions than *being seen*, especially for the very young; that is, relatively few drawings are directly about "me being watched while I'm dancing." Perhaps the discovery of Merleau-Ponty's (2010) recently translated *Child Psychology and Pedagogy*, with its attention to children's drawings as philosophical texts, opened my attention to the subtle yet abundant "eye statements" in the drawings mined to illustrate children's experience of dance for this chapter.

What I began to perceive, making the familiar strange (Sheets-Johnstone 2015), was the agency in these in/animate objects that perform and see, the inevitability of their seeing and performing and searching. I gathered a short list of 72 drawings onto a spreadsheet and immediately experienced a blinking "double take" as a myriad of eyes converged on me, some from impossibly rotated heads. Objects were "staring back," as art historian James Elkins (1996) puts it:

> Every object sees us; there are eyes growing on everythng. . . . To see is to be seen, and everything I see is like an eye, collecting my gaze, blinking, staring, focusing and reflecting, sending my look back at me. (51)

At the same time, "The world is full of things we do not see, even when they are right in front of us" (54).

I reminisce about a conversation with University of Melbourne botanist Jeremy Pickett-Heaps while viewing single-celled organisms captured by video microscopy, evenly spaced with all their eye spots turned toward a source of light. Jeremy said something like, "The usual explanations don't work; they are not seeking food or sex . . . this could be aesthetics." Human eyes also seek a kind of primary mutuality, which Emmanuel Levinas might describe as experientially engaged and ethically pre-ontological, expressing "infinite responsibility," a being-for Other that is unavoidable as soon as I encounter another face (1991).

Suddenly, this confab of seers proliferates into the many thousands (millions?) of eyes I have taken for granted, like the ubiquitious smiley face of the children's drawing genre. I find myself in epoché, wondering, do Syrian children draw themselves and others with smiley faces? I perform a Google image search and discover that there most do not; I feel a strong desire to travel to Syria to dance with children and families, to ease human pain, however briefly.

I see also that across the spread of dance drawings, eyes look like belly buttons. I think about Da Vinci's *Vetruvian Man* (c. 1490 ACE) whose navel is

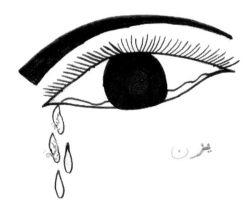

Figure 11.24. Eye on War.

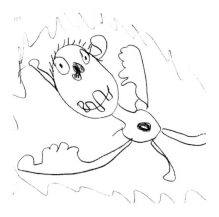

Figure 11.25. Vetruvian Child in Quantum Dance.

the center of his kinesphere and of the universe, along with all other unique, irreplaceable centers.

TRANSFORMATION

Finally, children's dance drawings show a propensity for experiences of transforming. Stinson (1990) observes that young children excel at transformation, shifting between "selves" and sense modalities more easily than adults do; they are able to "change their own identity instantly" (37). She adds, "When I look at most adults, it is easy to recognize that the capacities young children possess in such abundance practically disappear by adulthood" (37). Similar to Merleau-Ponty, Stinson highlights the young child's "sensory powers," which sometimes leave her "amazed" (37).

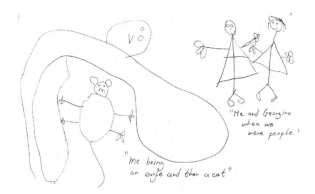

Figure 11.26. Transformations.

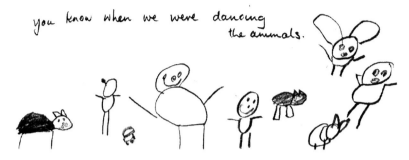

Figure 11.27. Dancing the Animals.

In my experience, when children are free to explore their unique rhythms, moves, and predilections in creative dance over time, they often "become animals" (Abram 1996), which continue to develop with nuance and novel variations. Figure 11.27 exemplifies a common response I have received when asking children what they remembered doing in creative dance.

Even in the ferment of a socially negotiated dance theme, children find ways to infuse their aesthetic agency, their personal style. The following set of drawings illustrates these phenomena: in a dance curriculum of eagles and reptiles, a young boy transitions from flying eagle to dancing bear; further, we caught the bear's eruption amid the collective rhythms of flying and swooping on video—the moment of transformation, along with his exclamation, "We need a bear in here!!" His drawings shift between first- and third-person description, the final one showing integration of lived experience and representation after his "transforming" occurs.

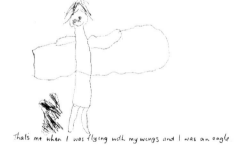

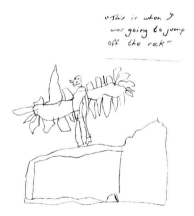

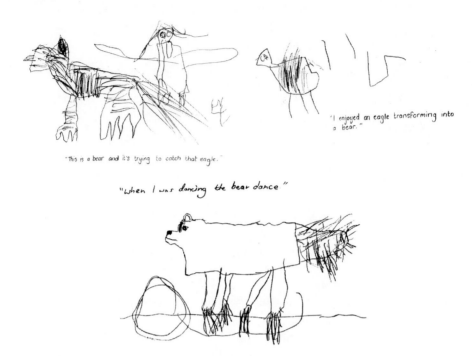

"This is a bear and it's trying to catch that eagle."

"I enjoyed an eagle transforming into a bear."

"When I was dancing the bear dance"

Figures 11.28–11.32. Becoming Bear.

The following series presents a variety of children's descriptions of "being animal" in dance, many of which burst forth independently of session themes and prompts, illustrating the phenomenon of *searching*, Feldstein's "universal rhythmic theme of personhood" (1979, 45). Further, children's search for novelty and variation in dance lends support for Louppe's (2010) assertion (cited earlier) that dance is "the art of extreme freedom" (135).

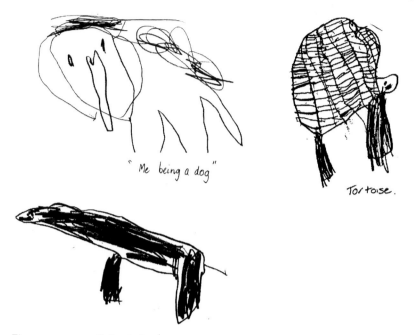

"Me being a dog"

Tortoise.

Figures 11.33–11.35. Being Animal.

Next, one of the group of running spinners finds a way to merge with a socially conceived session theme of spiders, illustrating holistic perception and thinking in movement: "We are spinning around and doing a very nice spider dance."

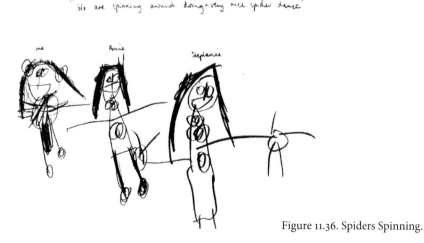

Figure 11.36. Spiders Spinning.

Descriptions of pleasure, agency, capability, and delight are plentiful in children's dance drawings and I close the chapter with one of my favorites, followed by a seven-year-old boy's logico-affective reflection on spinning. I hope you, the reader, have been engaged by the ideas, images, poetics, and possibilities in this chapter as "explained" by children, our species' natural phenomenologists of dance.

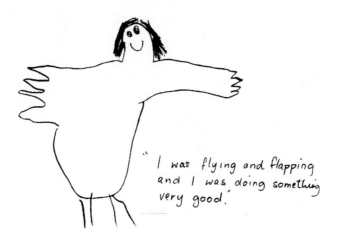

"I was flying and flapping and I was doing something very good."

Figure 11.37. "Doing Something Very Good."

I get dizzy when I spin on the floor
it is cool to spin on the floor
You have to spin on the floor
and see what it feels like
By by
I want to keep on dancing
the End

12

Dancing Epistemology, Situating Feminist Analysis

KAREN BARBOUR

Phenomenology, and particularly feminist phenomenology, has informed research and writing about women's lived experiences. The focus of this chapter is to briefly trace the weavings of philosophical and feminist engagements in phenomenology that have inspired dance scholarship and to illustrate embodied epistemology within dance performance. Philosophically and methodologically, feminist phenomenology provides a clear rationale for investigating embodied ways of knowing specific to dancers—who understand themselves, their relationship to others, and their relationship to the ecology of the planet—through moving. In this chapter, I consider the phenomenological notions of bracketing and variation, and of lifeworld and presence, relative to embodied ways of knowing in dance performance. I draw predominantly on feminists who have extended phenomenological work, including Simone de Beauvoir, Maxine Sheets-Johnstone, Iris Marion Young, Ann Cooper Albright, and Sondra Fraleigh. Throughout the chapter, I reflect on the lessons that breath and movement offer—juxtaposing intuitive descriptions of somatic phenomena with epistemological strategies—where feeling and knowing coalesce.

Phenomenology and Feminist Critique

Philosophically, as phenomenology unfolded it offered a crucial distinction between the everyday world and what Husserl called "the natural attitude," and the rigorous investigations of phenomenology (Husserl 1970, 1989; Sheets-Johnstone 1999; Van Manen 2014). According to Husserl, the basis of the natural attitude is our "inclination to believe that the world exists out there, independent of our personal human existence" (Van Manen 2014, 43). In the natural attitude, "We take the world as it presents itself, *and go from there* with our investigations and inquiries" (Sheets-Johnstone 1998, 188; italics original). While the natural world and we ourselves as lived bodies continue in a taken-for-granted sense as objects, "bracketing" offered phenomenologists a method to immediately engage with experiences and to suspend interpretations and meanings based on objective, scientific worldviews and on cultural, religious, social, historical, political, and other differences. Bracketing offered a method to suspend assumptions and attend anew to lived and embodied experiences in the world. Following from this method, we then derive meaning through the process known as *phenomenological reduction*. Maxine Sheets-Johnstone summarized this method:

> By bracketing we effect a suspension, an *epoche:* judgements and beliefs no longer have the potency they have in the natural attitude. Their modification frees us from epistemological constraints of the natural attitude such that we perceive things afresh. . . . Precisely because it is, we perceive it as strange and at the same time become aware of the presuppositions we ordinarily bring to its perception. By effecting such a move we have the possibility of elucidating how it is the thing comes to have meaning and the value it does for us in the natural attitude. In other words, we expose our own assumptions and prejudices such that we meet the object as if for the first time, on its own ground. (1999, 189)

So rather than pursuing the arguably futile endeavor of attempting to observe objects as external "things in themselves," phenomenologists highlight that we experience the world only as it appears to our consciousness, as experiences in consciousness. The effort to focus on our experience of "things in themselves" merely exposes our own assumptions about the natural world, and instead our focus should be on lived experiences and how we come to have knowledge (Bartky 2009; Sheets-Johnstone 1999; Van Manen 2014). Sheets-Johnstone's (1999) summary of the phenomenological project as paying attention to the taken-for-granted, and questioning the natural world and our embodied experiences to understand how we come to know, encapsulates the appeal of phenomenology for feminist philosophers and artists. Feminists and phenomenologists share a focus on embodied lived experiences, both questioning what we know and how we know, and asserting that women and artists can also be knowers (Code 1991).

While phenomenology had much appeal for feminists, particularly in situating the lived body and lived experience as crucial in philosophical understandings, feminist critiques also identified the way in which Husserl, his student Maurice Merleau-Ponty, and phenomenological peers continued to imagine the lived body as a male body and to universalize (mostly white) men's lived experiences to all human experiences (Butler 2011; Grosz 1994; Kruks 2014; Tidd 2004). Extending from the work of Husserl (1970, 1989), Merleau-Ponty (1962, 1964a, 1964b), and others, feminists created alternative understandings of women's lived bodies and women's lived movement experiences.

In the unfolding of phenomenological thinking, the work of Simone de Beauvoir (2010) offered gendered understandings of women's lived embodied experiences through her novels and key text *The Second Sex* (originally published in French in 1949 and translated to English in 1953). Her pivotal contributions to gender politics and feminist autobiographical writing asserted that women's sexual difference was an experiential reality and that women's embodiment is a lived situation—a woman's way of being (2010). She asserted that phenomenology had

> an epistemology and a descriptive method that resonate with many central feminist theoretical concerns: it eschews rationalism and objectifying mind-body dualism, and instead invites a focus on embodied, situated, immediate and often more affective forms of experience. (Kruks 2014, 76)

Following Beauvoir, feminist phenomenologists recognize that lived experience is always embodied, mediated, and situated culturally and historically, and that women's lived experiences are relevant in understanding human experience (Bartky 2009). While Beauvoir's work has been criticized as focusing on the experiences of white French intellectual women like herself, this may also be seen as the strength of her work (Kruks 2014). Beauvoir deliberately located her detailed consideration of women's experiences within her own community or "collectivity," and without expressing a masculinist intention to universalize to all women's (or all human) experiences. Beauvoir (2010) thus drew on Husserl's method of bracketing and variation in considering the unique experiences of many women "as a means also to explore what commonalities may persist among the many particular and highly diverse experiences of 'becoming a woman'" (Kruks 2014, 81). Beauvoir clarified:

> When I use the words "woman" or "feminine," after most of my statements one must understand "in the present state of upbringing and mores." There is no question here of pronouncing eternal truths, but of describing the common basis upon which all feminine existence arises. (2010, 279)

She chose to offer multiple and varied stories of women's individual embodied experiences and, in doing so, speaking to diverse women both within her collective and beyond. Her work drew attention to the common basis as well as the significant variations, even within the experiences of women like herself in her community, and without claiming to speak for other women in communities far different from her own (Kruks 2014). Simone de Beauvoir, together with Maxine Sheets-Johnstone, Iris Marion Young, and others, transformed phenomenology with feminist critique.

BREATHE

A deepening sense of rest and pleasure,
breathing easily as I lie on the sunlit wooden floor,
the nourishing presence of other women supporting me.
Waiting,
my breath comes to me, unhurried and unconstrained as my diaphragm
*   drops reflexively and air flows in.*
Arms gently wrapped around my torso, curled on my side,
I am aware of my breath but releasing control.
Breathe, embodied, in the present.

We had been working together for a week, immersed in the subtleties of
*   movement, improvising, dancing, meditating and investigating yoga.*
We talked and laughed and cried, allowing time for weaving loose strands
*   of friendships together after the fraying of the years, and creating*
*   new weavings. There was none of the competition and frustration I*
*   had experienced in my academic environment, or the unsustainable*
*   intensity of professional practice.*
Instead, we women shared dreams and farewelled past desires.
I watched beauty flowing through those around me.
Grateful to be embraced in community, I reflect on
the lessons that breath and movement offer.

Feminist Phenomenologies and Women's Movement

Simone de Beauvoir and Merleau-Ponty both provided inspiration for the work of Iris Young (1980, 1998b, 2005) as she sought to develop an understanding of women's lived movement experiences. Young's (1980) analysis reflected feminist understandings of the history of patriarchal oppression in Western societies (Foster 2009; Kruks 2014). Like Beauvoir, Young wished to articulate the specifics of women's lived embodied experiences and in one (now famous) example, she focused on achieving the specific movement task of throwing a ball. From her analysis of variations in experiences of "throwing like a girl," Young outlined basic modalities of feminine body comportment (1980). In achieving the task of throwing a ball, Young identified that a common experience for Western women involved being both an object as viewed by others and by simultaneously being a subject herself. As a consequence, women tended to imagine how they appeared as objects to others, while at the same time also experiencing their movement as intentional subjects (Foster 2009; Weiss 1999; Young 1980). Young surmised:

> An essential part of the situation of being a woman is that of living with the ever-present possibility that one will be gazed upon as a mere body, as shape and flesh that presents itself as the potential object of another subject's intentions and manipulations, rather than as a living manifestation of action and intention. (1998a, 270)

This experience resulted in discontinuity between a woman's intention in throwing a ball and seeing herself as an object from an external perspective.

In her sophisticated analysis, Young (1980) concluded that women did not use their full spatial and lateral potential in movement. Instead, women experienced their own movement, or feminine bodily comportment, as intentionally inhibited (by their perception of their own inability to achieve the task undertaken). Women's movement was also ambiguously transcendent (by concentrating her action in one part of the body while the rest remained uninvolved); and further, it had a discontinuous unity (by breaking connection between intention and action, between possibility and actual bodily achievement) (1980). Young's feminist study offered a strong analysis of women's movement experiences as distinct from men's movement experiences (1980, 1998b, 2005). As Susan Leigh Foster wrote, "It was Young's unique and perceptive insight to consider movement patterns as part of those structures and conditions that define the feminine" (2009, 69). Young later extended and critiqued her own work (1998b, 2005) and inspired further research on women's movement that considered how diverse women now move within (somewhat) different structures and conditions than when Young first undertook her analyses (for example, Chisholm 2008). In particular, Young inspired further research generating understandings of women's dance (such as Albright 1997; Barbour 2002, 2011a; Foster 2009).

Again, feminist attention to the uniqueness of individual women's lived experiences through phenomenological bracketing, and consideration of multiple variations of experiences, brought both richness to understandings and the prompt to consider how the experiences described do, or do not, resonate with diverse individual women in their lifeworlds. Recalling Beauvoir (2010), while there may be some shared experiences of feminine embodiment that relate to sociocultural context and to women's embodied differences, becoming a woman is also individually nuanced. Following Beauvoir's and Young's writings, other feminist writers developed different philosophies around embodiment (including Bartky 1990; Bordo 1993; Butler 2011), although not focused around movement analysis to the same extent (Foster 2009).

Focused on the epistemological significance of movement experience, Maxine Sheets-Johnstone extended Merleau-Ponty's (1962, 1964a) work on the primacy of perception, arguing instead for the primacy of movement (1999; Merritt 2015). Her analysis claimed that knowledge comes through moving. Young highlighted that experience in general has been devalued and repressed within Western societies (as have all women's ways of knowing), and that, instead, rational, logical thinking has been elevated in epistemology (Code 1991; Barbour 2011a). Sheets-Johnstone's (1966) influential description of thinking in movement in dance improvisation made clear that thinking and doing, that sensing and moving, are inseparable experiences; as Michele Merritt described simply, thinking is movement (2015).

Sheets-Johnstone (1999) developed an extensive account of human learning from infancy, demonstrating that we learn about ourselves and others initially through moving. We learn as babies by attending to our bodily sensations of movement, rather than by looking and seeing what is moving first:

> Coming to know the world in a quite literal sense means coming to grips with it—exploring it, searching it, discovering it in and through movement. There is no human culture in which movement is not epistemologically central in this way. There is, indeed, no culture in which movement is not our mother tongue. (226)

Through the kinesthetic sense, *kineasthesia* (Potter 2008) or *kinesthesis* (Husserl 1989; Pakes 2009; Stinson 1995), movement provides us with immediate information about space, time, movement, and objects, and the relationships between. The kinesthetic sense is fundamental to basic understanding of the world, to our ability to move knowledgeably in the world and to our knowledge of what we are (Sheets-Johnstone 1998). Thus, I assert that movement is of profound epistemological significance, as "the originating ground of our sense-makings" (1998, 161). Our kinesthetic sense provides that "dynamic sense of constantly shifting one's body in space and time in order to achieve a desired end"—the lived experience of a dancer (Fraleigh 1987, 2004; Potter 2008, 449). In Sheets-Johnstone's analysis of dance improvisation, she wrote:

A dynamically attuned body that knows the world and makes its way within it kinetically is thoughtfully attuned to the variable qualia of both its own movement and the movement of things in its surrounding world—to forceful, swift, slow, straight, swerving, flaccid, tense, sudden, up, down, and much more. Caught up in an adult world, we easily lose sight of movement and of our fundamental capacity to thinking in movement. Any time we care to turn our attention to it, however, there it is (1999, 516–517)

Sheets-Johnstone (1999) stimulated further phenomenological and feminist scholarship, particularly through her much-cited work on dance improvisation (including Albright 1997; Barbour 2002, 2011a, 2011b; Fraleigh 2004; Stinson 1995). Perhaps a phenomenological attitude and the methods of bracketing and variation appealed particularly to dance scholars because of the way in which these methods frame detailed description of a particular lived experience, rather as a performance frames aspects of embodied kinesthetic experience within the lifeworld (East 2015; Foster 2009; Fraleigh 1987; Franko 2011; Rothfield 2005). In paying attention to dance we describe the immediate embodied lived experiences of dancers (Fraleigh 1987; Rothfield 2005). In dancing, we each pay attention to our own embodied experiences that occur in relation to others around us and the world as a whole.

DANCE

A moving moment of living and performing,
boundaries dissolved between me and earth,
our community ecology
lived and danced.
Soul shared through feet into the earth, breath into the air,
movement into emotive, affective experience.
Walking the edge of the river, water and sand soothing my toes,
wind drying my skin, chattering birds and the rustle of leaves
accompanying the breath of my friends,
together stirring the world and the hearts of our audience.
A dance, in the embodied presence of the lifeworld.

Calling to memory these sensations from performing,
I reflect on my practice of suspending myself in presence.
Whether as an educator in the studio facilitating somatics, yoga or dance,
or as a performer in site-specific, place-responsive dance,
I find myself immersed,
simply being present.
And I wonder, if all the world is a stage, as Shakespeare said

*and if my preparation for dancing is my whole life as Deborah Hay
    proposed (2000),*
when am I performing and when am I not performing?
*My performing is an experience of bracketing presence, and I reflect on
the lessons dancing offers about presence in the lifeworld.*

Dancing Feminist Phenomenology

Feminist phenomenology has offered dance researchers a philosophical perspective and an epistemological understanding, a methodological focus for
describing specific instances of embodied experiences in dancing, and a
prompt to value and share the diversity of women's movement (Foster 2009;
Fraleigh 1987). While examples of detailed movement analysis are apparent
in dance research, particularly through the influential work of Rudolf von
Laban (1948) on movement attributes, Young's "insistence on the historically
constructed circumstances of feminine movement contributes a crucial argument to scholarship that attempts to resist the 'universal dance' and universals
in dance" (Foster 2009, 74). Thus, some dance researchers have developed
Young's work in detailed analyses of women's performance (such as Albright
1997; Barbour 2002, 2011a, 2011b; Foster 2009; Fraleigh 2004).

In researching women's contemporary dance specifically, Ann Cooper
Albright (1997) applied Young's analysis to other women's lived experiences
in dance performance. Albright argued that some dancers were able to expand the norms of feminine movement in their performance, rather than
remaining intentionally inhibited, ambiguously transcendent, and discon-
tinuously unified. Instead, Albright saw these women dancers as demonstrating clear, directed energy, clarity of weight, spatial intention, and movement
flow through intentional dancing (ibid.). Such women's movement was responsive, enduring, able to accommodate change, and could offer a more
profound experience for an audience (ibid.).

Albright's analysis provided inspiration for my phenomenological research
in women's solo contemporary dance (Barbour 2002, 2011a). Alongside
Young's (1998b, 2005) later suggestion that movement analysis might begin
with women's everyday experience of multiplicity rather than singularity, I
investigated other alternative feminine modalities. Researching solo contemporary dance performance with other women in my social-cultural context,
and in my own choreographic research, I found practices that allowed me
to develop movement that had multiple intentions. Multiplicity in intention
included developing kinesthetic empathy with my experiences through the

use of everyday, pedestrian, and gestural movement; subverting and resisting expectations of the dancer; challenging or changing stereotypical feminine movement and movement qualities; and ultimately, offering an embodied expression of lived experience (Barbour 2002, 2011a).

In solo contemporary dance performance I also valued the way in which I and the women I interviewed were able to be both receptive and responsive to lived experiences. Each of us aimed to receive and integrate information from multiple sources, including moment-to-moment changes and understandings developed during performing, audience responses, life events, and choreographed movement (Sheets-Johnstone 1999). In the moment of performance, it became possible to respond to these multiple sources in whatever manner felt appropriate. There were opportunities to improvise, adapt, and respond, both thinking *in* and *about* movement in dancing (ibid.). Instead of experiencing inhibited, partially expressive movement and feeling disconnection between intention and action, as described in Young's modalities of feminine movement, and instead of creating only a fixed singular plan, finding control, and developing singular intention (1980, 1998a), I experienced multiplicity in intention and receptivity and responsiveness in dancing. As I was thinking in movement, I experienced alternative modalities of feminine movement to those proposed in Young's analysis (Barbour 2002, 2011b). Thus, feminist phenomenology offered much insight into understanding the way in which women's movement had been shaped by patriarchal oppression (Bartky 2009; Foster 2009), as revealed through detailed analysis of different variations of lived embodied experience in solo dance performance. In particular, the phenomenological intent to suspend judgment and analysis, in the aspiration to be present in the moment of performance, brought into sharp focus assumptions, prejudices, and stereotypes about how women could and should dance. As a consequence of phenomenological inquiry, dance researchers have been able to explore alternative understandings of feminine movement and embodiment, including my articulation of embodied ways of knowing (Barbour, 2002, 2011a).

Embodied ways of knowing have been articulated in dance research in varied ways (for example, Foster 2009; Fraleigh 1987, 2004; Gardner 1999; Pakes 2009, 2011; Parviainen 2002; Rouhiainen 2008; Stinson 1995). From my own research, I have advocated for embodied ways of knowing as an epistemological strategy through which women dancers experience themselves as knowing subjects engaged in constructing knowledge within specific contexts and through embodied praxis (Barbour 2011a). Embodied knowledge arises in the intimate weaving of passion, experience, and varied knowledges. Embodied ways of knowing also arise in combining different ideas through improvisation, play, and experimentation, moving into gaps in understanding and articulating new connections between ideas and experiences. Thus, embodied ways of knowing foreground knowing as creatively living in the world (ibid.).

Feminist phenomenological scholarship and practice has continued to inform understandings of dance performance. In particular, the work of Sondra Fraleigh over many years continues to inspire deeper investigation of dancers' lived experiences, across a breadth of engagements in performance, pedagogy, and praxis (1987, 2000, 2004, 2010, 2015, 2016a, 2016b). Fraleigh's work has provided arguments for and examples of the significant understandings that may be gained from researching dancing from inside the aesthetic experience, from the unique artistic perspective of the dancer as simultaneously artist and art work. The potential of such feminist phenomenology of dance is to articulate embodied ways of knowing, demonstrating women's confident movement in the world drawing on cultivated kinaesthetic awareness and experiential knowledge, expressed in aesthetic performative, as well as in pedagogical contexts, and praxis. Fraleigh's work illustrates how feminist phenomenological inquiry does not take dance or performance for granted and instead returns us to the wonder of dancing anew. In particular, in writing about somatic dance practices Fraleigh and others articulate embodied methods that develop kinaesthetic awareness and somatic modes of attention that can expand beyond individual embodiment to embrace the world as a source of knowledge (Barbour in press; Csordas 1993; Fraleigh 2015; Rouhiainen 2008). Somatic attention, in brief, is about paying attention to felt life and the knowing that arises from it, including subjective and inter-experiences. Leena Rouhiainen wrote:

> Somatically informed dance can be a means to learn about ourselves, others and the world in a manner that offers us a chance to live with diversity and still maintain personal integrity. It is my belief that, by learning to listen to the body and by retrieving understanding of the messages it offers with a sense of phenomenological wonder, we can achieve valuable insight into who we are and how we relate to the situations we find ourselves in. (Rouhiainen 2008, 242)

Like phenomenological inquiry, somatic dance practices allow a return to the wonder of lived embodied experiences in the present moment and in the lifeworld. Lifeworld is an inclusive concept that encompasses concern for relationship, and recognizes our capacity for being in the world in "the flowing live present" (Fraleigh 2016a–c; Husserl 1989). Lifeworld considers humans embodied subjects in relation to the world, as beings in the world who are part of an interconnected ecological system of people, animals, plants, birds, rock, earth, water, weather, and so on. Dancers drawing on somatic modes of attention that support embodied ways of knowing may also cultivate attentiveness in the flowing live present, to embodied lived experience and to ecological and sociocultural systems as a whole (East 2015). Such practices may be interpreted as expressions of forms of ecological feminism (Warren 1996). "Because dance is of the human body, it is also of ourselves—of the times and spaces we live and move, as we live our world through our body in relation to others" (Fraleigh 1987, 208). In particular, cultivating presence in the flowing live present through somatic modes of awareness involves an openness to lived experience in the moment in the ecological and sociocultural context of place and time. Rather like the phenomenological method of bracketing, being present and dancing presence involves openness to the wonder of the world. Through embodied ways of knowing as living creatively in the world, I highlight my dancer's way of being in the world. In the flowing live present, dancing presence, I move between rising, suspension and falling—turning, rolling and gesturing. Dancing becomes an act of generating myself in the present. "It is when we are present centered—at one with the world and free of conflicting dualities—that we dance its grace" (Fraleigh 1987, 158). Crucially, I recognize my potential to be responsive to the lifeworld, and I experience how the lifeworld is also capable of responding to me. I am present, I am presence (see Plate 8).

SWAY

In me with mine, in Aotearoa New Zealand,
an unnerving sense of the world swaying affects my cells,
the fluids of my body slosh and the ground shifts beneath me.
Legs wide, arms wrapped around our son,
my love and I huddle in the doorway, riding the shifting tectonic plates.
Baby Rūaumoko rolls inside the belly of our earth mother Papatūānuku.
A sway, present in the moving lifeworld.

Writing in my home, my laptop framed by gentle rain on the luscious
     greens
of our overgrown garden,
the experience of the week's earthquakes is strong.
Unharmed in our home and our region of these "shaky isles,"
I nevertheless wonder if any moment there might be more,
today, tomorrow, next week.
There was none of the terrifying, loud, rock-wrenching

that I had briefly felt on a visit to the South Island of Aotearoa,
or the wave-like flow of an earthquake I recalled in the islands of
    Vanuatu years ago.
I watched the news reports from Kaikoura while we ate breakfast—
    interviews with tourists desperate for helicopter rescues,
photos of our coastal roads destroyed by gaping cracks and landslides,
footage of paua clinging to rocks exposed as the coast line rose out of the
    sea,
family members "marked as safe" on social media.
Deeply grateful to be unharmed,
I reflect on the lessons the earth is offering me and mine.

Sway—Presence

A number of writers on dance, performance, and the notion of presence have offered alternative understandings of presence, typically relating directly to time and the sense that the dance is repeated or leaves traces or is erased or disappears (Lepecki 2004a, 2004b). However, referring to Heidegger's understanding of presence, Andre Lepecki commented that "The imbrication of movement into ontology is choreographically specific. It is not just any movement that allows being to gain presence. Only a very particular movement-quality guarantees the full emerging of being as presence: a wavering, an oscillation, vibration" (Lepecki 2004a, 48). Lepecki's own analysis offers much interest as he proposes instead

> a politics of presence whose ontology is grounded neither on a quivering, nor on an oscillation, but on a non-Heideggerian stumbling. This is where general ontology, forced by the grooves of the ground and the ballistics of language, must be corrected by the contextual, political, historical, racial specificity of the stumble in the racist field. This is where general ontology must land on the historically and socially specific bumpy terrain where the choreo-political situation unfolds. (2004a, 59)

Both the experiences of stumbling and of falling can be seen as choreographically relevant movements in contemporary dance, as connected to key lived experiences of weight, suspension, and release (Ehrenberg 2015). In contemporary dance, we pay attention to all movement, even to the taken-for-granted movements of walking. As Shantel Ehrenberg wrote, dancers focus attention on the felt mechanics of walking and do not let the mechanics fall to the background of consciousness. In other words, contemporary dancers interrogate, in this instance of an exploration of walking (which has become very familiar movement to them since childhood), how the foot touches the floor; they sense detailed nuances of hip movements, notice the rhythmic pattern of the arm sway as they walk, and then respond to this sensing in their movement. They precisely interrogate those bodily experiences, sensations, perceptions, and habits that usually go "unnoticed" among non-dancers, and they simultaneously imagine and anticipate other ways of walking as they walk. (2015, 50)

Simple movements like walking encompass embodied experiences of weight, rising, suspension, release, and falling. All these experiences are related to presence, not only in relation to time, but also to our unique embodiments and to our specific location in the world (literally to the variable ground under our feet) (Lepecki 2004). Further, contemporary dance often explicitly attends to contact with the world; even in solo dance, we engage through the soles of our feet with the ground; through our skins with the surfaces of the world; with objects in the world; and with air, temperature, taste, sound, sight, and all the offerings of our senses. And when we dance with others, we engage in the immediate lived experiences of fleshy embodied relationships.

However, I wonder what happens when our lived embodied experiences of place and ground are not only of the bumpy grooves of the terrain that create stumbling, but when we experience the ground itself moving. I wonder how I might describe the choreographically specific movement that suspends me in the flowing live present. Like standing at the helm on a yacht, dancing on ground that has the potential to shift requires the capacity to sway, suspended in the flowing live present between upright stability, rising, stumbling, and falling. In swaying, I respond to uncertainty as I adjust my movement in place and time drawing on my kinaesthetic sense of my own movement dynamics. At the same time, I am able to respond somatically to movement beneath me as the earth quakes. Swaying requires continual embodied adaptation and change in response to place: sometimes rhythmic and graceful and perhaps as a subtle oscillation but not necessarily so and sometimes sharp and wrenching, perhaps as stumbling or falling but not necessarily so. Contemporary dance and somatic dance practices, through deepening awareness of the varied lived experiences of movement, enhance dancer's potential for embodied responsiveness and capacity to cope with multiplicity in experience. As Sondra Fraleigh wrote, "uncertainty is explored every day in the consciousness of dancers, in the studio and on stage . . . in the shifting thematics of their dances and in the precariousness of dancing itself" (2004, 142). Paying attention, we experience presence immediately, in the moment empathetically responsive to all of our lifeworld—in performance to other dancers; to audience members; to sociocultural assumptions and expectations; to birds, insects, trees, rivers; and to earth, weather, and geological change. This is an embodied lived experience; the basis of our sociability and our empathetic response to others and the world (Fraleigh 2004; Letiche 2012). As dancers, we deepen and extend our capacity to suspend ourselves in the moment in empathetic engagement and responsiveness with our lifeworlds.

Returning to the understandings of alternative modalities of feminine movement derived through my focus on women's lived experiences in solo contemporary dance, our lived experiences reveal the significance of our capacity to receive and integrate information from multiple sources, including moment-to-moment changes within our movement and the world around (Barbour 2011a; Sheets-Johnstone 1999). In the flowing live present, whether simply in life or bracketed in performance, responding improvisationally to multiple sources becomes possible. Lived embodied experiences offer moments to express multiplicity in intention, receptivity, and responsiveness, as happens the dancing moments of swaying. We dance epistemology in just such ways.

Bibliography

Abram, David. *Spell of the Sensuous: Perception and Language in a More-than-Human World.* New York: Vintage Books, 1996.

———. *Becoming Animal: An Earthly Cosmology.* New York: Pantheon Books, 2010.

Ahmed, Sarah. *Queer Phenomenology: Orientations, Objects, Subjects.* Durham: Duke University Press, 2006.

Albright, Ann C. *Choreographing Difference: The Body and Identity in Contemporary Dance.* Hanover, N.H.: Wesleyan University Press, 1997.

Alexander, F. M. *The Use of the Self.* London: Orion Books, 2001 [1932].

Atkins, Juan, Derrick May, and Kevin Saunderson. *Juan Atkins and Derrick May.* Panel Discussion. Museum of Contemporary Art Detroit. May 28, 2016.

Augros, Robert, and George Stanciu. *The New Biology: Discovering the Wisdom in Nature.* Boston: Shambala, 1988.

Bachelard, Gaston. *La Poétique de l'Espace.* Paris: Presses Universitaires de France, 1958.

———. *The Poetics of Space.* Trans. Maria Jolas. Boston: Beacon, 1994.

Bainbridge Cohen, Bonnie. *Sensing, Feeling, and Action: The Experiential Anatomy of Body-Mind Centering.* Northampton, Mass.: Contact Editions, 1993.

Bakewell, Sarah. *At the Existentialist Café: Freedom, Being, and Apricot Cocktails with Jean-Paul Sartre, Simone de Beauvoir, Albert Camus, Martin Heidegger, Karl Jaspers, Edmund Husserl, Maurice Merleau-Ponty and Others.* New York: Other Press, 2016.

Ball, David. "The New Anthropocene Epoch Has Dawned, and It's 'Very Worrisome.'" *Vancouver Metro News.* Sept. 14, 2016. Web.

Barad, Karen. *Meeting the Universe Halfway: Quantum Physics and the Entanglement of Matter and Meaning.* Durham: Duke University Press, 2007.

Barbour, Karen N. "Embodied Ways of Knowing: Women's Solo Contemporary Dance in Aotearoa, New Zealand." PhD thesis. Faculty of Education. University of Waikato, New Zealand, 2002.

———. *Dancing across the Page: Narrative and Embodied Ways of Knowing.* Bristol, U.K.: Intellect Books, 2011a.

———. "Writing, Dancing, Embodied Knowing: Autoethnographic Research." *Fields in Motion: Ethnography in the Worlds of Dance.* Ed. Dena Davida. Waterloo, Canada: Wilfrid Laurier University Press, 2011b. 101–117.

———. "Embodied Ways of Knowing: Revisiting Feminist Epistemology." *The Palgrave Handbook of Feminisms in Sport, Leisure and Physical Education.* Eds. L. Mansfield, Jayne Caudwell, R. Watson, and Belinda Wheaton. Hampshire, U.K.: Palgrave Macmillan (in press).

Bartenieff, Irmgard, with Dori Lewis. *Body Movement: Coping with the Environment.* Newark, N.J: Gordon and Breach, 1980.

Bartky, Sandra L. *Femininity and Domination: Studies in the Phenomenology of Oppression.* New York: Routledge, 1990.

———. "Iris Young and the Gendering of Phenomenology." *Studies in Feminist Philosophy: Dancing with Iris: The Philosophy of Iris Marion Young.* Eds. Ann Ferguson and Mechthild Nagel. Cary, U.K.: Oxford University Press, 2009. 41–67.

Bateson, Glena, with Margaret Wilson. *Body and Mind in Motion: Dance and Neuroscience in Conversation.* Bristol, U.K.: Intellect Ltd., 2014.

Bateson, Gregory. *Steps to an Ecology of Mind: Collected Essays in Anthropology, Psychiatry, Evolution, and Epistemology.* San Francisco: Chandler, 1972.

Beardsley, John, et al. *Connecting the Dots: Tyree Guyton's Heidelberg Project.* Detroit: Wayne State University Press, 2007.

Beauvoir, Simone de. *The Ethics of Ambiguity.* Trans. Bernard Frecthman. New York: Carol Publishing, 1994 [1948].

———. *The Second Sex*, Trans. Constance Borde and Shelia Malovany-Chevallier. New York: Knopf, 2010 [1949].

———. *The Second Sex.* Trans. H. M. Parshley. New York: Vintage, 2011 [1949].

Behar, Ruth. *The Vulnerable Observer: Anthropology That Breaks Your Heart.* Boston: Beacon, 1996.

Behnke, Elizabeth A. "Edmund Husserl's Contribution to Phenomenology of the Body in *Ideas II*." *Issues in Husserl's Ideas II.* Eds. Thomas Nenon and Lester Embree. Dordrecht: Springer Science + Business Media, 1996. 135–160.

———. "Working Notions: A Meditation on Husserlian Phenomenological Practice." *Advancing Phenomenology: Essays in Honor of Lester Embree, Contributions to Phenomenology.* Eds. Thomas Nenon and Philip Blosser. Dordrecht: Springer Science + Business Media, B.V., 2010. 45–70.

Bennett, Jane. *Vibrant Matter: A Political Ecology of Things.* Durham: Duke University Press, 2010.

Blackwood, Michael. *Butoh: Body on the Edge of Crisis.* Coprod. BBC, BRT, and DR, 1990. DVD. *Vimeo.* https://vimeo.com/ondemand/butohfilm. Accessed Jan. 13, 2018.

Bogost, Ian. *Alien Phenomenology, or What It's Like to Be a Thing.* Minneapolis: University of Minnesota, 2012.

Bohm, David. *Wholeness and the Implicate Order*. London: Routledge, 1980.

Bond, Karen. "Receiving the Dance of the Child: An Application of Developmental and Humanistic Learning Theories to Teaching Dance." World Congress, International Society for Education through the Arts, Adelaide, South Australia, July 1978.

———. *Dance for Nonverbal Children with Dual Sensory Impairments*. PhD thesis. 1991. La Trobe University, Bundoora, Australia.

———. "Personal Style as a Mediator of Engagement in Dance: Watching Terpsichore Rise." *Dance Research Journal* 26.1 (1994): 15–26.

———. "'I'm Not an Eagle, I'm a Chicken'—Young Children's Perceptions of Creative Dance." *Early Childhood Connections* 7.4 (2001): 41–51.

———. "The Human Nature of Dance: Towards a Theory of Aesthetic Community." *Communicative Musicality: Exploring the Basis of Human Companionship*. Eds. Stephen Malloch and Colwyn Trevarthen. Oxford: Oxford University Press, 2008. 401–422.

———. "Recurrence and Renewal: Enduring Themes in Children's Dance." *Revisiting Impulse: A Contemporary Look at Writings on Dance, 1950–1970*. Eds. Thomas K. Hagood and Luke C. Kahlich. Youngstown: Cambria, 2013. 161–192.

———. "Susan W. Stinson: Teacher, Scholar, Advocate." *Focus on Dance: The Art and Craft of Teaching—Proceedings of the 2013 National Dance Education Organization Conference*. Ed. Kirsten Harvey. Bethesda: NDEO, 2014. 36–43.

———. *Dance and Quality of Life*. Dordrecht: Springer, forthcoming.

Bond, Karen E., and Susan W. Stinson. "'I Feel Like I'm Going to Take Off!': Young People's Experiences of the Super Ordinary in Dance." *Dance Research Journal* 32.2 (2000/01): 52–87.

Bordo, Susan. *Unbearable Weight: Feminism, Western Culture and the Body*. Berkeley: University of California Press, 1993.

Braude, Hillel D. "Radical Somatics." *Moving Consciously: Somatic Transformations through Dance, Yoga, and Touch*. Ed. Sondra Fraleigh. Urbana: University of Illinois Press, 2015. 124–134.

———. "Between Psychology and Philosophy: A Review of Thinking and Doing by Moshe Feldenkrais." *International Feldenkrais Federation Journal*, 2016. www.iffresearchjournal.org/volume/5/braude. Accessed Aug. 5, 2017.

Brennan, Mary Alice. "Every Little Movement Has a Meaning All Its Own: Movement Analysis in Dance Research." *Researching Dance: Evolving Modes of Inquiry*. Eds. Sondra Fraleigh and Penelope Hanstein. Pittsburgh: University of Pittsburgh Press, 1999. 283–308.

Brown, Charles S., and Ted Toadvine. Eds. *Eco-Phenomenology: Back to the Earth Itself*. Albany: State University of New York Press, 2003.

Bruzina, Ronald. "Translators Introduction," Fink and Husserl, *Sixth Cartesian Meditation*. Trans. Ronald Bruzina. Bloomington: Indiana University Press, 1995. vii–xcii.

———. *Edmund Husserl and Eugen Fink*. New Haven: Yale University Press, 2004.

Buber, Martin. *I and Thou*. Trans. W. Kaufmann. Edinburgh: T. and Clark, 1970.

Butler, Judith. *Bodies That Matter: On the Discursive Limits of "Sex."* New York: Routledge, 1993.

———. *Gender Trouble: Feminism and the Subversion of Identity.* New York: Routledge, 2011 [1990].

Capra, Fritjof. *The Turning Point.* New York: Simon and Schuster, 1982.

Casey, Edward S. *Getting Back into Place: Toward a Renewed Understanding of the Place-World.* Bloomington: Indiana University Press, 1993.

———. *The Fate of Place: A Philosophical History.* Berkeley: University of California Press, 1997.

———. "Taking a Glance at the Environment: Preliminary Thoughts." *Eco-Phenomenology: Back to the Earth Itself.* Eds. Charles S. Brown and Ted Toadvine. Albany: State University of New York Press, 2003, 187–210.

Certeau, Michel de. *The Practice of Everyday Life.* Berkeley: University of California Press, 1984.

Cevallos, Kirmaya, and Dennis Scholl, dirs. *Acres of Diamonds: The Story of the Knight Arts Challenge in Detroit (Special edited Jitterbug version).* Online video clip. *YouTube.* YouTube, Feb. 24, 2013. Web, Aug. 16, 2016.

Chakrabarti, Meghan. *Bringing Back: Detroit's "Jit" Dance.* Here and Now; wbur. Interview of Tracy McGhee and Haleem Rasul. Jan. 2, 2014. http://www.wbur.org/hereandnow/2014/01/02/detroit-jit-dance. Accessed July 16, 2016.

Cheetham, Thomas. *Imaginal Love: The Meanings of Imagination in Henry Corbin and James Hillman.* London: Sage, 2015.

Chisholm, Dianne. "Climbing Like a Girl: An Exemplary Adventure in Feminist Phenomenology." *Hypatia* 23.1 (Jan.–Mar. 2008): 9–40.

Chödrön, Pema. *Start Where You Are.* Boston: Shambhala Publications, 1994.

Code, Lorraine. *What Can She Know? Feminist Theory and the Construction of Knowledge.* New York: Cornell University Press, 1991.

Colin, Noyale. "Becoming Plural: The Distribution of the Self in Collaborative Performance Research." *Choreographic Practices* 6.2 (Spring 2016): 279–296.

Conrad, Emile. *Life on Land: The Story of Continuum.* California: North Atlantic Books, 2007.

Crowther, Paul. *Art and Embodiment: From Aesthetics to Self-Consciousness.* Oxford: Clarendon, 1993.

Csordas, Thomas J. "Embodiment as a Paradigm for Anthropology." *Ethos* 18.1 (1990): 5–47.

———. "Somatic Modes of Attention." *Cultural Anthropology* 8.2 (1993): 135–156.

———. "Cultural Phenomenology: Embodiment, Agency, Sexual Difference, and Illness." *A Companion to the Anthropology of the Body and Embodiment.* Ed. Frances E. Mascia-Lees. Chichester: Blackwell Publishing, 2011. 137–156.

Cull, Laura. *Theatres of Immanence: Deleuze and the Ethics of Performance.* Great Britain: Palgrave Macmillan, 2013.

Daly, Anya. *Merleau-Ponty and the Ethics of Intersubjectivity.* London: Palgrave Macmillan, 2016.

Damasio, Antonio. *Descartes Error: Emotion, Reason, and the Human Brain*. New York: G. P. Putnam's Sons, 1994.

———. *The Feeling of What Happens: Body, Emotion and the Making of Consciousness*. London: Heinemann, 1999.

———. *Self Comes to Mind: Constructing the Conscious Brain*. New York: Vintage Books, Random House Inc., 2012.

Daniel, Yvonne. *Dancing Wisdom: Embodied Knowledge in Haitian Vodou, Cuban Yoruba, and Bahian Condomble*. Urbana: University of Illinois Press, 2005.

Davis, Heather, and Etienne Turpin, Eds. *Art in the Anthropocene*. London: Open Humanities Press, 2015.

Deans, Catherine E., Doris McIlwaine, and Andrew Geeves. "The Interpersonal Development of an Embodied Agency." *Psychology of Consciousness: Theory, Research and Practice* 2.3 (2015): 315–325.

Deleuze, Gilles. *Difference and Repetition*. Trans. Paul R. Patton. New York: Columbia University Press, 1994.

Deleuze, Gilles, and Felix Guattari. *Kafka: Toward a Minor Literature*. Trans. Dana Polan. Minneapolis: University of Minnesota Press, 1986.

———. *A Thousand Plateaus: Capitalism and Schizophrenia*. Trans. Brian Massumi. Minneapolis: University of Minnesota Press, 1987.

———. *What Is Philosophy?* Trans. Hugh Tomlinson and Graham Burchell. New York: Columbia University Press, 1994.

Delkeskamp, Corinna. "Body, Mind, and Conditions of Novelty: Some Remarks on Leonard C. Feldstein's Luminosity." *Mental Health: Philosophical Perspectives 4*. Eds. H. Tristram Englehardt Jr. and Stuart F. Spicker. Dordrecht: Springer, 1978. 191–198.

De Man, Paul. "Semiology and Rhetoric." *Diacritics* 3.3 (1973): 27–33.

Dissanayake, Ellen. *What Is Art For?* Seattle: University of Washington Press, 1988.

———. *Homo Aestheticus: Where Art Comes From and Why*. Seattle: University of Washington Press, 1995.

Dreyfus, Hubert L. "The Mystery of the Background qua Background." *Knowing without Thinking: The Background in Philosophy of Mind*. Ed. Zdravko Radman. Basingstoke, U.K.: Palgrave, 2012. 1–10.

Dunbar, Robin. *Grooming, Gossip, and the Evolution of Language*. Cambridge: Harvard University Press.

Duncan, Isadora. *Art of the Dance*. Theatre Arts Books, 1928. Cambridge: Harvard University Press, 1998.

Eagleton, Terry. *The Significance of Theory*. Cambridge: Blackwell, 1990.

East, Alison. "Performing Body as Nature." in *Moving Consciously*. Ed. Sondra Fraleigh. Urbana: University of Illinois Press, 2015. 164–179.

Ehrenberg, Shantel. "A Kinesthetic Mode of Attention in Contemporary Dance." *Dance Research Journal* 47.2 (Aug. 2015): 43–62.

Elkins, James. *The Object Stares Back: On the Nature of Seeing*. New York: Houghton Mifflin Harcourt, 1996.

Farias, Victor. *Heidegger and Nazism*. Philadelphia: Temple University Press, 1987.

Feldenkrais, Moshe. *Practical Unarmed Combat*. New York: Frederick Warne, 1942.
———. *The Potent Self: A Guide to Spontaneity*. Ed. Michaeleen Kimmey. New York: Harper and Row, 1985.
Feldstein, Leonard. *The Dance of Being: Man's Labyrinthine Rhythms*. New York: Fordham UP, 1979.
Fink, Eugen, and Edmund Husserl. *Sixth Cartesian Meditation: The Idea of a Transcendental Theory of Method*. Textual notations and appendix by Edmund Husserl. Trans. with intro., Ronald Bruzina. Bloomington: Indiana University Press, 1995.
Flam, Jack, Ed. *Robert Smithson: The Collected Writings*. Berkeley: University of California Press, 1966.
Fortin, Sylvie, and Darrell Siedentop. "The Interplay of Knowledge and Practice in Dance Teaching: What We Can Learn from a Non-traditional Dance Teacher." *Dance Research Journal* 27.2 (1995): 3–15.
Foster, Susan Leigh. "Kinesthetic Empathies and the Politics of Compassion." *Continents in Movement: Proceedings of the International Conference, The Meeting of Cultures in Dance History*. Ed. Daniel Tércio. Lisbon: FMH Editions, 1998.
———. "Throwing Like a Girl, Dancing Like a Feminist Philosopher." *Studies in Feminist Philosophy: Dancing with Iris: The Philosophy of Iris Marion Young*. Eds. Ann Ferguson and Mechthild Nagel. Cary, U.K.: Oxford University Press, 2009. 69–78.
———. *Choreographing Empathy: Kinesthesia in Performance*. New York: Routledge, 2011a.
———. "Hired Bodies and Dancing Nomads." Lecture at Spring Dance Salons. Theatre Studies, Utrecht University, The Netherlands, 2011b.
Fraleigh, Sondra. *Dance and the Lived Body: A Descriptive Aesthetics*. Pittsburgh: University of Pittsburgh Press, 1987.
———. "A Vulnerable Glance: Seeing Dance through Phenomenology." *Dance Research Journal* 23.1 (1991): 11–16.
———. "Witnessing the Frog Pond." *Researching Dance: Evolving Modes of Inquiry*. Eds. Sondra Horton Fraleigh and Penelope Hanstein. Pittsburgh: University of Pittsburgh Press, 1999a. 188–244.
———. *Dancing into Darkness: Butoh, Zen, and Japan*. Pittsburgh: University of Pittsburgh Press, 1999b.
———. "Consciousness Matters." *Dance Research Journal* 32.1 (Summer 2000): 54–62.
———. *Dancing Identity: Metaphysics in Motion*. Pittsburgh: University of Pittsburgh Press, 2004.
———. *BUTOH: Metamorphic Dance and Global Alchemy*. Urbana: University of Illinois Press, 2010.
———. "Permission and the Making of Consciousness." in *Dance, Somatics and Spiritualities: Contemporary Sacred Narratives*. Eds. Amanda Williamson, Glenna Batson, Sarah Whatley, and Rebecca Weber. Bristol: Intellect Press, 2014. 239–260.
———, Ed. *Moving Consciously: Somatic Transformations through Dance, Yoga, and Touch*. Urbana: University of Illinois Press, 2015.

———. "Phenomenologies in the Flowing Live Present." Ed. Amanda Williamson. *Dance, Movement and Spiritualities* 2.2 (Fall 2016a): 141–158.

———. "On Dance and Phenomenology: An Essay Interview with Professor Sondra Fraleigh." Interview by editor Amanda Williamson. *Dance, Movement and Spiritualities* 2.2 (Fall 2016b): 199–217.

———. "Butoh Translations and the Suffering of Nature." *Performance Research. Routledge* 21.4 (2016c): 61–71.

———. *Tidal Space, Elemental Time.* Music Video. https://youtu.be/0VDD4QoHUoc. June 11, 2017. Accessed Sept. 4, 2017.

———. "A Philosophy of the Improvisational Body." *The Oxford Handbook of Improvisation in Dance.* Ed. Vida Midgelow. Oxford: Oxford UP, forthcoming.

Fraleigh, Sondra, and Penelope Hanstein. Eds. *Researching Dance: Evolving Modes of Inquiry.* Pittsburgh: University of Pittsburgh Press, 1999.

Fraleigh, Sondra, and Tamah Nakamura. *Hijikata Tatsumi and Ohno Kazuo.* London: Routledge, 2006.

Franko, Mark. *The Work of Dance: Labor, Movement and Identity in the 1930s.* Middletown, Conn.: Wesleyan University Press, 2002.

———. "Editor's Note: What Is Dead and What Is Alive in Dance Phenomenology?" *Dance Research Journal* 43.2 (Winter 2011): 1–4.

Freire, Paulo. *Pedagogy of Hope: Reliving Pedagogy of the Oppressed.* New York: Continuum, 1994.

Friedman, Jeff. "Muscle Memory: Performing Oral History." *Oral History* 33.2 (Autumn 2005): 35–47.

Gadamer, Hans-Georg, and Robert Bernasconi. *Truth and Method.* New York: Seabury Press, 1975.

———. "Practical Philosophy as a Model of the Human Sciences." *Research Phenomenology* 9.1 (1980): 74–86.

———. *The Relevance of the Beautiful and Other Essays.* Cambridge: Cambridge University Press, 1986.

Gallagher, Shaun. "Direct Perception in the Intersubjective Context." *Consciousness and Cognition* 17 (2005): 535–543.

Gardner, Howard. *Intelligence Reframed: Multiple Intelligences for the 21st Century.* New York: Basic Books, 1999.

Gendlin, Eugene T. *Focusing-Orientated Psychotherapy: A Manual of the Experiential Method.* London: The Guilford Press, 1996.

———. *Experiencing the Creation of Meaning.* Evanston: Northwestern University Press, 1997.

———. *Focusing: How to Gain Direct Access to Your Body's Knowledge.* New York: Rider, 2003 [1978].

George, Doran. *A Conceit of the Natural Body: The Universal-Individual in Somatic Dance Training.* PhD dissertation. Los Angeles, University of California, 2014.

Gilman, Robert. "The Next Great Turning." *Context* 34 (1993): 11.

Ginsburg, Carl. *The Intelligence of Moving Bodies: A Somatic View of Life and Its Consequences.* AWAREing Press, 1970.

Goldman, Daniel. *I Want to Be Ready: Improvised Dance as a Practice of Freedom.* East Lansing: University of Michigan Press, 2010.

Goode, David. *A World without Words: The Social Construction of Children Born Deaf and Blind.* Philadelphia: Temple University Press, 1994.

Grosz, Elizabeth. *Volatile Bodies. Toward a Corporeal Feminism.* Crows Nest, Australia: Allen and Unwin, 1994.

Guigot, André. *Focus sur Sartre: L'existentialisme est un humanisme et L'être et lenéant.* Paris: Éditions Ellipses, 2013.

Günzel, Stephan. "Deleuze and Phenomenology." *Metodo. International Studies in Phenomenology and Philosophy* 2.2 (2014): 31–45.

Hallam, Elizabeth, and Tim Ingold, Eds. *Creativity and Cultural Improvisation.* Oxford: Berg, 2007.

Halprin, Daria. *The Expressive Body in Life, Art and Therapy: Working with Movement, Meaning and Metaphor.* London: Jessica Kingsley Publishers, 2003.

———. "Body Ensouled, Enacted and Entranced: Movement/Dance as Transformative Art." *Dance, Somatics and Spiritualities: Contemporary Sacred Narratives.* Eds. Amanda Williamson, Glenna Batson, Sarah Whatley, and Rebecca Weber. Bristol: Intellect Press, 2014. 87–114.

Hamp, Amanda E. "Their Hands in the Dirt: How Kazuo Ohno and Stephanie Skura Cultivate Dance Practices and Alterity from Nature." *Choreographic Practices* 4.1 (2013): 9–28.

Hannah, Barbara. *Encounters with the Soul: Active Imagination as Developed by C. G. Jung.* Wilmette, Ill.: Chiron Publications, 2013.

Harman, Graham. *Prince of Networks: Bruno Latour and Metaphysics.* Prahran, Australia: re-press, 2009.

Hartley, Linda. *Wisdom of the Body Moving: An Introduction to Body-Mind Centering.* Berkeley: North Atlantic Books, 1995.

Hay, Deborah. *My Body, the Buddhist.* Middletown, Conn.: Wesleyan University Press, 2000.

Hayes, Jill. *Soul and Spirit in Dance Movement Psychotherapy.* London: Jessica Kingsley, 2013.

———. "Dancing in the Spirit of Sophia," in *Dance, Somatics and Spiritualities: Contemporary Sacred Narratives.* Eds. Amanda Williamson, Glenna Batson, Sarah Whatley, and Rebecca Weber. Bristol: Intellect Press, 2014. 61–86.

Heidegger, Martin. *Being and Time.* Trans. John Macquarrie and Edward Robinson. New York: Harper and Row, 1962 [1927].

———. *Basic Writings.* Trans. D. F. Krell. San Francisco: Harper San Francisco, 1977.

———. *Contributions to Philosophy (From Enowning).* Trans. Parvis Emad and Kenneth Maly. Bloomington: Indiana University Press, 1999 [1938].

Hillman, James. *Re-Visioning Psychology.* New York: Harper and Row, 1975.

———. *Blue Fire: Selected Writings by James Hillman*. New York: Harper and Row, 1989.

———. *The Soul's Code: In Search of Character and Calling*. London: Bantam Books, 1996.

———. *Alchemical Psychology*. New York: Spring Publications, 2015.

Hobson, Will. "Releasing Sensibilities: William Hobson Eavesdrops on a Conversation between Joan Skinner and Gaby Agis." *Dance Theatre Journal* 13.3 (Spring 1997): 34–37.

Husserl, Edmund. *Husserliana*. Den Haag, Dordrecht: Martinus Nijhoff/Kluwer Academic Publishers/Springer, 1950ff.

———. *Husserliana Materialien*. Dordrecht: Kluwer Academic Publishers/Springer, 1950ff.

———. *Cartesian Meditations*. Trans. Dorion Cairns. Dordrecht: Martinus Nijhoff, 1960.

———. *Ideas: General Introduction to Pure Phenomenology*. Trans. W. R. Boyce Gibson. New York: Collier Books, 1962 [1913].

———. *Formal and Transcendental Logic*. Trans. Dorion Cairns. Dordrecht: Martinus Nijhoff, 1969.

———. *Logical Investigations*. Trans. J. N. Findlay. London: Routledge and Kegan Paul, 1970a [1900].

———. *The Crisis of European Sciences and Transcendental Phenomenology: An Introduction to Phenomenological Philosophy*. Trans. David Carr. Evanston: Northwestern University Press, 1970b [1936].

———. *Ideas: General Introduction to a Pure Phenomenology*. Trans. F. Kersten. The Hague: Nijhoff, 1982 [1913].

———. *Ideas Pertaining to a Pure Phenomenology and to a Phenomenological Philosophy*, Book 2 (Ideas II). Trans. R. Rojcewicz and A. Schuwer. Boston: Kluwer Academic Publishers, 1989 [1952].

———. "Appendices." in Fink and Husserl, *Sixth Cartesian Meditation*. Trans. Ronald Bruzina. Bloomington: Indiana University Press, 1995 [first prepared in 1932]. 163–198.

———. *Logical Investigations*. Ed. Dermot Moran. London: Routledge, 2001 [1900].

———. *Cartesian Meditations: An Introduction to Phenomenology*. Trans. Dorion Cairns. Dordrecht: Springer, 2013 [1931].

Isozaki, Arata. *MA: Space-Time in Japan*. Exhibition Catalogue by Cooper-Hewitt Museum, Smithsonian Institution and Japan Foundation, 2001 [1979].

———. "Ma (Interstice) and Rubble." *Japan-ness in Architecture*. Cambridge: MIT Press, 2011 [2006], 81–100.

Johnson, Don Hanlon. "Body Work and Being: The Deeper Significance of Somatics."*New Realities*. (Sept./Oct. 1987): 20–23.

———. *Body: Recovering Our Sensual Wisdom*. Berkeley: North Atlantic Books, 1992.

———. *Body, Spirit, and Democracy*. Berkeley: North Atlantic Books, 1994.

———. *Bone, Breath, and Gesture*. Berkeley: North Atlantic Books, 1995.

———. *Groundworks: Narratives of Embodiment*. Berkeley: North Atlantic Books, 1997.

———. *Everyday Hopes, Utopian Dreams: Reflections on American Culture*. Berkeley: North Atlantic Books, 2006.

———. "Preface." in *Dance, Somatics and Spiritualities: Contemporary Sacred Narratives*. Eds. Amanda Williamson, Glenna Batson, Sarah Whatley, and Rebecca Weber. Bristol: Intellect Press, 2014. xii–xxi.

Kasulis, Thomas P. *Shinto: The Way Home*. Honolulu: University of Hawai´i Press, 2004.

Keeney, Bradford. "Reentry into First Creation: A Contextual Frame for the Ju|'hoan Bushman Performance of Puberty Rites, Storytelling, and Healing Dance." *Journal of Anthropological Research* 69 (2013): 65–86.

Keeney, Bradford, and Hillary Keeney, Eds. *Way of the Bushman: Spiritual Teachings and Practices of the Kalahari Ju|'hoansi*. Rochester, Vt.: Bear and Co., 2015.

Klaver, Irene. "Always Already Rhythm: Merleau-Ponty's Movement toward Ontology." *Studies in Practical Philosophy* 5.1 (2005): 41–49.

Kloetzal, Melanie. *Site Dance*. Gainesville: University Press of Florida, 2011.

Kozel, Susan. *Closer: Performance, Technologies, and Phenomenology*. Cambridge: MIT Press, 2007.

———. "The Virtual and the Physical: A Phenomenological Approach to Performance Research." *The Routledge Companion to Research in the Arts*. Eds. Michael Biggs and Henrik Karlsson. London: Routledge, 2011. 204–222.

———. "Process Phenomenologies," in *Performance Phenomenology: Traditions and Transformations*. Eds. Maaike Bleeker, Sherman Jon Foley, and Nedelkopoulou. London: Routledge, 2015. 54–74.

Kruks, Sonia. "Women's Lived Experience: Feminism and Phenomenology from Simone de Beauvoir to the Present." *The SAGE Handbook of Feminist Theory*. Eds. Mary Evans, Clare Hemmings, and Marsha Henry. London: Sage Publications, 2014. 75–92.

Kurath, Gertrude, Jane Ettawageshik, and Fred Ettawageshik. *The Art of Tradition: Sacred Music, Dance, and Myth of Michigan's Anishinaabe, 1946–1955*. Ed. Michael McNally. East Lansing: University of Michigan Press, 2009.

Laage, Joan E. "Embodying the Spirit: The Significance of the Body in Contemporary Japanese Dance Movement of Butoh." PhD dissertation. Texas Woman's University: UMI, 1993. PDF/Microfilm.

Laban, Rudolph von. *Modern Educational Dance*. London: MacDonald and Evans, 1948.

LaMothe, Kimerer L. *Nietzsche's Dancers: Isadora Duncan, Martha Graham and the Reevaluation of Christian Values*. New York: Palgrave Macmillan, 2006.

———. *Family Planting: A Farm-fed Philosophy of Human Relations*. U.K.: Changemakers Books, John Hunt Publishing, 2011.

———. "Transformation: An Ecokinetic Approach to the Study of Ritual Dance," *Journal of Dance, Movement, and Spiritualities* 1.1 (2014): 57–72.

———. *Why We Dance: A Philosophy of Bodily Becoming.* New York: Columbia UP, 2015.

Laszlo, Ervin. *Science and the Akashic Field.* Rochester, Vt.: Inner Traditions, 2007.

Lawrence, Nathaniel, and Daniel O'Connor, Eds. *Readings in Existential Phenomenology.* Englewood Cliffs, N.J.: Prentice Hall, 1967.

Leder, Drew. *The Absent Body.* Chicago: University of Chicago Press, 1990.

Legrand, Dorothée, and Susanne Ravn. "Perceiving Subjectivity in Bodily Movement: The Case of Dancers." *Phenomenology and the Cognitive Sciences* 8 (2009): 389–408.

Lepecki, Andre. "Stumble Dance." *Women and Performance: A Journal of Feminist Theory* 14.1 (2004a): 47–61.

———, Ed. *Of the Presence of the Body.* Middletown, Conn: Wesleyan University Press. 2004b.

———. "Reciprocal Topographies," *Eiko and Koma.* Minneapolis: Walker Arts Center, 2011. 48–53.

———. *Singularities.* London: Routledge, 2016.

Letiche, Hugo. "Research Ethics: Dance, Presence, Performance and Performativity." *Culture and Organization* 18.3 (2012): 177–193.

Levinas, Emmanuel. *Otherwise than Being.* Trans. A. Lingis. Dordrecht: Nijhoff, 1974.

———. *Totality and Infinity.* Dordrecht: Kluwer Academic, 1991 [1961].

Llewelyn, John. "Prolegomena to Any Future Phenomenological Ecology." Eds. Charles S. Brown and Ted Toadvine. *Eco-phenomenology: Back to the Earth itself.* Albany: State University of New York Press, 2003. 51–72.

Louppe, Laurence. *Poetics of Contemporary Dance.* Trans. Sally Gardner. Alton, U.K.: Dance Books, 2010.

Manning, Erin. *Relationscapes: Movement, Art, Philosophy.* Cambridge: MIT Press, 2009.

Margulis, Lynn, and Dorion Sagan. *Microcosmos: Four Billion Years of Microbial Evolution,* New York: Summit Books, 1986.

———. *What Is Life?* Berkeley: University of California Press, 1995.

Markula, Pirkko. "The Dancing Body without Organs: Deleuze, Femininity, and Performing Research." *Qualitative Inquiry* 12.1 (2006): 3–27.

Martin, John. *The Modern Dance.* New York: Dance Horizons, 1933.

McCoubrey, Catherine. "Intersubjectivity vs Objectivity: Implications for Effort Observation and Training." *Movement Studies: A Journal of the Laban/Bartenieff Institute of Movement Studies* 2 (1987): 3–6.

McHose, Caryn, and Kevin Frank. *How Life Moves: Explorations* in Meaning and Body Awareness. Berkeley: North Atlantic Books, 2006.

McNamara, Joanna. "Dance in the Hermeneutic Circle," *Researching Dance: Evolving Modes of Inquiry.* Eds. Sondra Fraleigh and Penny Hanstein. Pittsburgh: University of Pittsburgh Press, 1999. 162–187.

Merleau-Ponty, Maurice. *The Phenomenology of Perception.* Trans. Colin Smith. London: Routledge and Kegan Paul, 1962 [1945].

———. *The Primacy of Perception and Other Essays.* Ed. James M. Edie. Trans. Charles Dallery. Evanston: Northwestern University Press, 1964a.

————. *Signs*. Trans. R. C. McCleary. Evanston: Northwestern University Press, 1964b.

————. *The Visible and the Invisible*. Ed. Claude Lefort. Trans. Alphonso Lingis. Evanston: Northwestern University Press, 1968a[1964].

————. "Reflection and Interrogation." *The Visible and the Invisible*. Ed. Claude Lefort. Trans. Alphonso Lingus. Evanston: Northwestern University Press, 1968b. 3–49.

————. *Phenomenology of Perception*. Trans. Colin Smith. New York: Routledge Classics, 2002 [1945].

————. *Child Psychology and Pedagogy: The Sorbonne Lectures 1949–1952*. Trans. Talia Welsh. Evanston: Northwestern University Press, 2010.

————. *Phenomenology of Perception*. Trans. Donald A. Landes. London: Routledge and Taylor Francis Group, 2012 [1945].

Merritt, Michele. "Thinking-Is-Moving: Dance, Agency, and a Radically Enactive Mind." *Phenomenology and the Cognitive Sciences* 14 (2015): 95–110.

Meschonnic, Henri. "The Rhythm Party Manifesto." *Thinking Verse* I (2011): 161–173.

Mesle, C. Robert. *Process-related Philosophy: An Introduction to Alfred North Whitehead*. West Conshohocken, Pa.: Templeton Foundation Press, 2008.

Midgelow, Vida L. "Some Fleshy Thinking: Improvisation and Experience." *The Oxford Handbook of Dance and Theater*. Ed. Nadine George-Graves. New York: Oxford University Press, 2015. 109–122.

————. "Improvising Dance: A Way of Going About Things." *Oxford Handbook of Improvisation in Dance*. Ed. Vida Midgelow. New York: Oxford University Press, in press.

Miller, Alice. *For Your Own Good: Hidden Cruelty in Child-Rearing and the Roots of Violence*. 3rd ed. Trans. Hildegard Hannem and Hunter Hannem. New York: Farrar, Strauss, and Giroux, 1990 [1983].

Mohanty, J. N. "Husserl on 'Possibility.'" *Husserl Studies* 1 (1984): 13–29.

Moran, Dermot. *Introduction to Phenomenology*. New York: Routledge, 2000.

Morris, Michael. "Towards a Posthuman Ethics: Moving with Others in Karl Cronin's Natural History Archive." *Choreographic Practices* 6.2 (Spring 2015): 201–217.

Morton, Timothy. "The Biosphere Which Is Not One: Towards Weird Essentialism." *Journal of the British Society for Phenomenology* 46.2 (2015): 141–155.

Moustakas, Clark. *Heuristic Research: Design, Method, and Applications*. Newbury Park, Calif.: Sage Publications, 1990.

Mowe, Sam. "Signs of Intelligent Life: Carl Safina's Evidence That Other Animals Think and Feel." *The Sun* 488 (2016): 4–11.

Mueller-Vollmer, K., Ed. *The Hermeneutic Reader*. New York: The Continuum Publishing Company, 1985.

Murphy, Michelle. "Alterlife in the Ongoing Aftermath." *Toxic: A Symposium on Exposure, Entanglement and Endurance*. New Haven: Yale University. Conference Presentation, Mar. 3, 2016.

Nagatomo, Shigenori. *Attunement through the Body*. Albany: State University of New York Press, 1992.

Nancy, Jean-Luc. *Listening*. Trans. Charlotte Mandell. New York: Fordam University, 2007.

Ness, Sally Ann. "Bouldering in Yosemite: Emergent Signs of Place and Landscape." *American Anthropologist* 113.1 (2011): 71–87.

Nietzsche, Friedrich. *On the Genealogy of Morals and Ecce Homo*. Ed. and Trans. Walter Kaufmann. New York: Vintage Books, 1989.

———. *The Portable Nietzsche*. Ed. Walter Kaufmann. New York: Penguin, 1954.

Nishida, Kitaro. *An Inquiry into the Good*. New Haven: Yale University Press, 1990 [1921].

Nitschke, Günter. "Ma, The Japanese Conception of Space." *Architectural Design* 36 (Mar. 1966): 115–116, missing pages.

———. *From Shinto to Ando: Studies in Architectural Anthropology in Japan*. New York: Wiley, 1993.

———. Nixon, Rob. *Slow Violence and the Environmentalism of the Poor*. Cambridge: Harvard University, 2011.

Olsen, Andrea. *Body and Earth: An Experiential Guide*. Middlebury, N.H.: Middlebury College Press, 2002.

Olsen, Andrea, and Caryn McHose. *Bodystories: A Guide to Experiential Anatomy*. Lebanon, N.H.: University Press of New England, 1998.

———. *How Life Moves: Explorations in Meaning and Body Awareness*. Lebanon, N.H.: University Press of New England, 2006.

O'Shea, Janet. "Roots/Routes of Dance Studies." *The Routledge Dance Studies Reader*. 2nd ed. Eds. Alexandra Carter and Janet O'Shea. London: Routledge, 2010 [1998]. 1–16.

Oxford English Dictionary. "Power." http://www.oed.com.libproxy.temple.edu/view/Entry/149167?rskey=ribAZS&result=1&isAdvanced=false#eid. Accessed Oct. 29, 2016.

Pakes, Anna. "Knowing through Dancing-making: Choreography, Practical Knowledge and Practice-as-Research." *Contemporary Choreography: A Critical Reader*. Eds. Joanne Butterworth and Lisbeth Wildschut. London: Routledge, 2009. 10–22.

———. "Phenomenology and Dance: Husserlian Meditations." *Dance Research Journal* 43.2 (Winter 2011): 33–49.

Parviainen, Jaana. "Bodily Knowledge: Epistemological Reflections on Dance." *Dance Research Journal* 34.1 (2002): 11–26.

———. "Dwelling in the Virtual Sonic Environment: A Phenomenological Analysis of Dancers' Learning Processes." *The European Legacy* 16.5 (2011): 633–647.

Pearce, Fred. *The New Wild: Why Invasive Species Will Be Nature's Salvation*. Boston: Beacon Press, 2015.

Pirsig, Robert M. *Zen and the Art of Motorcycle Maintenance*. New York: HarperCollins, 1974.

Potter, Caroline. "Sense of Motion, Senses of Self: Becoming a Dancer." *Ethnos* 43.4 (2008): 444–465.

Ramachandran, V. K. *The Tell-Tale Brain: A Neuroscientist's Quest for What Makes Us Human.* New York: W. W. Norton and Co., 2011.

Rasul, Haleem, dir. . *The Jitterbugs: The Pioneers of the Jit.* Hardcore Detroit, 2013. DVD.

Ravn, Susanne, and Helle P. Hansen. "How to Explore Dancers' Sense Experiences: A Study of How Multi-sited Fieldwork and Phenomenology Can Be Combined." *Qualitative Research in Sport, Exercise and Health* 5.2 (2013): 196–213.

Reason, Matthew, and Dee Reynolds. "Kinesthesia, Empathy, and Related Pleasures: An Inquiry into Audience Experiences of Watching Dance." *Dance Research Journal* 42.2 (2010): 49–75.

Reese, Mark. *Moshe Feldenkrais: A Life in Movement, Volume One.* Berkeley: Reese-Kress Somatics Press, 2015.

Rei, Delta. "Butoh Meets Contemporary Dance eX . . . it' 03." Dokumentation von Bernd Terstegge. eX . . . it! 2003—part 1, *3rd International Butoh Dance-eXchange and Performance Festival at Schloss Bröllin, Germany.* Vimeo. Jan. 3, 2015, vimeo.com/115846827. Accessed Jan. 13, 2018.

Richardson, Laurel. "Writing: A Method of Inquiry." *Handbook of Qualitative Research.* Eds. Norman K. Denzin and Yvonna S. Lincoln. Thousand Oaks, Calif.: Sage, 1994. 516–529.

Robin, Libby. "How Do People Live in the Anthropocene?" *Geophysical Research Abstracts* (2016): 18.

Rothfield, Philippa. "Differentiating Phenomenology and Dance." *Topoi* 24 (2005): 43–53.

———. "Dance and the Passing Moment: Deleuze's Nietzsche." *Deleuze and the Body.* Eds. Laura Gillaume and Joe Hughes. Edinburgh: Edinburgh University Press, 2011. 203–223.

Rouhiainen, Leena. "Somatic Dance as a Means of Cultivating Ethically Embodied Subjects." *Research in Dance Education* 9.3 (2008): 241–256.

Ryan, Robert. *Shamanism and the Psychology of C. G. Jung: The Great Circle.* London: Chrysalis books, 2002.

Saint-Exupéry, Antoine de. *The Little Prince.* Trans. Katherine Woods. 1943. http://www.hilpro.com.br/wp-content/uploads/2015/11/Pequeno-Pri%CC%81ncipe-Ingle%CC%82s.pdf.3. Accessed Jan. 12, 2018.

Sartre, Jean Paul. *Existentialism.* Trans. Bernard Frechtman. New York: Philosophical Library, 1947.

———. *La nausée.* Paris: Gallimard, 1963a [1938].

———. *L'existentialisme est un humanisme.* Genève: Nagel, 1963b [1946].

———. *Being and Nothingness.* 3rd ed. Trans. Hazel Barnes. New York: Citadel, 1965.

Schwendener, M. "New Jersey Images, Unbound by Galleries: A Review of 'Robert Smithson's New Jersey' at the Montclair Art Museum." *New York Times,* Mar. 7, 2014.

Sheets-Johnstone, Maxine. *The Phenomenology of Dance.* Milwaukee: University of Wisconsin Press, 1966.

———. *The Primacy of Movement.* Amsterdam: John Benjamins, 1999.

———. "Existential Fit and Evolutionary Continuities." *The Corporeal Turn: An Interdisciplinary Reader.* Exeter, U.K.: Imprint Academic, 2009a. 64–90.

———. "Man has Always Danced: Forays into an Art Form Largely Forgotten by Philosophers." *The Corporeal Turn: An Interdisciplinary Reader.* Exeter, U.K.: Imprint Academic, 2009b. 306–327.

———. *The Primacy of Movement.* 2nd ed. Amsterdam: John Benjamins, 2011.

———. "From Movement to Dance." *Phenomenology and the Cognitive Sciences* 11 (2012): 39–57.

———. *The Phenomenology of Dance.* 50th Anniversary Edition. Philadelphia: Temple University Press, 2015.

Shubin, Neil. *Your Inner Fish: A Journey into the 3.5-Billion-Year History of the Human Body.* New York: Vintage, 2008.

Siegfried, Wolfgang. "Dance, the Fugitive Form of Art: Aesthetics as Behavior." *Beauty and the Brain: Biological Aspects of Aesthetics.* Eds. B. Rentschler, B. Herzberger, and D. Epstein. Basel: Birkhauser Verlag, 1988. 117–145.

Simon, Steven, Andre Bouville and Charles Land. "Fallout from Nuclear Weapons Tests and Cancer Risks." *American Scientist* (Jan.–Feb.) 2006.

Skinner, Joan. www.skinnerreleasing.com. Accessed Oct. 12, 2016.

———, with Bridget Davis, Sally Metcalf, and Kris Wheeler. "Notes on Skinner Releasing Technique." *Contact Quarterly* (Fall 1979): 8–14.

Sklar, Deidre. *Dancing the Virgin: Body and Faith in the Fiesta of Tortugas, New Mexico.* Los Angeles: University of California Press, 2001.

Skura, Stephanie. www.opensourceforms.com. Accessed Oct. 12, 2016.

Smyth, Cliff. "Feldenkrais Method and Health: Phenomenological Perspectives." *IFF Feldenkrais Research Journal,* vol. 5. www.http://iffresearchjournal.org/volume/5/smyth. Accessed Sept. 25, 2016.

Stafford, Barbara. *Visual Analogy: Consciousness as the Art of Connecting.* Chicago: University of Chicago Press, 2001.

St. Denis, Ruth. "Seeds of a New Order," Clippings file at New York City Public Library, 1950–1959.

Stinson, Susan W. "Dance Education in Early Childhood." *Design for Arts in Education* 91.6 (1990): 34–41.

———. "Body of Knowledge." *Educational Theory* 45.1 (1995): 43–54.

Strenski, Ivan. *Thinking about Religion: An Historical Introduction to Theories of Religions.* Oxford: Blackwell Publishing, 2006.

Stromsted, Tina. "The Alchemy of Authentic Movement: Awaking Spirit in the Body." *Dance, Somatics and Spiritualities: Contemporary Sacred Narratives.* Eds. Amanda Williamson, Glenna Batson, Sarah Whatley, and Rebecca Weber. Bristol: Intellect Press, 2014. 35–61.

Takenouchi, Atsushi. *Jinen Butoh: Atsushi Takenouchi. Artist website.* http://www.jinen-butoh.com. Accessed Jan. 13, 2018.

———. *Skin. Seattle Butoh Festival 2012 YouTube*. DAIPAN Butoh Collective, Feb. 17, 2013. http//www.youtube.com/watch?v=ntWXnXOIubk. Accessed July 15, 2015.

Taylor, Paul. *Normative Discourse*. Englewood Cliffs, N.J.: Prentice-Hall, 1961.

———. *Respect for Nature. A Theory of Environmental Ethics*. Princeton: Princeton University Press, 1986.

Tidd, Ursula. *Simone de Beauvoir*. London: Routledge. 2004.

Todres, Les. *Embodied Enquiry: Phenomenological Touchstones for Research, Psychotherapy and Spirituality*. New York: Palgrave Macmillan, 2007.

UNICEF. www.unicef.org/statistics/. Accessed Oct. 15, 2016.

Ursprung, Philip. "The Architecture Performances of Gordon Matta-Clark," in *Performance and the Politics of Space*. New York: Routledge Press, 2013. 239–250.

Vagle, Mark D. *Crafting Phenomenological Research*. Walnut Creek, Calif.: Left Coast Press, 2014.

Van der Leeuw, Gerardus. *Sacred and Profane Beauty: The Holy in Art*. Trans. David Green. New York: Henry Holt, 1963.

———. *Religion in Essence and Manifestation*. Trans. J. E. Turner. Princeton: Princeton University Press, 1986.

Van Manen, Max. "Pedagogical Text as Method: Phenomenological Research as Writing." *Saybrook Review* 7.2 (1989): 23–45.

———. *Researching Lived Experience: Human Science for an Action-Sensitive Pedagogy*. London, Ont.: Althouse, 1990.

———. "Professional Practice and 'Doing Phenomenology,'" in *Handbook of Phenomenology and Medicine*. Ed. S. Kay Toombs. London: Kluwer Publishers, 2000.

———. "Phenomenology of Practice." *Phenomenology and Practice* 1.1 (2007): 11–30.

———. *Phenomenology of Practice: Meaning Giving Methods in Phenomenological Research and Writing*. Walnut Creek, Calif.: Left Coast Press, 2014.

Varela, Francisco. "Neurophenomenology: A Methodological Remedy for the Hard Problems." *Journal of Consciousness Studies* 3.4 (1996): 330–349.

Vasquez, Manuel A. *More than Belief: A Materialist Theory of Religion*. London: Oxford University Press, 2011.

Veillette, Mario. "Danse Butô et éducation somatique: caractéristiques communeset spécificités." (2005): Unpublished paper.

Viale, Martine. *Action / Installation*. Artist website. https://martinviale.wordpress.com. Accessed Jan. 13, 2018.

Wang Hongyuan. *Aux sources de l'écriture Chinoise*. Beijing: Sinolingua, 1997.

Warren, Karen J. *Ecological Feminist Philosophies*, Bloomington: Indiana University Press. 1996.

Weiss, Gail. *Body Images. Embodiment as Intercorporeality*. New York: Routledge, 1999.

Welsh, Talia. *The Child as Natural Phenomenologist: Primal and Primary Experience in Merleau-Ponty's Psychology*. Evanston: Northwestern University Press, 2013.

Williamson, Amanda. "Reflections and Theoretical Approaches to the Study of Spiritualities within the Field of Somatic Movement Dance Education." *Journal of Dance and Somatic Practices* 2.1 (2010): 35–36.

———. "Somatically Inspired Movement and Prepatriarchal Religious Symbolism." *Journal of Dance, Movement and Spiritualities* 2.3 (2015a): 323–335.

———. "Reflections on Existential Phenomenology, Spirituality, Dance and Movement-Based Somatics." *Journal of Dance and Somatic Practices* 8.2 (2015b): 275–301.

Williamson, Amanda, Glenna Batson, Sarah Whatley, and Rebecca Weber, Eds. *Dance Somatics and Spiritualities: Contemporary Sacred Narratives*. Bristol: Intellect, 2014.

Willis, Peter. "The Scholarly and Pathic Cavalier: Max van Manen's *Phenomenology of Practice.*" *Phenomenology and Practice* 8.2 (2014): 64–67.

Wilshire, Bruce. *Wild Hunger: The Primal Roots of Modern Addiction*. Lanham: Rowman and Littlefield, 1998.

Wiskus, Jessica. *The Rhythm of Thought: Art, Literature, and Music after Merleau-Ponty*. Chicago: The University of Chicago Press, 2008.

Woolf, Virginia. *The Death of the Moth and Other Essays*. New York: Harcourt, Brace, Jovanovich, 1974.

Working Group on the "Anthropocene." "What Is the 'Anthropocene'?"—Current Definition and Status. *Subcommission on Quaternary Stratigraphy, 2016*. www.quaternary.stratigraphy.org/workinggroups/anthropocene/. Accessed Nov. 12, 2016.

Yeatman, Anna. "A Feminist Theory of Social Differentiation." *Feminism/Postmodernism*. Ed. Linda J. Nicholson. New York: Routledge, 1990.

Yeats, William Butler. *The Collected Poems of W. B. Yeats*. Basingstoke, U.K.: Macmillan, 1956.

Young, Iris M. "Throwing Like a Girl." *Throwing Like a Girl*. Ed. Iris Young. Bloomington: Indiana University Press, 1980. 141–159.

———. "Situated Bodies. Throwing Like a Girl." *Body and Flesh. A Philosophical Reader*. Ed. Donn Welton. Oxford: Blackwell. 1998a. 259–273.

———. "'Throwing Like a Girl': Twenty Years Later." *Body and Flesh. A Philosophical Reader*. Ed. Donn Welton. Oxford: Blackwell, 1998b. 286–290.

———. *On Female Body Experience: "Throwing Like a Girl" and Other Essays*. Oxford: Oxford University Press. 2005.

Yuasa, Yasuo. *The Body, Self-Cultivation and Ki-Energy*. Albany: State University of New York Press, 1993.

Zahavi, Dan. *Husserl's Phenomenology*. Stanford: Stanford University Press, 2003.

Zaner, Richard. *The Context of Self: A Phenomenological Inquiry Using Medicine as a Clue*. Athens: Ohio University Press, 1981.

———. *At Play in the Field of the Possibles*. Bucharest: Zeta Books, 2012.

Zen Sourcebook: Traditional Documents from China, Korea, and Japan. Ed. Stephen Addiss, with Stanley Lombardo and Judith Roitman. Indianapolis: Hackett Publishing, 2008.

Index

becoming: being and, 3, 66, 76, 99; in butoh, 110, 115; in dance, 178; global, 114–16;
other, 101; phenomenologies of, 208–22;
through movement, 21, 173
becoming, bodily, 17, 115, 123–40; being and,
3; in dance, 133, 139; empathy and, 137;
movement patterns in, 127–28, 135; nature
and, 5; philosophy of, 126–28, 134; rhythm
of, 136
Behar, Ruth, 208
Behnke, Elizabeth, 185
being: as agency, 216; becoming and, 3, 66,
76, 99, 176; dance of, 215; embodying and,
81; history of movement in, 128; ontological study of, 163; for Other, 227; presence
as, 244; relationship to practice, 62; as
rhythm, 216; vulnerability in, 69; wom-
en's, 235. See also existence
Bellerose, Christine, 6; Healing My Mother,
175, 176, plate 7; on ma, 29; on relationship to land, 175
belonging, worlding and, 107
Bennett, Jane, 55; Vibrant Matter, 38–39, 104
Bingham, Robert, 4; on Anthropocene, 28;
on eco-phenomenology, 31; heuristic research of, 42; Snow Canyon dance, 44–45,
45, 48–49, 52–53, plate 3; study with Nagatomo, 15
body: as alchemical vessel, 91; being and
becoming of, 3; biases concerning,
113–14; ecological, 25, 31; environment
and, 190; felt sense of, 193; in hermeneutics, 143; of images, 90; improvisatory, 67; of language, 90; life-energy of,
50–51; mineralization of, 53; the "more"
of, 82; nondualistic philosophy of, 2–3;
and place, 6, 142; portal of, 164–71, 173;
potentiality of, 188; in quantum physics,
49; relationship with environment, 51;
self and, 11; somatic attunement of, 47;
subjectivity of, 189, 190; without organs
(BwO), 34; and world, 11; world's, 161.
See also lived body
body, women's: comportment of, 237; lived,
235, 237
Body-Mind Centering, 97
Body Weather Farm, butoh performance
at, 169
bodywork, somatic, 85; neutrality in, 103;
trust in, 117; verbal communication in, 86
Bogost, Ian, 214
Bohm, David, 49

Bond, Karen, 7, 17; "Receiving the Dance of
the Child," 209
bracketing, 8, 235; in dance, 36, 39; engagement with experience, 234; of kinetic
preferences, 138; lived body concept in,
36; of lived experience, 239; of movement
patterns, 136; suspending of judgment in,
29; in tabula rasa thinking, 17; of women's
experience, 237. See also epoché
Braude, Hillel, 7, 29, 197
break'n (dance), 153
Brunsvold, Megan, plate 1
Buber, Martin, 80
Buddhism: ma and, 163; nonattachment in,
107; phenomena in, 52. See also Zen Buddhism
Bush, Amy, 118
Bushmen, Kalahari: dance of, 135, 136
Butler, Judith, 210; on performativity, 33
butoh (Japanese dance form), 6, 7, plate 6;
aesthetic of, 177; appearance and disappearance in, 170; becoming in, 110, 115;
becoming other in, 101; engagement with
the nonhuman, 41; as experience, 178;
global phenomenality of, 116; hokotai
walk of, 111; improvisational, 111; intersubjectivity of, 41; metamorphosis in, 115;
performance of nature, 108–9; place-
dances of, 108; slow-flow in, 177; Takenouchi's, 31; therapeutic modes of, 111;
and World War II, 18, 25

capitalism, neoliberal, 55
Capitolene era, 40
Casey, Edward, 13; on built space, 156; concept of place, 108, 141, 142; ecological perspectives of, 143
Cass, Howard, 142
center: children's knowledge of, 224; phenomenologies of, 223–24
change: anthropogenic, 40–41; as performance, 99; somatic, 21
Cheetham, Thomas, 79, 80, 93
chi (life-energy), 110
chiasm, 12, 165; of body, 12; in ma, 176–77
childhood, qualia of, 222
children: aesthetic perceptions of, 224;
agency of, 220; dialogic relation to, 210;
essentialism of, 221, 222; holistic perception of, 221; intelligence of, 205–6; lived
experience of, 208; nonverbal, deaf-blind,
214, 224, 225–26; as phenomenologists, 7,

improvisation, dance, 4; decision-making in, 64; feedback-loop process of, 74; folding imagery in, 71; "I can" in, 194; listening in, 64; phenomenology and, 63–76; possibility in, 189; scores for, 73–74; shared practices of, 64; in Snow Canyon, 44–49, *45, 48*, 52–53, 56, *plate 1*; somatically informed, 59–60, 64; thinking in, 238–39; vulnerability in, 65, 75; ways of knowing in, 242

Institute of Early Childhood Development (State College of Victoria), 208

intelligence: children's, 205–6; of kinesthesia, 192; somato-cognitive, 220

intentionality: in attention, 114; in dance, 204n1; multiplicity in, 240, 241, 246; phenomenology and, 59, 100; purposeful, 30

intersubjectivity: agency in, 208; of butoh, 41; ethics of, 20; genesis of, 221; lifeworld and, 19; as perceptual field, 209; in phenomenology, 24; in researcher/researched relationships, 61; somatic engagement in, 208

Isozaki Arata, 166; *Angel Cage*, 167; "Ma (Interstice) and Rubble," 167–71

Iwase Kanako, 172, 173, 178

Japan: history with West, 116; phenomenology of, 15, 110. *See also* butoh

Jit, Detroit (urban street dance), 141–60; acclaim for, 153; body of, 150–55; competition in, 154; Heidelberg Project and, 145–59; history of, 151–53; originators of, 151–53; resurrection of, 158; styles of, 154; and techno music, 154; women Jitters, 154. *See also* Detroit

Jitdance: Detroit Redux (screendance), 6, 141–60, *155, 157*; collaborators in, 142; at Heidelberg Project, 149; night shoots of, 156–59; settings of, 144; spontaneity of, 158; theme of, 144, 158

Jit'n, at front of Soul Never Dies House, *152*

Jitterbugs (dancers), 152–53; at auto shows, 153; legacy of, 154

Johnson, Charles, 155

Johnson, Don Hanlon, 80; on language, 88; somatics work of, 79

Jung, Carl, 5, 30, 79; alchemical hermeneutics of, 94, 96

Jung, Joori, 144

kami (Japanese divinities), 6–7, 166–67, 171; in dance creativity, 167; flow in, 177; *hi-morogi* and, 166, 172; ruling of ebb and flow, 166; temporary bodies of, 166–67; in void, 168

Kanji ma, collage of, 164, *165*

Kao, Peiling, 18

Kasulis, Thomas P., 163–64

ki (life-energy), 50–51, 110

Kierkegaard, Søren, 163

kinesthesia, 26; corporeality in, 204; experience of movement in, 138, 194, 202, 238, 245; in FFV, 198–99, 201; groundedness of, 202; imagery of, 35; intelligence of, 192; knowledge of, 73; language and, 5; of listening, 195; phenomenology of, 202; possibility in, 191; practical possibility in, 203; tactile, 104; of touch, 195; in understanding of world, 238

Klaver, Irene, 220

Kleist, Heinrich von: "On the Marionette Theater," 54

Knight Arts Challenge, awards in Detroit, 144, 150

knowledge: bodily-participant, 83; children's contributions to, 205; disjunctive models of, 88; embedded in dance, 28, 134; embodied, 241–43; as historical consciousness, 152; improvisational, 61–62; kinesthetic, 73; pre-linguistic, 61; sites of, 56; vulnerability in, 88

Kozel, Susan, 74, 105–6

Kresge Foundation, awards in Detroit, 144, 150

Kuramata Shiro, 166

Laage, Joan, 178

Laban, Rudolph, 174

LaMothe, Kimerer, 5; on bodily becoming, 17; *Moon Rock*, 124; rural residence of, 123–27, 130, 131; *White Rose, 130; Why We Dance*, 139n1, 139n4

Langer, Suzanne, 72

language: affective, 5; alchemical, 80, 96–97; body of, 90; conceptual, 96; dance and, 4–5, 80; literalism of, 95; movement and, 18; nominalism of, 79, 92; repersonification of, 98; resonating with, 84; sharing, 84; somatic enactment in, 78, 79, 80, 84; somatic perspectives on, 4–5, 81, 88. *See also* words

language formulation: Abrams's, 86–88; focusing in, 82; somatic, 80, 95

Laszlo, Ervin, 50

SONDRA FRALEIGH is a professor emeritus of the Department of Dance at State University of New York College at Brockport. She is the editor of *Moving Consciously: Somatic Transformations through Dance, Yoga, and Touch* and the author of *Butoh: Metamorphic Dance and Global Alchemy*.

The University of Illinois Press
is a founding member of the
Association of American University Presses.

—————————————————————————

University of Illinois Press
1325 South Oak Street
Champaign, IL 61820-6903
www.press.uillinois.edu